Communication Assessment and Intervention Strategies for Adolescents

Communication Assessment and Intervention Strategies for Adolescents

Vicki Lord Larson, Ph.D.
Nancy L. McKinley, M.S.

THINKING PUBLICATIONS
A Division of McKinley Companies, Inc.

International Standard Book Number: 0-930599-07-1

Library of Congress Catalog Card Number: 86-51418

Cover Photograph by Michael Joles

Printed in the United States of America

Thinking Publications®

A Division of McKinley Companies, Inc.
P.O. Box 163
Eau Claire, WI 54702-0163

DEDICATION

In loving memory of our mothers

Stella Mae Hilton Lord
and
Grace Lorraine Reichmann Mrnak

who guided us through our adolescence

FOREWORD

Communication disorders as an academic discipline is still young. Clinical efforts for the remediation of communication disorders has had a somewhat longer life. Neurologists, other physicians, and psychologists first identified and worked with persons with communication disorders, particularly fluency disorders and the language disorders associated with aphasia. Initially it was the adult who was the focus of interest to these practitioners. Later an interest in the "developmental aphasia" of children came about. With the publication of case studies of children who did not learn to talk and the recognition that some children were displaying other communication disorders, data became available on the mentally retarded, autistic, and learning-disabled child. Since it was not possible to specify what was abnormal without knowing what was normal, there was an increase in interest in the way normal language was acquired. Although the theories of language acquisition reflected different perspectives, they made a similar basic assumption, that almost all the interesting things related to language acquisition, and therefore, to language disorders, happened very early in life; the usual time brackets were birth to about five years of age. Both researchers and practitioners acted as though there was little linguistic development after this early period, except continued vocabulary growth. There was also the suggestion that even if something were happening, because of a likely critical period for development, there was little to be done to help the older child or adolescent.

It is curious that research and clinical interests in communication disorders have developed in apparent parallelism to research and clinical interests in several other areas. Examples may be found in theories of development and in the practice of medicine. Most early developmental theory focused on the infant and young child; only after a period of time was adolescence found to be an interesting and unique period of development. Pediatricians have practiced medicine as a specialty for many years, but it has only been in recent years that specialists in adolescent medicine have practiced. Before that time, the adolescent was treated either by a pediatrician or by an internist with mainly adult clientele. One may speculate why the adolescent and the period of adolescence are only now receiving appropriate attention. Perhaps it is due to the increased census of persons in this developmental period, or perhaps researchers and clinicians recognize the need to understand and to provide services to all persons as individuals in the total continuum of life. Whatever the reason, it is clear that the adolescent's time has come.

This book is a trailblazer within the literature of communication sciences and disorders. It is the first to present a comprehensive description of adolescent development and communication disorders. It also is unique in its presentation of the integration of assessment and intervention for the adolescent with communication disorders. Finally, it stands out because of its insistence on the use of theory, where it exists, and on a systematized approach and on data gathering where information is needed. The knowledge base of communication sciences and disorders must be expanded; the use of a systematic and theoretical perspective will facilitate that endeavor. Adolescents deserve appropriate services to aid them in meeting their communication needs. The authors of this book have a combination of academic training and professional experience which have allowed them to produce a book with vision and practicality. It will serve well the academic discipline, the practitioner, and ultimately, the adolescent with communication disorders.

Delores Kluppel Vetter, Ph.D.
University of Wisconsin-Madison

PREFACE

Many adolescents with communication disorders have remained undetected, unserved, and thus unable to realize their complete human potential. The intent of this book is to review the current information on adolescent development and communication disorders, and to present a prototype service delivery model. The book integrates theoretical knowledge with practical ideas for serving adolescents with communication disorders, and summarizes effective assessment and intervention strategies for adolescents. This book is primarily for practicing speech-language pathologists providing services to adolescents, but it could also be adopted as a text for university classes emphasizing services for school-age students.

This volume expands on our workshop manual (Boyce and Larson, 1983), and presents a conceptual framework to accommodate emerging data on adolescents with communication disorders. As awareness of the adolescent population heightens, new tests and programs are evolving at a rapid rate. This text provides a comprehensive prototype model into which new data can be organized.

Chapter One considers definitions of adolescence, dispels common myths about adolescents, and presents what is currently known about disordered communication development during adolescence. Chapter Two summarizes theories of adolescence and normal physical, psychological, and communication development. These two chapters serve as the background on adolescents for the remaining chapters of the book, which present the prototype delivery model.

Chapter Three gives an overview of the prototype service delivery model that we advocate and discusses the first two components of the model in detail. The model includes six components: Information dissemination, identification, assessment, program planning, intervention, and follow-up. Each component consists of working with the adolescent directly, and working through the educational and environmental systems to reach the adolescent indirectly. A diagram of this prototype service delivery model is displayed on the inside back cover of the book.

Chapter Four emphasizes an integrative assessment process to evaluate the adolescent's communication behaviors. An extensive description of what behaviors to assess are considered: Cognition, comprehension and production of linguistic features, discourse (narrations and conversations), nonverbal communication, and survival language. This information is followed by a discussion of informal procedures to use to evaluate the adolescent's communication behaviors. The informal procedures proposed are: Case history forms, learning style questionnaire, analysis procedures for conversations and narrations, and directed tasks. In addition, formal tests that might be useful to evaluate the adolescent's communication behaviors are summarized.

Chapter Five presents parameters to consider and ways to evaluate these parameters when indirectly assessing the adolescent through the educational and environmental systems. We strongly contend that a communication problem may not always lie within the adolescent. At times the educational and/or environmental systems may be the problem.

Chapter Six underscores the need to engage in program planning. Program planning is viewed as the connecting link between assessment and intervention. Included within this chapter is information on what to consider and how to engage in program planning with the adolescent (direct program planning) as well as interacting with the people in the educational and environmental systems who are involved with the adolescent (indirect program planning). Our contention is that program planning should not be glossed over, since it is essential to the establishment of a comprehensive intervention program.

Chapter Seven provides data on what to consider and how to engage in direct intervention with the adolescent. Specifically, data are presented on what to modify in the adolescent's performance regarding thinking, listening, speaking, nonverbal communication, and survival language behaviors. How to modify these behaviors is presented through a discussion of general and specific intervention procedures. Commercial resources appropriate to use with adolescents to enhance their communication performance are summarized. We emphasize using a strategies approach during intervention with adolescents.

Chapter Eight considers indirect intervention for adolescents. This is accomplished by describing appropriate supportive modifications within the educational and environmental systems. Also, major vehicles for modifying these systems are presented. The major vehicle described to modify the educational system is consultation, while within the environmental system the vehicle is counseling.

Chapter Nine presents a rationale for and ideas about engaging in direct and indirect follow-up activities. Currently, this component is implemented the least of all the components of the prototype delivery model. Follow-up allows the professional to demonstrate the efficacy of services to the adolescent. Accountability is critical to the development and maintenance of services for adolescents.

The Appendices of this book contain numerous forms and charts that can be used to establish and implement the various components of the prototype delivery model. Throughout Chapters Three through Nine, which detail what to consider and how to implement each of the six components of the delivery model, is information about using the microcomputer and specified software. Having entered the information age, the professional must accommodate the technology to serve adolescents with communication disorders more effectively and efficiently. We maintain that we need to position ourselves to act, rather than to react, to the challenging era of technology ahead.

We hope you will read, study, enjoy, and most of all, question this book. It is a beginning in an area that has insufficient research. This book compiles our personal clinical experiences, research endeavors, consultantships, and workshops on various topics related to service delivery, assessment, and intervention with adolescents. It attempts to integrate these domains with available information housed in various disciplines such as psychology, sociology, anthropology, special education, and English, to name a few. Admittedly, it is a wedding of insufficiencies until a broader knowledge base is gained by the discipline of communication sciences and disorders. As you use our prototype service delivery model, we hope that you will find working with adolescents to be as exciting, challenging, and fulfilling as we have.

The authors gratefully acknowledge those who have helped in the completion of this book. Delores Kluppel Vetter was a positive source for influencing and challenging our thinking. Delesa Boley, Susan Schultz, Freda Adashek, and Jean Dorward contributed generously of their time to field test various forms and to offer insight from the perspective of the public school speech-language pathologist.

We are indebted to Vivian Joubert who served as a technical and editorial adviser on the manuscript. We thank Yvonne McCarty, Rosanne Vonasek, Shelley Sweeny, and Mary Holte for their countless hours at the word processor over the past several years. We appreciate the library work of Julie Kosikowski, Kari Kalewski, and the many others who have assisted us.

A special thanks to the workshop participants and the graduate students over the past ten years who have questioned, challenged, supplied ideas, and stimulated our thinking about adolescents with communication disorders. To the adolescents with whom we have worked — you have taught us and continue to teach us about adolescence.

Finally, we are grateful to James Larson and Michael McKinley, our husbands, for their encouragement, sense of humor, support, patience, tolerance, and love. Because of them, this book was completed.

Vicki Lord Larson
University of Wisconsin-Eau Claire

Nancy L. McKinley
University of Wisconsin-Eau Claire

CREDITS

TABLES 2.2, 2.3, and 2.4
Average Number of Words per Communication Unit-Oral Language, Maze Words as a Percentage of Total Words-Oral Language, and Average Number of Words per Maze-Oral Language from *Language Development: Kindergarten through Grade Twelve* by Walter Loban (1976). Reprinted with permission of National Council of Teachers of English, Urbana, IL.

TABLES 4.2 and 7.2
Cognitive Functions and Thinking Behaviors from *The Dynamic Assessment of Retarded Performers: The Learning Potential Assessment Device, Theory, Instruments, and Techniques* by Reuven Feuerstein (1979). Adapted with permission of the original publisher of the text, University Park Press, Baltimore, MD.

TABLE 5.2
Minimum Competencies: Speaking and Listening by Speech Communication Association of America (1979). Reprinted with permission of Speech Communication Association, Annandale, VA.

FIGURE 7.1
Problem Solving Model Chart by Thinking Publications (1983). Reprinted with permission of Thinking Publications, Eau Claire, WI.

APPENDIX N
Consultation Feedback Forms from *Collaborative Consultation* (Appendix 8-A and Exhibit 8-6) by Idol, N., Paolucci-Whitcomb, P., and Nevin, A. (1986). Reprinted with permission of Aspen Publishers, Inc.

TABLE OF CONTENTS

Page

LIST OF TABLES AND FIGURES

CHAPTER 1

Adolescence: A Concept in Transition

GOALS:

To present definitions of adolescence

To dispel common myths about adolescents

To cite prevalence of communication disorders during adolescence

To describe characteristics of adolescents with communication disorders

To challenge the need to label adolescents

In western society, the time span between the ages of approximately twelve to twenty years is called adolescence. Adolescence, derived from the Latin word "adolescere," means "to grow into maturity" (Turner and Helms, 1979). In workshops across the country when we have asked, "What images does the word 'adolescence' bring to mind?" professionals have tended to list negative characteristics (e.g., rebellious, inconsistent, impulsive, moody). Yet the vast majority of adolescents are thriving, healthy beings who feel confident, happy, and self-satisfied (Offer, Ostrov, and Howard, 1981a). Adolescents are individuals who are establishing their identities, making career choices, learning how to think about their thinking, and realizing the potential of adult communication.

DEFINITIONS OF ADOLESCENCE

An extensive review of the literature reveals numerous definitions of adolescence. Adolescence has been defined as a transitional period between childhood and adulthood (Lewin, 1939; Turner and Helms, 1979); as a rite of passage into adulthood (Kett, 1977); as a time of identity crisis and psychosocial moratorium (Erikson, 1968); as a coming of age (Freeman, 1983; Mead, 1950); and as the age of commitment and a move toward interdependence (Konopka, 1973). However, at the root of these definitions is the heated debate on whether adolescence is a natural developmental stage, or purely sociologically determined, and thus a product of western society (Konopka, 1971). Elder (1975) emphasized that adolescence must be discussed from a socio-historical perspective, that is, relative to the current decade or to a specific moment in time. Lipsitz (1980) stated, "Any global statement about adolescence may hold for a decade; if one is lucky" (p. 6).

How do these definitions concur with professionals who work with adolescents? Adolescents are often stereotyped by professionals as rebellious, irrational beings to be tolerated and endured. They are looked upon as a homogeneous age group, discontinuous from the remainder of the life cycle (Lipsitz, 1980).

We view adolescence, as do Konopka (1971) and Lipsitz (1980), as just one of the developmental periods within the overall life cycle. Adolescents must be perceived first as unique individuals, and second as people going through a period of development called adolescence. Adolescence involves biological, socio-cultural, and psychological aspects, and each interacts with the others. No single aspect is sufficient to explain adolescence, but all are necessary; collectively, they may describe adolescence.

Biologically, adolescence spans the years between the onset of puberty and the completion of bone growth (Lipsitz, 1980). Puberty, according to Tanner (1974), may be divided as follows: (1) adolescent growth spurt, which can occur in the individual with various onset, intensity, magnitude, and duration, resulting in an increase in the skeleton, muscles, and viscera; (2) changes in body composition such as bone, fat, and muscles; (3) sex specific growth rate, varying between the sexes, and leading to differences in body dimensions; and (4) development of the adult reproductive system and secondary sex characteristics.

Socio-culturally, adolescence is influenced by cultural values, attitudes, and beliefs, as well as by socioeconomic class, and by western society's laws on compulsory education, child labor, and juvenile proceedings (Bakan, 1971). Most societies use functional criteria (e.g., ability to support one's self) or status criteria (e.g., voting rights) to mark the end of adolescence. These socio-cultural dimensions influence society's tolerance range for what is the time length for "typical adolescence." Researchers note that the more sophisticated a society's technology, the more prolonged is the period of adolescence (Eisenberg, 1965).

Psychologically, adolescents attain the ability to think at an abstract level (Inhelder and Piaget, 1958) and to establish a personal identity (Erikson, 1968). Thus, this is a time of accelerated cognitive growth (Alley and Deshler, 1979; Epstein, 1978) and of personality formation (Ferguson, 1970). Both of these domains will continue to evolve in later stages of adulthood, but at a lesser rate.

The critical aspect of a definition of adolescence is that it emphasizes an interrelationship among biological, socio-cultural, and psychological dimensions. For example, as people mature physically and thus sexually, they learn, through their culture and social class, a specific sex role, which in turn is made a part of their personality; or it is rejected and may result in some personal confusion.

In summary, any cohesive definition of adolescence must accommodate the fact that adolescence as a developmental period is constantly changing, contingent upon the socio-cultural environment and upon the function of time. Adolescence, therefore, must be perceived as a concept in transition.

MYTHS ABOUT ADOLESCENTS

The failure to perceive adolescence as a concept in transition can lead to myths about adolescents that may impair perception and consequently lead to erroneous assumptions about this period of development. The following myths may be evident:

1. The "continuous growth" myth implies that development is uniform and synchronized during adolescence (Lipsitz, 1979). Frequently, however, a mismatch occurs in development. Physical growth may spurt without a corresponding psychological change. Rather than being uniform, growth tends to be characterized by spurts, troughs, and plateaus. Adolescent growth and development should be considered neither continuous nor stagelike, since both patterns are considered possible (Muuss, 1975).

2. The "generation gap" myth states that vast differences exist between youth and adults (Mitchell, 1979). But generational differences are often differences in outlook for achieving the same goal, and they have to do with specific preferences rather than general beliefs. In other words, parents may struggle with the adolescent over dress code, curfew, and peer group choice, but these conflicts are fundamentally the same as when that child was a toddler and conflict arose over bedtime and bath time, i.e., the struggle for independence. The change is that all participants are a decade or so older. Adult-adolescent conflict is no more unusual than adult-adult conflict, or conflict arising between adolescents. In fact, the rift between early and late ado-

lescents is often much stronger than between adolescents and adults (Mitchell, 1979).

3. The "life skills incompetence" myth promotes the image of adolescents who are incompetent in performing important tasks (Mitchell, 1979). However, competence may be difficult to determine because adolescents have been excluded from any important work where competence might be demonstrated: Laws prohibit most jobs before age sixteen; even after that age, business and labor usually refuse to hire adolescents for anything except menial jobs. Half of the unemployed in America are between sixteen and twenty-four years of age (National Commission on Youth, 1980). Few adolescents, particularly those in early adolescence, are trained in a specific skill area that would make them marketable to business and labor. Mitchell (1979) argues that many constructive uses of youth talent in the community are currently being ignored. He cites exemplary community work projects such as "Share and Repair," in Sacramento, where adolescents repaired houses for low income families, and "Operation Venus," in Philadelphia, where youth organized and opened a venereal disease hot line.

4. The "turmoil" myth suggests that adolescents are in constant psychological turmoil. Mitchell (1979) believes that this myth may stem from the negative way that many social scientists describe the adolescent experience. A quick check of article and book titles containing information about adolescents carries through the turmoil theme: *The Turbulent Teens* (Gardner, 1982), "The Age of Insolence: Those Terrible Teens" (Coles, 1983), *The Transition of Youth to Adulthood: A Bridge Too Long* (National Commission on Youth, 1980).

Not all adolescents experience turmoil; yet adults may expect it. Mental health professionals were asked to complete the Offer Self-Image Questionnaire (Offer, Ostrov, and Howard, 1977) the way they thought normal adolescents would complete it. In seven out of ten scales, professionals described the normal adolescent as significantly more disturbed than normal adolescents viewed themselves (Offer, Ostrov, and Howard, 1981a). Much of the turmoil appears to be created in the minds of adults, although some adolescents do experience turmoil. Adults might consider assuming some responsibility for whatever problems these youth are encountering. For example, by age fourteen, the average adolescent has witnessed 11,000 murders on television (National Commission on Youth, 1980). The "throw away population," those adolescents disposed of by parents who can no longer cope, is on the increase (Wellborn, 1981). Today's adolescents, growing up in a crowded world, are in strong competition with the baby boom generation of adults who are demanding jobs, goods, and services at record levels. Although the majority of adolescents are not in turmoil, those who are should not go unnoticed by adults.

5. The "in trouble" myth stems from the assumption that adolescents are in more trouble than ever before: There is more suicide, more juvenile delin-

quency, more violent crimes. However, the data to confirm or to refute this myth are varied and contradictory (Peck, 1982). While there should be concern about suicide and crimes among adolescents, all is not totally grim. Holinger (1980) pointed out that the emergence of violent deaths as a leading cause of adolescent mortality is not due to the *increase* in the rate of violent deaths, but is due to the *decrease* in the incidence of other causes of death. Holinger's (1980) evidence indicates that the percentage of violent deaths among adolescents by suicide, homicide, and accident has stayed constant over the past eighty years.

Upon examining the suicide rate, Holinger and Offer (1981) found a significant correlation between adolescent suicide rates and the proportion of adolescents in the nation's total population. Thus, as the population of adolescents increases, so does the suicide rate, and vice versa (Offer, Ostrov, and Howard, 1981b). In contrast, Colt (1983) reported that adolescent suicide has tripled over the past twenty-five years, despite expanding prevention efforts. Although statistics on adolescent suicide vary, it may be more helpful to consider whether certain types of youth are more suicidal than others. The Los Angeles Suicide Prevention Center found that fifty percent of young victims (ten to fourteen years of age) were diagnosed as learning disabled. They were diagnosed as hyperactive, perceptually impaired, and dyslexic. Some researchers suggest that being learning disabled is accompanied by feelings of low self-esteem; thus these researchers suggested another reason for placing this population in a high risk category (Peck, 1982). Furthermore, the majority of case studies have shown that suicide victims feel that they have no one with whom they can talk. This lack of a friend, of someone who will listen, can be a major concern for adolescents with learning or language disorders. Their communication problems often interfere with making and keeping friends (Donahue and Bryan, 1984), and with expressing their feelings; both are potentially contributing factors in the total despair preceding suicide (Peck, 1982). Talking and listening are major attempts at preventing suicide, as evidenced by the increasing number of hot lines available across the country. When oral language skills are impaired, and the adolescent is suicide-prone, there is cause for concern.

While the media promotes the myth that adolescents are in more trouble than ever before, adults can be reminded of one hundred years ago when ". . . whole areas of New York were held in the grip of street gangs . . . These gangs fought savage battles in the streets. A death toll of fifteen or twenty was not uncommon. Even the police feared to enter some neighborhoods" (Morris and Hawkins, 1970, p. 140). News about teens seems to be sensationalized by journalists. For example, the death of two adolescents today can provoke national alarm and prolonged, agonized debate (Offer, Ostrov, and Howard, 1981b). As Naisbitt (1984) has stated so well, "Satellites have turned the earth inward, upon itself" (p. 12). Today's mass production of information does not always help the image of adolescents. More is known now about the few deviant individuals who, before instant news, went undetected except by those people around them.

The professional's belief in any one of these common myths can lead to erroneous assumptions about adolescents. Professionals must examine their beliefs about and attitudes toward adolescence and then determine whether objective evidence substantiates or contradicts their beliefs and attitudes. This examination of beliefs will ensure a more objective approach to working with adolescents.

6. Finally, we believe that a sixth myth needs to be dispelled. The "there's nothing more to do" myth is an additional myth about adolescents that has been held by speech-language pathologists. This widespread assumption holds that little can be done past the fourth grade for the student with an oral language disorder. Many developmental charts for language end at ten years; thus speech-language pathologists may question what more can be accomplished if the child has not already been "cured" by that age.

This myth is fueled by current diagnostic batteries. Many times formal tests seem to indicate that the student's language deficit has been cured, when in fact it has not. While clinical intuition might suspect continuation of certain language deficits into the middle school grades and beyond, many formal tests are not sensitive to the functional aspects of communication which affect the older student (Damico, 1985). Current assessment instruments overemphasize superficial aspects of language and artificially fragment language into separate parts (Damico, 1985).

The "discrete point" testing approach, i.e., evaluating isolated finite aspects of language, contributes to the disparity between formal test observations and what students do in actual conversation. Older students may perform within norms on standardized tests, but may display deficits in discourse which severely impede them academically, socially, or vocationally. "As a function of this testing procedure, these older children [are] classified according to a different set of guidelines and [are] labeled as having learning disorders rather than language disorders. They [are], in effect, taken out of our professional domain." (Damico, 1985, p. 167). It is not that speech-language pathologists *cannot* do anything more for older students, but that frequently they *have not* done anything more. In the past, other professionals have served adolescents with language disorders, or these individuals have been unserved. Yet the prevalence of adolescents with communication disorders is sufficiently documented to warrant speech-language pathologists' attention as service providers to this population. Adolescents should no longer go unserved or underserved.

PREVALENCE OF COMMUNICATION DISORDERS IN ADOLESCENTS

Statistics on the number of adolescents with impairments of speech, language, or hearing are scattered because specific data on this age group have not often been gathered. The one exception has been data gathered in juvenile detention centers. In these centers, a disproportionately large number of adolescents with communication disorders were evident. Taylor (1969) found that eighty-four percent of the incarcerated youth she studied had communication disorders.

Gillespie and Cooper (1973) reported the prevalence of speech problems in junior and senior high schools to be 5.5 percent. A report from the American Speech-Language-Hearing Association (ASHA) (Fein, 1983) documented that 1.94 percent of individuals five to fourteen years and 0.67 percent of individuals fifteen to twenty-four years were speech-language impaired. These data excluded cleft palate cases, deaf people who cannot speak, and any institutionalized individuals. Based on available data, researchers cannot derive a specific prevalence figure for the entire adolescent population.

In late 1983, we attempted a national survey of state consultants for speech-language programs to determine the prevalence of communication disorders among adolescents. The return rate of the questionnaires was twenty-six percent. The majority of the surveys returned indicated that consultants had no means to retrieve statistics specifically for adolescents with communication disorders. Thus, we could not compute a national prevalence figure. However, one reporting state, Florida, computed prevalence figures and reported that 1.4 percent of students aged thirteen to twenty-one years were receiving services. Florida recently implemented Project Adolang (Task Force on Secondary Programs for the Speech-Language Impaired, 1983) to identify adolescent language problems and their implications for education.

To obtain additional data on prevalence, we surveyed two hundred speech-language pathologists who were randomly sampled from an original pool of six hundred people who had attended one of our 1983–1985 workshops (Larson and McKinley, 1985a). The original pool of six hundred people was selected because they had demonstrated an interest in serving adolescents. There was a fifty-five percent return rate of the questionnaires. The average prevalence of secondary school students being served by these speech-language pathologists was two percent. The range of adolescents being served was from .04 percent to ten percent of the secondary-level population. Sixty-one percent of these secondary-level students were receiving dual services (e.g., services from both a speech-language pathologist and a learning disabilities specialist) and thirty-nine percent were receiving speech-language services exclusively.

After reviewing the literature on prevalence of communication disorders among adolescents, and then attempting to collect data specific to that population, we have concluded that perhaps as many youths as the five percent figure often quoted by ASHA are in need of services. However, wide discrepancies exist in the provision of those services.

CHARACTERISTICS OF ADOLESCENTS WITH COMMUNICATION DISORDERS

Weiner (1974) was one of the first researchers to report on an adolescent with a communication disorder. He observed that journals in communication sciences and disorders were nearly devoid of reference to the adolescent population. Although information since then has become more plentiful, it remains sparse compared with the wealth of empirical research that has been conducted with preschool and elementary children. Presently, much of what is known about adolescents with communication disorders comes from related literature in learning disabilities and deaf education. Yet communication problems during adolescence may have any number of etiological bases. These adolescents with communication disorders may be housed in residential schools, hospitals, juvenile detention centers and jails, or institutions for the developmentally disabled. They may be high school drops-outs living at home, or earning their graduation equivalency degrees (GED's) from vocational-technical schools or within the military system. Many more are in regular junior and senior high schools.

A growing number of secondary students in the public school system fit the category of "everyone's problem and no one's responsibility" (National Youth Workers Conference, 1982). They are not deviant enough for criminal justice services, not deprived enough for social service programs, and not disabled enough for special educational services. These students are described as having a high incidence of problems related to reasoning and communication skills, yet they may be receiving no help from established systems, including no speech-language services in the schools.

Increasing evidence shows that children who were language impaired during their early years experience a "continuum of failure" as they mature into adolescents (Aram, Ekelman, and Nation, 1984; DeAjuriaguerra et al., 1976; Garvey and Gordon, 1973; Griffiths, 1969; King, Jones, and Lasky, 1982; Strominger and Bashir, 1977; Weiss, Hansen, and Heubelein, 1979). A fifteen year follow-up study of fifty speech-language students ranging in age from thirteen years, ten months, to twenty years, five months was conducted by King et al. (1982). At the time of the investigation, forty-two percent of the students still had some form of a communication problem. These students' spoken language disabilities frequently underlie and interact with reading failures that persist into adolescence and adulthood (Allington and Fleming, 1978; Johnson, 1985; Rees, 1974; Velluntino, 1978). The Committee on Language Learning Disorders of ASHA (1982) emphasized the importance of identifying and serving school-age speech-language impaired children. Important changes in language occur beyond age five as the demands of the school curricula increase. Therefore, communication disorders have a profound effect on school performance and frequently exist concomitantly with other disabilities (e.g., learning disabilities, retardation).

How do speech-language pathologists recognize adolescents who need speech-language services? Most of the time, professionals rely on their clinical experience and their knowledge of normal development. However, within the past decade or two, a growing body of research literature in communication sciences and disorders and in related disciplines has attempted to describe the communication (i.e., the meeting of meaning between two or more people) of adolescents with cognitive deficits and language disorders. Characteristics of these adolescents are summarized below.

Cognition

Cognition is the mental organization of experience. Cognition subsumes thinking, which is the application of cognition for a purpose. These purposes may include reasoning, judging, analyzing, recalling, inferring, imagining, problem solving, and so forth. Labels such as propositional thinking, reflective thinking, and abstract thinking have emerged. We recommend the use of the term "thinking," rather than cognition, with adolescents because thinking is a term with which they are familiar.

Many studies have found that adolescents with cognitive deficits often fail to attain higher levels of abstract reasoning (Feuerstein, 1980; Hains and Miller, 1980; Havertape and Kass, 1978; Neimark, 1980). In other words, these adolescents remain concrete thinkers and do not use organized, efficient strategies for solving problems. While it might be tempting to blame hereditary or environmental factors, Feuerstein (1980) argues that errors in methods of teaching are frequently the cause of low levels of abstraction in adolescents. Indeed, some adolescents with hearing impairments have achieved age-appropriate cognitive behaviors, even with inadequate verbal encoding skills (Furth, 1966; Furth and Youniss, 1971). Johnson (1977), using the *Torrance Tests of Creative Thinking* (1974), found that deaf adolescents performed significantly better than hearing adolescents on several creative thinking subtests such as fluency, flexibility, originality, and elaboration. The hearing-impaired adolescents did better on the fluency, flexibility, and elaboration subtests than the hearing adolescents.

Comprehension and Production of Linguistic Features

Comprehension of linguistic features includes the understanding of morphological, syntactic, and semantic components of language. Comprehension deficits during adolescence may be demonstrated by the lack of understanding of the figurative uses of language (Blackwell et al., 1978) and of semantic concepts, including relationships that are comparative, familial, passive, spatial, or temporal (Brenza, Kricos, and Lasky, 1981; Schmitt, 1968; Wiig and Semel, 1974). Riedlinger-Ryan and Shewan (1984), using a series of standardized tests, investigated the auditory comprehension of linguistic features by learning-disabled and academically achieving adolescents. This study supported the findings presented in previous studies that documented the persistence of auditory language comprehension deficits in learning-disabled adolescents. While some deficits in auditory comprehension were clearly demonstrated, deficits in comprehension of supersegmental features remain controversial. Furthermore, evidence conflicts regarding the ability of adolescents with learning disabilities to comprehend stress and intonation patterns (Vogel, 1974; Wiig et al., 1977).

The production of linguistic features includes the appropriate expression of morphological, syntactic, and semantic components during speaking. The term "speaking" is being used in this book because adolescents understand the term, since it is part of the secondary curriculum. Production deficits during adolescence may be evident in (1) agrammatical sentences (Wiig and Semel, 1975), (2) sentences of shorter length (Donahue, Pearl, and Bryan, 1982; Wiig and Semel, 1975), and (3) sentences that are less syntactically complex than normal peers' (Donahue, Pearl, and Bryan, 1982; Geers and Moog, 1978). Word retrieval problems, the inability to call up an intended word from memory, are common (Blalock, 1981; Wiig and Becker-Caplan, 1984; Wiig and Semel, 1975). Wiig and Semel (1975) noted longer response lags in producing sentences. Asking questions may be difficult (Bryan, Donahue, and Pearl, 1981) and may occur with low frequency in specific situations (Larson and McKinley, In preparation). In addition, adolescents with language disorders have problems expressing themselves concisely (Wiig and Semel, 1976), and they tend to overuse a limited and concrete vocabulary (Wiig and Semel, 1975; 1976).

Donahue and Bryan (1984) have suggested that there is a strong relationship between the learning-disabled adolescent's knowledge and use of slang and the amount of interaction with and acceptance from the normal peer group. Thus, ". . . failure to conform to peer group norms for appropriate language use may have increasingly negative consequences" (p. 18) for learning-disabled students in terms of establishing and maintaining friendships and enhancing self-esteem.

Discourse

According to Austin (1962), discourse is composed not of words or sentences but of speech acts. Austin maintained that speech acts can be analyzed into three parts: (1) locutions, or propositions; (2) illocutions, or the speaker's intentions; and (3) perlocutions, or the listener's interpretation. "The ways in which normally developing children link consecutive utterances within discourse to maintain coherency and to clarify messages" (Craig, 1983, p. 106) is referred to as "pragmatics." This definition of pragmatics considers the integrated nature of structural and conversational rules. Hymes, writing in 1971 before the popularity of the term "pragmatics," discussed the importance of sentence acceptability, or ". . . who can say what, in what way, where, and when, by what means and to whom?" (p. 15). His insight into "sentence acceptability" in the 1970s paved the way to pragmatics in the 1980s.

There are two types of discourse: Narrations and conversations. Several primary differences exist between narrations and conversations (Roth and Spekman, 1986):

1. Narrations have more extended or elaborated units of text than conversations.
2. Narrations are expected to have story markers (e.g., an introduction and closing) and an orderly presentation of events leading to a logical resolution.
3. Narrations carry the expectation that the speaker will engage in an oral monologue and that the listener's role can be more passive. More responsibility is placed on the speaker to be organized, coherent, and interesting.

Narrations Structurally, narrations are midway between oral and literary language (Westby, 1985; 1984). "Narrations may be viewed as suprasentential discourse units with underlying organizational rules, or *story grammars*; as conceptual units which reveal the speaker's expectations about event sequences, or *scripts*; as linguistic expressions requiring specific formal devices to bind them into coherent *texts*; and as *communication events* which demand thoughtful assessment of the listener's needs" (Johnston, 1982, p. 144). Narrations can be viewed as extended monologues, in contrast with conversations, which are interactive dialogues.

Studies investigating story recall in children and adults with language disorders and learning disabilities have revealed that these individuals tend to preserve the order of events in a story and recall the patterns of story organization with the same degree of accuracy as their normally achieving counterparts; but they tend to recall significantly less information from stories (Weaver and Dickinson, 1982; Worden, Malmgren, and Gabourie, 1982). Researchers found these same differences in quantity of information within spontaneous story production by learning-disabled students (Roth and Spekman, 1986).

Differences were found when rating stories on the importance of their idea units (Worden and Nakamura, 1982). Older students with a learning disability had more difficulty rating the stories on the importance of the idea unit in the story than did their normal counterparts. Worden and Nakamura (1982) suggested that the lower agreement on ratings by learning-disabled students may reflect a deficit in comprehension of the story or in remembering it.

Blalock (1982), summarizing persistent auditory language deficits, reported that young adults had difficulty in conveying extended explanations and narratives; in relating experiences; in explaining ideas or problems; in retelling stories; and in organizing the narrative. They also had difficulty comprehending narrations such as classroom lectures (Blalock, 1981). Some studies report no differences in story telling or retelling between normal and learning-disabled students, but these findings may be the result of applying story grammar analysis procedures that are insensitive to subtle developmental changes (Weaver and Dickinson, 1982).

Conversations The term "conversation" frequently ". . . is used loosely and non-technically to refer to any interactional stretch of talk involving at least two participants, and taking place in a non-formalized setting" (Edmondson, 1981, p. 6). During conversational speech, production deficits may include a lack of sustaining and monitoring conversations (Bryan, Donahue, and Pearl, 1981); a lack of requesting clarification of inadequate or ambiguous messages (Donahue, Pearl, and Bryan, 1980); and a lack of arguing for or against a position (Bryan et al., 1981). No significant differences have been found between normal adolescents and those with learning disabilities regarding the number of conversational turns (Bryan et al., 1981), the number of times they engaged in conversations with peers (Schumaker, Sheldon-Wildgen, and Sherman, 1980), or the number of times they were targets of peer initiation (Schumaker et al., 1980). Furthermore, some studies have found a lack of evidence that these adolescents, despite their social communication hindrances, are any more withdrawn, rejected, or isolated than normal adolescents (Bryan et al., 1981; Deshler and Schumaker, 1983).

Blalock (1981) argued that the adolescent's oral language deficits and social imperceptions prevent *quality* interactions with others and impede close friendships. Nisbet, Zanella, and Miller (1984) found that adolescents with moderate handicaps are less talkative when conversing with nonhandicapped peers than with fellow handicapped peers.

For some adolescents, listening to conversational speech may also be impaired. We are using the term "listening" because of its predominance in textbooks used by adolescents and in professional literature involving adolescents. Listening is difficult to define because of the complexity of the behavior. As many definitions of listening exist as persons who have written about the topic (Barker, 1971; Nichols and Lewis, 1954; Weaver, 1972; Wolff et al., 1983). According to Wolvin and Coakley (1982), a definition of listening is still being developed, since research on the topic is in an exploratory stage. Although we agree that additional research in the area is needed, listening must be considered an integral part of the total communication process: The function of the listener is to derive meaning from the speaker's intent. Blalock (1981) also observed that listening to fast-paced conversations is difficult for older students with learning disabilities and language disorders.

During referential communication tasks, oral descriptions of an item or activity by adolescents with learning disabilities tend to be less informative for listeners than those provided by normal adolescents (Knight-Arest, 1984; Noel, 1980; Spekman, 1981). Knight-Arest (1984) found that learning-disabled boys talked more but conveyed less information than their normal peers. The learning-disabled boys appeared more comfortable when doing than when describing a task to a listener. Furthermore, they were less effective at adapting messages to the needs of the listener than their normally achieving peers (e.g., repeating rather than reformulating what they said). They often appeared to be oblivious to the listener's needs.

Nonverbal Communication

Nonverbal communication refers to communication that transcends spoken words, and includes six categories: Kinesic behaviors, physical characteristics, touching behavior, paralanguage (including voice quality and vocalizations), proxemics, and artifacts (e.g., perfume, clothes) (Knapp, 1978). While we recognize that the discipline of communication sciences and disorders typically has not included paralanguage within nonverbal communication, we have selected to use Knapp's comprehensive definition of nonverbal communication. Edmondson (1981) defined paralanguage features as purposeful, directed, and controllable behaviors that may accompany or substitute for language, and thus contribute to the development of a conversation. Nonverbal factors are major determinants of meaning in the interpersonal context. Birdwhistell (1970) asserted that only thirty to thirty-five percent of the social meaning of a conversation is carried by words, while Mehrabian (1968) estimated that nonverbal factors are even more important. According to Knapp (1978), nonverbal communication serves these purposes: Repetition, contradiction, substitution, complementation, accentuation, regulation.

Although our clinical experiences indicate that many adolescents with language disorders have deficits in nonverbal behavior, little formal research confirms or refutes these observations. Wiig and Harris (1974) found that students with learning disabilities may have an inability to recognize nonverbal emotional expressions. Bryan (1977) also found that students with learning disabilities were less skillful at understanding nonverbal behavior when compared with their normal counterparts. Blalock (1981) documented inappropriate use of proxemics, i.e., social distance, during conversational speech.

Our own observations of adolescents with language disorders have indicated these nonverbal communication problems:

1. Frequent failure to interpret accurately the facial expression accompanying a spoken message
2. Inconsistent understanding of gestures used by others
3. Occasional failure to inhibit socially unacceptable gestures
4. Significantly less eye contact than that of normal adolescent communicators
5. Inappropriate maintenance of distance during various conversational situations.

Survival Language

"Survival language" is a term used to denote those language behaviors needed because of their functional relevance within and across typical daily living situations. These language behaviors allow people to function successfully and independently with their families and in their communities and jobs. Survival language behaviors include two types (Boyce and Larson, 1983):

1. *Situational language*, which includes the comprehension and production of the language necessary to survive a specific daily living experience such as shopping in a supermarket or eating in a restaurant.

2. *Multi-situational language*, which includes the person's ability to comprehend and produce the language needed across a number of daily living situations such as appropriately using money, telling time, or understanding warning signs.

Deficits in survival language behaviors are most common among adolescents who have moderate to severe cognitive deficits (e.g., adolescents who are mentally retarded). However, even mildly impaired adolescents may have problems in language needed for daily living situations. For example, Mathews, Whang, and Fawcett (1982) found that learning-disabled adolescents in high school lacked important basic skills to participate in a job interview. In addition, these adolescents did not have the basic language abilities to survive a series of employment-related skills such as accepting criticism, providing constructive criticism to co-workers, and explaining a problem to a supervisor.

Summation of Characteristics of Adolescents with Language Disorders

Using the data from studies just presented, and drawing upon our clinical experience with adolescents, we have constructed Table 1.1, Characteristic Problems of Adolescents with Communication Disorders. Within each of five areas (cognition, comprehension and production of linguistic features, discourse, nonverbal communication, and survival language skills), expectations for adolescents are listed, followed by a summary of the data describing problems observed when expectations are not met. The expectations are derived from the type of communication demands that educators, parents, and peers place upon junior/senior high-school students. The problems are derived from the review of the literature presented above, and from our clinical experience with adolescents with language disorders.

Note when reviewing Table 1.1 that typically a single problem would not result in an adolescent's being placed on the caseload, although there may be an exception (e.g., a severe word retrieval problem). Usually, a number of concomitant problems would exist before an adolescent would become a candidate for the services of a speech-language pathologist. Candidates for services have communication deficits that interfere with achieving academic progress, developing personal-social skills, or reaching vocational potential.

This book focuses on adolescents who display the problems listed in Table 1.1, regardless of etiology or setting. When speech-language pathologists examine the multitude of problems that can interfere with the academic, social, and vocational well-being of the adolescent, they realize that they cannot afford to ignore students with communication disorders after the elementary years. Special compensatory programs, for grades K–6 only, might make sense if sixth-grade level skills were the end goal of intervention. Early childhood and elementary speech-language programs have not failed, but by themselves they perform only a portion of the task. Some students, without continued intervention, will regress to previous levels of functioning by the time they enter junior high school (Larson and Dittman, 1975). Other adolescents need continued assistance to learn the language skills demanded for higher grade levels. Still other adolescents surface for the first time during early adolescence when they have not acquired the necessary communication skills to survive the verbal and social demands of higher grade levels.

By using the expectations and problems listed in Table 1.1, speech-language pathologists can begin to determine where a given adolescent matches or mismatches with educators', parents', and peers' expectations. Table 1.1 is a skeletal outline, which will be elaborated and illustrated later in the book in terms of how it can be used for assessment and intervention.

Americans traditionally evaluate an educational program by the contribution that it makes to the richness and productivity of the lives people lead after they leave school. Communication skills are a basic component of produc-

TABLE 1.1 CHARACTERISTIC PROBLEMS OF ADOLESCENTS WITH COMMUNICATION DISORDERS

Expectations	Problems
A. Cognition	
1. To be at the formal operational level (Inhelder and Piaget, 1958).	They often remain concrete operational thinkers (Hains and Miller, 1980; Neimark, 1980).
2. To observe, organize, and categorize data from an experience (Feuerstein, 1980).	They make chaos out of order (Havertape and Kass, 1978).
3. To identify problems, suggest possible causes and solutions, and predict consequences (Alley and Deshler, 1979).	They may not recognize the problem when it exists; if they do, they do not know how to develop alternative solutions (Havertape and Kass, 1978).
4. To place concepts into hierarchial order (Feuerstein, 1980).	They often cannot place concepts in a hierarchy (Boyce and Larson, 1983; 1981).
5. To find, select, and utilize data on a given topic (Vermont, 1979).	They have limited strategies for finding, selecting, and utilizing data (Havertape and Kass, 1978).
B. Comprehension and Production of Linguistic Features	
1. To comprehend all linguistic features and structures (Duker, 1971).	They misunderstand advanced syntactical forms (Wiig and Semel, 1974; 1973).
2. To follow oral directions of three steps or more after listening to them one time (Vermont, 1977).	They do not always realize that they are being given directions (Boyce and Larson, 1983; 1981).
3. To use grammatically intact utterances (Simon, 1979).	They often use sentences that are fragmented and that do not convey their messages (Boyce and Larson, 1983; 1981).
4. To have a vocabulary capable of expressing ideas and experiences (Simon, 1979).	They have word-retrieval problems as well as a high frequency of low informational words (Wiig and Semel, 1975).

TABLE 1.1 Continued

Expectations	Problems
5. To give directions with clarity and accuracy (Vermont, 1977).	They often leave their listeners confused (Spekman, 1981).
6. To get information or assistance by asking questions and to respond appropriately to questions asked of them (Simon, 1979).	They may know what question or answer to give, but they do not know how to do so tactfully (Wiig, 1983).
7. To comprehend and produce the slang and jargon of the hour (Donahue and Bryan, 1984).	They do not comprehend or produce slang/jargon, thus they are ostracized from the group they most desire to be a member (Boyce and Larson, 1983; 1981).
C. Discourse	
1. To produce language that is organized, coherent, and intelligible to their listeners (Grice, 1975).	They use many false starts and verbal mazes (Simon, 1979).
2. To follow adult conversational rules for speakers (e.g., maintaining a topic, initiating conversation, turn taking) (Rees and Wollner, 1982).	They consistently violate the rules (Bryan, Donahue, and Pearl, 1981).
3. To be effective listeners during conversation without displaying incorrect listening habits (Nichols and Stevens, 1957).	They often have poor listening skills (Boyce and Larson, 1983; 1981).
4. To make a report, tell or retell a story, and explain a process in detail (Vermont, 1977; Westby, 1985; 1984).	They often leave their listeners confused (Spekman, 1981).
5. To listen to lectures and to select main ideas and supporting details (Duker, 1971; Roeber, 1980).	They often do not grasp the essential message of a lecture (Blalock, 1981).
6. To analyze critically other speakers (Duker, 1971; Roeber, 1980).	Their judgements are arbitrary, illogical, and impulsive (Boyce and Larson, 1983; 1981).

TABLE 1.1 Continued

Expectations	Problems
7. To express their own attitudes, moods, and feelings and to disagree appropriately (Wiig, 1982a).	They have abrasive conversational speech (Wiig, 1983).
D. Nonverbal Communication	
1. To follow nonverbal rules for kinesics (Knapp, 1978).	They violate the rules and misinterpret body movements and facial expressions (Bryan, 1977; Wiig and Harris, 1974).
2. To follow nonverbal rules for proxemics (Knapp, 1978).	They violate the rules for social distance (Blalock, 1981).
E. Survival Language	
1. To comprehend and produce situational phrases and vocabulary required for survival in our society (Valletutti and Bender, 1982).	They do not have the necessary concepts and vocabulary needed in places such as banks, grocery stores, and employment agencies (Boyce and Larson, 1983; 1981).
2. To comprehend and produce concepts and vocabulary required across daily living situations (Valletutti and Bender, 1982).	They do not have the necessary concepts and vocabulary needed across daily living situations such as telling time, using money, and understanding warning signs (Boyce and Larson, 1983; 1981).

tivity. Adolescents growing up without adequate speech-language skills risk becoming part of the sixty percent of the unemployed adult population who have handicaps and live in poverty (Biklen and Bogdan, 1976).

WHY NOT LABELS?

Adolescents who exhibit a number of the problem behaviors listed in Table 1.1 are often labeled as language disordered or learning disabled. These labels supply no information about the nature of the communication problem. Instead, labels set up negative expectations for performance. Therefore, affixing a label that indicates a diagnostic category may be the most powerful determining force in the individual's personality and social interactions, virtually guaranteeing the formulation of a prognosis that will continue to justify the diagnosis and the continued application of the label (Feuerstein, 1979). As such, labels are a disservice. Although only specific aspects of the person's behavior lead to a label, in practice the whole person is labeled, and treated accordingly. Unfortunately, ". . . the process of labeling is a formal procedure, [but] the removal of labels is not" (Goldstein et al., 1975, p. 36). Mercer (1975) found, in the community she studied, that public schools were the predominant label users among 241 agencies serving people with retardation. This may be because state and federal laws mandate the use of these labels for reimbursement purposes.

A whole series of behavioral expectations, beliefs, and images operate under the rubric of the label. "Normal" people develop an explicit set of negative expectations, beliefs, and images about "disabled" people, especially those with physical, mental, or emotional disorders. Often, "disabled" people develop similar beliefs about themselves that restrict their potential to overcome or to accept their limitations. When this set of beliefs is operating, the "disabled" view themselves as "handicapped." These labels, and others, undermine one of the essential premises of categorizing youth, i.e., that students are benefited. Findings suggest that adverse categorization stigmatizes students and reduces both their self-image and their worth in the eyes of others (Kirp, 1974). Categorizing also tends to separate students along racial and social class lines, and this segregation may cause educational injury to minority students (Rivers et al., 1975).

While the labels of "language disordered" and "speech impaired" may not carry the emotional impact of the labels of "mentally retarded" and "emotionally disturbed," we have chosen to use labels cautiously; to talk instead about adolescents with communication disorders rather than about "the communicatively-disordered adolescent." Emphasis is placed first upon the normality of the individual, and second upon the communication disorder manifested by one or more of the problems listed in Table 1.1. Although labeling may be necessary in certain agencies, to procure funding or to ensure services under P.L. 94–142, it serves no utility in education past that point.

SUMMARY

This chapter defined adolescence as a concept in transition in western society during the late twentieth century. Common myths of adolescence were discussed and, we hope, dispelled. These myths ("continuous growth," "generation gap," "life skills incompetence," "turmoil," "in trouble," and "there's nothing more to do"), if strictly adhered to by professionals, may interfere with establishing and maintaining effective programs for adolescents.

Based upon a review of the literature, characteristics of adolescents with communication disorders were described for these areas: Cognition, comprehension and production of linguistic features, discourse (narrations and conversations), nonverbal communication, and survival language. From these data and our clinical experiences, the adolescent population addressed in this book was described by listing expectations of normal adolescents and problems of adolescents with communication disorders. This information will be used in future chapters that address assessment and intervention. Finally, professionals were urged to apply cautiously categorical labels to adolescents with communication disorders. Labels may actually be a disservice to adolescents, i.e., they may lower professionals' expectations and create negative self-images.

DISCUSSION QUESTIONS

1. In what additional myths of adolescence do you believe? Are there any cited in this chapter with which you disagree?
2. What expectations and problems of adolescents' communication listed in Table 1.1 have you observed? Should any be added? If so, which ones?
3. What advantages and disadvantages do you see in labeling adolescents by categories?

SUGGESTED READINGS

Lipsitz, J. Adolescent development: Myths and realities. *Children Today*. 8(5): 2–7, 1979.

National Commission on Youth. *The Transition of Youth to Adulthood: A Bridge Too Long*. Westview Press, Boulder, CO, 1980.

Offer, D., Ostrov, E., and Howard, K. *The Adolescent: A Psychological Self-Portrait*. Basic Books, New York, 1981.

CHAPTER 2

Adolescence: Theories and Development

GOALS:

To describe theories of adolescence

To present a theory of adolescence as it relates to adolescents with communication disorders

To summarize information on normal development:

* physical
* cognitive
* communication

Knowles (1973) isolated the most salient features of a theory when he stated, "A theory is a comprehensive, coherent, and internally consistent system of ideas about a set of phenomena" (p. 6). A theory should unify, relate, and explain diverse phenomena that were previously viewed as separate, unrelated, and unaccountable (Eisner, 1965). Theories provide an explanation of phenomena and guidelines for action (Knowles, 1973). In communication sciences and disorders, theories should provide the framework upon which rigorous research and clinical assessment and intervention procedures are based. In summary, a theory provides a basis for action, a rationale for practice, and a roadmap for exploring unfamiliar terrain.

THEORIES OF ADOLESCENCE

A number of theorists and theoretical positions have contributed to professionals' knowledge of adolescence. In turn, how these theorists impact upon the speech-language pathologist's work with adolescents with language disorders will be discussed later in this chapter. Muuss (1975) considered various theories of adolescence and isolated the following theoretical viewpoints: biological, anthropological, sociological, and psychological. The major theoretical positions and their theorists, or major contributors are presented in Table 2.1. Each of these theoretical positions has influenced how adolescents are viewed in the latter part of the twentieth century.

Biological Theory

In 1904, Hall perceived adolescence as a period of Sturm und Drang (storm and stress), a myth that remains to the present day. Hall's (1904) recapitulation theory (i.e., ontogeny recapitulates phylogeny) presented adolescence as a genetically predetermined time which corresponds to a turbulent transitional stage in the human race. Today, many people continue to view adolescence as "turbulent" and "transitional," due mainly to the major physiological changes that teen-agers experience.

Anthropological Theories

Anthropologists (Benedict, 1954; Mead, 1950) have argued that adolescence is culturally determined. Stress and turmoil, if experienced during adolescence, are the result of one's culture, not of biological changes in the body. Mead (1950), for example, argued that cultures, such as the Samoan, perceived the overall cycle from birth to death as gradual and continuous, because the adolescent girls she studied did not experience stress and turmoil. Benedict (1954), supporting Mead's position, maintained that growth was a gradual, continuous process from infantile dependence to adult independence, unless altered by the culture. The implication in Benedict's and in Mead's work is that western society, unlike the Samoan culture, has created a phenomenon called "adolescence" and has decreed that this time is filled with stress and turmoil. It should be noted that Mead's work has recently received severe criticism from Freeman (1983), who believes that Mead's cultural determinism ideology biased her observations.

TABLE 2.1 THEORIES OF ADOLESCENCE

BIOLOGICAL	ANTHROPOLOGICAL	SOCIOLOGICAL	PSYCHOLOGICAL
Hall (1904)	Mead (1950)	Davis (1944)	Central European Theories
	Benedict (1954)	Havighurst (1953)	Kroh (1944)
	Freeman (1983)		Kretschmer (1951)
			Zeller (1952)
			Spranger (1955)
			Remplein (1956)
			Psychoanalytic Theory
			Rank (1945)
			Freud, A. (1948)
			Freud, S. (1953)
			Field Theory
			Lewin (1939)
			Social Learning Theory
			Miller and Dollard (1941)
			Bandura and Walters (1963)
			Stage Theories
			General Development
			Gesell, Ilg, and Ames (1956)
			Mitchell (1979)
			Identity Development
			Erikson (1968)
			Cognitive
			Inhelder and Piaget (1958)
			Elkind (1978; 1974)
			Feuerstein (1980; 1979)
			Moral
			Kohlberg (1975)

Sociological Theories

In contrast with the biologists and anthropologists, sociologists have not concerned themselves with whether adolescence is biologically or culturally determined. Instead, the primary contribution of sociologists (Davis, 1944; Havighurst, 1953) has been their description of social development occurring during adolescence. Davis (1944) emphasized the emergence of "internalizing socialized anxiety" during adolescence. He postulated that adolescents control their behavior because of their anticipation and fear of punishment. Havighurst (1953) emphasized developmental tasks of adolescents, such as achieving a masculine or feminine social role, achieving emotional independence from parents and other adults, desiring and achieving socially responsible behavior, and so forth. Both Davis and Havighurst emphasized how social class differences affect expectations of social development, an ongoing topic of interest in the late twentieth century.

Psychological Theories

Like the sociologists, psychologists (see Table 2.1 Theories of Adolescence) have not debated whether adolescence is primarily determined by biological or cultural factors; instead, psychologists have attempted to document theories of psychological development, both personality and cognitive, during adolescence. Psychological theories of adolescent development have been grouped according to Central European theories, psychoanalytic theory, field theory, social learning theory, and stage theory. Each of these theoretical groups will be discussed, except for Central European theories (Kretschmer, 1951; Kroh, 1944; Remplein, 1956; Spranger, 1955; Zeller, 1952), which have had minimal influence upon American psychologists and educators.

Sigmund Freud (1953) catalyzed American inquiry into psychoanalytic theory by documenting universal psychosexual stages that are genetically, not environmentally, determined. Freud believed that character formation during adolescence has resulted from a struggle between two forces—the id (i.e., the biological-instinctual force) and the superego (i.e., the socially oriented force). Anna Freud (1948) placed greater emphasis on adolescent development and the role of puberty in character formation than did her father. Rank (1945), unlike Sigmund and Anna Freud, placed more emphasis on positive human dimensions of creativity and productivity, the conscious ego, and the present, than on human repression and neurosis, the unconscious ego, and the past.

An alternate explanation of psychological development during adolescence has been offered by field theory (Lewin, 1939). In this theory, adolescence is viewed as a period of transition during which the individual changes group membership. The adolescent belongs partly to the child group and partly to the adult group, without belonging to either. It should be noted that this viewpoint of adolescence has been expressed frequently during the last decade by speech-language pathologists attending our workshops. Lewin believes that various cultures differ regarding their requirements for changing from the child to the adult group. Muuss (1975), who offered an interpretation of Lewin, noted that the greater the differentiation between the adult group and the child group in a given culture or social class, the more difficult the transition.

A third alternative to explain psychological development during adolescence has been offered by social learning theorists (Bandura and Walters, 1963; Miller and Dollard, 1941). These theorists attempted to integrate psychoanalytic and behavioristic theory by stressing a reliance upon environmental events (e.g., imitation of parents, teachers, peers) rather than biological factors to explain development. They seem to agree with the anthropologists in that they view adolescence as part of the continuous development from childhood to adulthood, not as a separate stage of development.

Finally, stage theories attempted to explain psychological development during adolescence (Elkind, 1978, 1974; Erikson, 1968; Feuerstein, 1983, 1980; Gesell, Ilg, and Ames, 1956; Inhelder and Piaget, 1958; Kohlberg, 1975; Mitchell, 1979). Some theories concentrated attention on general development (Gesell, Ilg, and Ames, 1956; Mitchell, 1979) while others focused on specific aspects of development, notably identity development (Erikson, 1968), moral development (Kohlberg, 1975), and cognitive development (Elkind, 1978, 1974; Feuerstein, 1983, 1980; Inhelder and Piaget, 1958). From these stage theories in particular, information on adolescents has been extrapolated by speech-language pathologists. For this reason, these theories will be discussed in greater depth than preceding theories.

General Development Stage Theories According to Muuss (1975), Gesell's theory of adolescence drew heavily from his general theory of recapitulation. Gesell's theory incorporated the concept that developmental trends and behavioral traits are biologically determined. The environment can only stimulate, modify, and support growth; it cannot sequence it. Gesell was mainly interested in studying overt behaviors as they are manifested in gradual stages or cycles of development. He studied both mental and physical growth from a normative, descriptive, and chronological age perspective. Gesell explained that his sequential patterns of development oscillate along a spiral course toward maturity: The child begins to master a skill, then reverts to earlier forms of behavior, and then may plateau before totally mastering the new skill and moving forward.

Gesell considered adolescence to be a transitional period from childhood to adulthood. The adolescent period appears at approximately eleven years and ends in the early twenties, although he believes that girls go through this period more rapidly than boys, and that the most important changes occur in the first five years of adolescence. Gesell et al. (1956) described the specific aspects of adolescence through a series of maturity profiles at each age level.

Gesell, unlike Hall (1904), did not see adolescence as a time of "storm and stress," but as a process of enrichment with some inconsistencies. Although Gesell stated that the chronological ages used are only age approximates, his tables of averages are frequently under criticism. His critics believe that these tables do not take into account the diversity and variability in human behavior and development. Also, the subjects used to derive the behavioral characteristics at each age level were from one geographical area and from a high average to a superior intellectual population.

Mitchell (1979), who is not a theorist per se, advocated that adolescence covers too many years and too much growth to be considered one developmental period. Instead, Mitchell subdivided adolescence into three stages: the early adolescence or child-adolescence stage, the middle adolescence or adolescence stage, and the late adolescence or adult-adolescence stage. He emphasized that the differences between early and late adolescence are profound, and that professionals should treat these differences with more respect. Mitchell used chronological age clusters for each stage, but emphasized the overlap between the upper limits of one age group and the lower limits of the next. This was done intentionally, to indicate that general age clusters are more important than rigid chronological years. The major characteristics in each of the three stages of adolescence are as follows:

Stage I—Early adolescence or child-adolescence. Chronological ages for Stage I are twelve, thirteen, and fourteen years for boys; and eleven, twelve, and thirteen years for girls. This stage is dominated more than the other stages by body growth spurts in height and weight, and in primary and secondary sex characteristics. As a result of the rapid body growth, the psychological response of the adolescent is one of being concerned about how the body looks and feels. These individuals are child-like and limited in their emotional range. Of the three stages, this is the time the adolescent is the most egocentric. Socially, the peer group exerts influence, but the home and family still remain the most important social and emotional factors in the adolescent's life. Moral outlook is at the conventional level (Kohlberg, 1975). (Conventional level is explained in the forthcoming section entitled "Moral Stage Theory.") During this stage, the future carries less importance than it does during the next two stages.

Stage II—Middle adolescence or adolescence. This stage most closely resembles the typical image of adolescents. Mitchell maintains that the individual in this stage is neither a child nor an adult. Chronological ages for both boys and girls include thirteen, fourteen, and fifteen years. Physical growth continues, but not at as rapid a pace as during early adolescence. Mental growth increases dramatically: It is now more abstract, theoretical, and idealistic. Because of the mental growth factor, the person shows more awareness of the outside world, engages in introspection, and experiences an increase in self-doubt. Along with this, idealism is tested. The person is more interested in the opposite sex, and dating is more common than during early adolescence. The individual's social life is primarily with peers. This is the time in which

Erikson's (1968) psychosocial moratorium, explained in the next section, "Identity Development Stage Theory," is most likely to take place.

Stage III—Late adolescence or adult-adolescence. The ages for both boys and girls are sixteen, seventeen, and eighteen years. Physically and mentally, these individuals are adults and have achieved most of their adult growth. However, in terms of their social roles they remain primarily adolescents. Stage III is more a social phenomenon than a biological fact. During this stage, sexual intimacy increases and the person is more capable of dealing with interpersonal complexities. In addition, the individual becomes increasingly concerned about the future.

Identity Development Stage Theory Erikson (1968) studied with Sigmund and Anna Freud and he was influenced by their psychoanalytic training. However, his theory of identity development went beyond their theories by encompassing socialization. The main concept in Erikson's theory was the acquisition of an ego-identity, and the most important characteristic of adolescence was identity crisis. Erikson (1968) maintained that the adolescent must search out an identity by asking, "Who am I?" Identity, then, is not given by society, nor is it a maturational phenomenon. Identity can be found only through interaction with, and feedback from, other people; thus, peer group conformity is a means of testing roles. Erikson also noted that pubescence is a time of rapid body changes; hence the identity crisis is partly the result of psychophysiological factors. In other words, personal identity is achieved during adolescence through acceptance of the past, integration of the present, and orientation toward the future in terms of a decision about a career.

Another phenomenon occurring during adolescence is that of a *psychosocial moratorium*, or an *as if* period when the adolescent can try on different roles as if not fully committed and accountable. Experimentation with various roles in life can occur without penalty. The moratorium is an essential prerequisite for identity achievement.

Cognitive Stage Theories Piaget's theory of cognitive development (Piaget, 1970) has two interrelated aspects: A description of the four periods of development, which are sensorimotor, preoperational, concrete operational, and formal operational; and an explanation of concepts such as assimilation, accommodation, and equilibrium, which are as applicable to the sensorimotor period as to the formal operational period. The formal operational period is the most relevant to adolescence. According to Inhelder and Piaget (1958), this period has two stages: IIIA (approximately age eleven or twelve to fourteen or fifteen years) and IIIB (approximately age fourteen or fifteen years and upward). Stage IIIA appears to be a preparatory stage in which the adolescent can handle some formal operations, but in a cumbersome way, and with systematic, rigorous proof. However, in Stage IIIB the adolescent is capable of performing formal operational tasks in a spontaneous, systematic, rigorous way. Some of the characteristics of adolescents in the formal period are that they can reason on the basis of verbal propositions; leave the world of reality behind and enter the world of ideas; and think about their thinking.

The formal operational period is characterized by propositional and combinatorial operations: (1) combine by conjunction, i.e., both A and B make a difference; (2) combine by disjunction, i.e., it has to be this or that; (3) combine by implications, i.e., if it is this, then that happens; (4) combine by incompatibility, i.e., when this happens, then that does not (Inhelder and Piaget, 1958). A second set of formal groupings, in the propositional logic of the adolescent, is the INCR group. Each of the four letters stands for one of the logical transformations that can be performed on a propositional operation (Inhelder and Piaget, 1958): I=identity transformation, in which the original proposition retains its identity; N=negation transformation, in which everything in a given proposition is changed into the opposite of the original proposition; R=reciprocal transformation, in which the reciprocal of a proposition is transformed without modifying the conjunction or disjunction that joins the parts of the proposition; and C=correlative transformation, in which the reciprocal is inverted, or C is to R as N is to I.

David Elkind (1978; 1974) has written extensively on children and adolescents, and has done much to popularize Inhelder and Piaget's theory in the United States. He has described several developmental phenomena that emerge at adolescence as a result of higher levels of thinking. One is the *imaginary audience.* Adolescents, with their newly acquired skill of thinking about what others are thinking of them, act as though they are constantly on stage performing for everyone. The imaginary audience phenomenon is a new form of egocentrism through which adolescents must pass. The second phenomenon is the *personal fable* that maintains adolescents think that they are not like other people. Others might die in a car accident, but they could not; nothing bad could happen to them. Elkind's ideas supplement, rather that supplant, Inhelder and Piaget's theory of cognitive development.

Feuerstein (1980), who worked with Piaget, has made a significant contribution to adolescents with learning problems. His theory of cognitive modifiability held that the human organism, even one judged to be severely impaired, is capable of change at any age. This is true even if adolescents had inadequate development earlier in life or were exposed to conditions typically considered as barriers to change. Some of these barriers are exogenic (e.g., poverty, lack of stimulation at early ages), and others are endogenic (e.g., genetic defects, sensory impairments). Cognitive modifiability results from direct exposure to stimuli and mediated learning experience. However, while direct exposure to stimuli may explain some learning, it does not explain the diversity of learning that occurs within different individuals given the same situation. People who have the same biological parents, and similar environmental stimuli, turn out to be very different individuals. According to Feuerstein, differences in mediated learning experiences are the primary way to explain this phenomenon.

In a mediated learning experience, an adult selects and organizes stimuli for the adolescent. An experience becomes mediated when there is an intention on the part of the adult to focus an experience and to transmit the meaning of the object or event. An attempt to generalize the learning should occur. The adult needs to think continually, "How can I make the adolescent acquire *alone* what I now need to facilitate?" The cognitive structure of the individual is affected through this process of mediation, and as learning sets are acquired, the capacity to become modified through direct exposure to stimuli increases in efficiency. According to Feuerstein (1980), the more and the earlier that children are subjected to mediated learning experience, the greater will be their capacity to be affected by and to learn from direct exposure to stimuli. Normal adolescents have had consistent mediated learning experience, according to Feuerstein, and have benefited from direct exposure to stimuli. In essence, they have learned how to continue learning on their own. Feuerstein's theory maintained that when barriers obstruct learning, they can be overcome or bypassed; thus making it possible to restore a normal pattern of cognitive growth during adolescence.

Moral Stage Theory Kohlberg's (1975) theory of moral development was greatly influenced by Piaget's cognitive-developmental approach. Kohlberg advanced three levels of moral development: the preconventional or premoral level, the conventional or moral level, and the postconventional or autonomous level. Each level is divided into two stages. The conventional level is where most adolescents and many adults function. At this level, the person conforms to authority and obeys laws and social rules.

Kohlberg's theory of moral development (1975) incorporated the following principles: Moral stages form an invariant sequence of development; moral development can terminate at any stage. Kohlberg maintained that the advancement through the stages of moral reasoning depends upon the interplay of three factors: Cognitive developmental level, ability to empathize, and cognitive disequilibrium. He also maintained that these stages are universal and cut across cultures and socio-economic levels.

Kohlberg's theory has been criticized by several of his colleagues. Siegal (1980) questioned the invariant sequence of the early stages and the methodology which posed moral dilemmas outside the subjects' personal experiences. Gilligan (1982) criticized Kohlberg's theory for failing to consider differences in stages of moral development between boys and girls during early adolescence. In Gilligan's research, young girls have not adhered to the stages postulated by Kohlberg.

Summary of Theories of Adolescence

This section summarized the viewpoints of the major contributors to the theoretical positions on adolescent development. With this summary, professionals should have a better understanding of how these theoretical positions have influenced, historically and currently, the concept of normal adolescence.

Muuss (1975) compared and contrasted the various theoretical positions. He noted disagreements in definitions, characteristics, and general patterns of adolescent development among the different theories. However, once the older and more extreme theoretical positions are eliminated, agreement does exist. All theorists agree on the existence of endocrinological changes during early adolescence and on behavioral changes due to an increase in sexual interests, awarenesses, and tensions. They disagree on the amount of importance placed on the endocrine changes, and on the extent to which the behavioral changes are caused by physiological or sociological events. Most theorists discuss physiological changes that result in the individual's need to adjust to a new body image, and they view adolescence as a transitional period. The exceptions are those social learning theorists who view human development as a continuous process. A few theorists agree that adolescence is a period of development with stages within it, but disagree as to the number, characteristics, and psychological meaning of each of the stages. Lipsitz (1980) stated that all theories of adolescence emphasize physical growth, sexual maturation, increased autonomy, and cognitive sophistication. The various theoretical positions collectively postulate that adolescence is a time of rapid physiological and psychological changes influenced by socio-cultural determinants.

COPING WITH DIFFERENT THEORIES

When confronted with varying theoretical perspectives, a professional might select one of the following options.

Ignore All Theories

This option has been advocated by some professionals who believe theories are too impractical, abstract, and obtuse to be of any clinical value. Perhaps this attitude is responsible for the lack of a theoretical framework in many tests and educational materials. For example, when critiquing standardized tests and commercial intervention programs used with adolescents, we discovered how frequently professionals either do not state, or do not have, a theoretical model on which they base their test or program. However, the theory or theories upon which a test or program is developed is essential for providing a rationale as to why it is being used. "There is a cliche in the applied social sciences, often attributed to Kurt Lewin, that nothing is as practical as a good theory to enable you to make choices confidently and consistently, and to explain or defend why you are making the choices you make" (Knowles, 1973, p. 93).

Select One Theory

Another option is to conclude that one theory is the most appropriate, regardless of any conflicting evidence. Picking one theory may be initially advantageous in that one theory might minimize confusion. The disadvantage is that this option reflects a rigid position, and may be erroneous, and thus result in negative consequences. The state of the art is such that concepts, assumptions, and hypotheses about adolescents are constantly changing; therefore, a single theoretical position may result in a narrow perspective of the problem, and the assessment and intervention procedures.

Select One Theory for Research and Another for Clinical Application

This option is selected by professionals who view research and clinical application as opposing or mutually exclusive entities. Individuals are seen not as whole people, but as fragments to be either investigated or treated. Selecting one theory for research and another for clinical application creates false dichotomies within a discipline. This results in researchers and clinicians failing to communicate and work cooperatively for the benefit of the person with a communication disorder.

Select Precepts From a Variety of Theories and Develop a More Comprehensive, Synthesized Perspective

Currently, no one theory exists to account for the wide array of adolescent behaviors that require the speech-language pathologist's assessment and intervention. For example, cognitive functions of adolescents may be accounted for by one theory, while syntactic and semantic features may be accounted for by other theories. Although selecting precepts from a variety of theories may prove to be time consuming, this alternative may ultimately prove to be the most effective. The selection of precepts, when thought through carefully, avoids a superficial eclecticism. If professionals select this option of incorporating features from a variety of prevailing theories into a unified whole, they must do this in a systematic fashion to guarantee compatibility and consistency among the various theoretical constructs. For example, according to Lipsitz (1980), one of the problems of categorizing adolescence into a biological, anthropological, or sociological camp is that there is little dialogue among these disciplines. Each theoretical position is insufficient by itself, but each may be necessary when developing a comprehensive theoretical perspective of adolescence.

In conclusion, nothing is as practical as a good theory to provide a rationale as to why professionals are doing what they are doing. If professionals do not spend the necessary time on building a theoretical perspective into research and clinical services, the result will be a confusing, invalid, and unreliable data base.

THE AUTHORS' THEORETICAL POSITION

We chose the comprehensive option, i.e., "select precepts from a variety of theories and develop a more comprehensive, synthesized perspective" when developing the theoretical base for this text. No one theoretical position adequately explains what we believe about adolescents.

Our theory of adolescence holds that both biological and environmental factors influence adolescent development, although environmental factors may be stronger. This viewpoint has been influenced by Feuerstein (1980), who has documented bringing some individuals to near normal levels of functioning, despite negatively loaded genetics, by bombarding them with mediated learning experiences.

Adolescence involves unique and genetically predetermined bodily changes (e.g., puberty) to which the American culture has had different responses across racial and socio-economic stratas. For example, in some lower and middle socio-economic stratas, adolescence marks the time when children are expected to contribute significantly to finances of the family by getting a job or working in the family business; in some middle and higher socio-economic stratas, adolescents are not expected to work, but rather are sent away to private high schools to better prepare themselves for future careers. These responses constantly change as new generations of adults seek to improve their communication with adolescents.

We view the life cycle as a series of developmental phases of which adolescence is one period. To us, adolescence is no more "transitional" than are the periods from infancy to toddlerhood to childhood. It can be said that any period of time in human development is transitional (Sheehy, 1981). Furthermore, we concur with Muuss (1975) who has argued that adolescence manifests *both* continuous and stagelike patterns. Adolescence is continuous, i.e., part of a continuum from infancy to adulthood, but there are stages within the adolescent period, i.e., early, middle, and late.

We also question whether adolescence is filled with more stresses than other periods. We believe that adolescence is a major developmental period within the life cycle, filled with its own unique challenges and stressful moments.

We concur with Mitchell (1979) that adolescence is an extended time period encompassing several stages. We believe that speech-language pathologists should be guided in their assessment and intervention decisions by the stage of adolescence the student is in, i.e. Stage I—early; Stage II—middle; Stage III—late. We also extrapolate from the psychological theories of Inhelder and Piaget (1958) and Feuerstein (1980) when making decisions about cognitive functioning of adolescents. This cognitive functioning in turn influences intervention procedures. Adolescents at lower cognitive levels will probably need more concrete, hands-on activities; adolescents at higher levels may participate in communication activities requiring abstract reasoning.

Finally, we have observed that the physical development of adolescents influences their psychosocial development, and in turn, these two domains impact upon communication development. It would be artificial to assume that only biological, or only environmental, factors affect the adolescent's overall development. Rather, a combination of developmental factors occur simultaneously. These developmental milestones are highlighted in the remainder of the chapter. Specifically, information will be presented on physical, psychological, and communication development.

PHYSICAL DEVELOPMENT

Lipsitz (1979) observed that early adolescence involves a more rapid period of growth than any other period in life, including infancy and early childhood. These rapid bodily changes have a profound effect on how adolescents perceive themselves and communicate with others. Professionals working with adolescents need to be cognizant of how preoccupied adolescents can be with their own bodily changes. For example, the adolescent who is late in making bodily changes (described later in this section) may feel very uncomfortable being grouped with peers who have already begun developmental changes. Adolescents, desiring peer conformity, do not easily tolerate noticeable developmental differences. The adolescent with an obvious physical disability or delayed development or accelerated development is often at a disadvantage when it comes to peer acceptance and peer popularity. While the differences in physical development during adolescence may not seem important to adults, those differences may be of singular importance to some adolescents. Failure by professionals to recognize the impact of physical development can undermine attempts to communicate with adolescents. Professionals need to empathize with their growing pains.

During adolescence, pronounced bodily changes take place because of the presence of testosterone in males and estrogen in females. This time of rapid biological growth, which gives way to the first indications of sexual maturity, is known as puberty (Turner and Helms, 1979). The adolescent growth spurt is characterized by a sharp increase in height in girls, usually between eleven and thirteen years, and in boys between thirteen and fifteen years (Papalia and Olds, 1975). Weight follows a similar curve, but may not be as informative, because weight reflects a combination of developmental events such as skeletal growth, increased muscles and fat tissue, or size of various organs (Conger, 1973). Almost all skeletal and muscular dimensions are growing, but not to an equal degree, with greater changes in males than in females (Tanner, 1974).

Epstein (1978; 1974) studied brain growth stages and concluded that the first four stages of brain growth (i.e., three to ten months; two to four, six to eight, and ten to twelve years) coincide with mental growth (i.e., Piaget's four periods of cognitive development). Epstein hypothesized a fifth stage of brain growth (i.e., fourteen to sixteen plus years) that has no identifiable counterpart in Piaget's periods of cognitive development. Arlin (1975) investigated this notion and reported that such a cognitive period does exist, having its onset in the fourteen-to-sixteen-year period.

Epstein (1978; 1974) suggested that brain growth data may reveal why some children fail to learn in certain intervention programs such as Head Start: The four-to-six year age period is one of minimal brain and cognitive growth. Therefore, for biological reasons, the results do not indicate intellectual development for children in those programs. Epstein and Toepfer (1978) also speculated that the adjustment problems and the social and educational difficulties of junior high students may be tied to a brain-related growth plateau. These difficulties have been commonly blamed on sexual maturation.

Sex differences in body composition (sexual dimorphism) are evident prior to adolescence, even during fetal development. However, some of the most notable differences arise during adolescence: The male's greater height and width of his shoulders, and the female's wider hips (Tanner, 1974). Adolescent males show a decrease in adipose mass as a percentage of body weight whereas females do not lose any fat, but show a slower accumulation (Adams, 1980).

In addition to these physical changes, the body undergoes changes in primary and secondary sex characteristics. Primary sex characteristics involve those physiological features related to the sex organs (Turner and Helms, 1979); secondary sex characteristics serve to distinguish mature males from mature females. Hair growth is one of the obvious secondary sex characteristics of adolescence. Papalia and Olds (1975) state that one of the meanings of the Latin word *pubescere* is "to grow hairy." Other secondary sex characteristics are breast development and increased width and depth of the pelvis in females, and voice changes in males. Voice changes in both males and females will be discussed under communication development.

One needs only to observe an eighth or ninth grade class to realize the physical variability in the students. According to Papalia and Olds (1975), "the normal age range for puberty is ten to sixteen years for girls, with an average age of twelve, and twelve to eighteen years for boys, with an average age of fourteen" (p. 554). Although individual variability is normal, the sequence of pubertal events is similar.

In addition to individual variability, changes are observed in adolescents from one century to another. The trend is toward larger size and earlier maturation of adolescents. This trend, of adolescents being slightly taller and heavier than their parents, and females experiencing menarche ten months earlier than their mothers, is probably influenced by a higher standard of living today than a century ago (Papalia and Olds, 1975).

In summary, a discussion of adolescent physical development is incomplete without acknowledging the interaction of physical and psychological development. Adolescents appear to be self-conscious about their bodily changes whether they mature early or late. Generally, early maturers are found to be more adept in overall social adjustments than late maturers (Turner and Helms, 1979). Boys appear to be more affected by the timing of maturation than girls (Papalia and Olds, 1975).

PSYCHOLOGICAL DEVELOPMENT

Personality

Ferguson (1970) defined personality as the sum total of the ways in which one characteristically reacts to and interacts with others, as well as one's conception and feelings about oneself. Researchers have stated that it is during adolescence when the person establishes an identity and achieves an emotional personal autonomy. Erikson (1968) maintained that to achieve self-identity and autonomy, adolescents must experience conflict and crises. However, other writers (Bandura and Walters 1963; Douvan and Adelson, 1966) asserted that autonomy is achieved on a more gradual, continuous basis.

A study by Offer, Ostrov, and Howard (1981b) has suggested that the model American teen-ager exhibits feelings of confidence, happiness, and self-satisfaction. They achieve personal autonomy and identity as part of a continual, gradual process. Research by Offer, Ostrov, and Howard (1981b) indicated that girls report a worse self-concept (psychological self) than boys; in contrast, the girls report a more positive self-image (social self) than boys. They found no age differences for either sex in self-image. However, major differences were noted across the decades, i.e., adolescents of the 1960s had greater self-esteem than those of the 1970s and early 1980s. Cross-cultural differences were small and may suggest universal characteristics in western culture.

The adolescent's personality appears to be influenced by a number of variables. Among these variables are patterns of interaction between family members, peer group members, and important other persons such as educators, movie and television stars, and community members.

Cognition

Current empirical studies on cognitive development during adolescence have focused on these issues:

1. The use of formal operational thought based upon replication or expansion of Piaget's work
2. The relationship between cognitive development and language skills
3. The development of concepts.

An abundance of research studies and journal articles have debated the existence of formal operational thought during adolescence, as well as who engages in such thinking, when, and under what experimental conditions (Bart, 1971; Berzonsky, 1978; Broughton, 1977; Elkind, 1975; Hains and Miller, 1980; Lawson and Wollman, 1976; Leadbeater and Dionne, 1981; Martorano, 1977; Modgil and Modgil, 1976; Neimark, 1979; Overton and Meehan, 1982). Several studies found that adolescents apply formal operational thought in some contexts but not in others (Bart, 1971; Martorano, 1977). For example, formal operational thought may be applied in English literature, but not in chemistry. Some researchers found that the transition from concrete to formal operational thought may never be complete across all content areas; that as many as half of the adults in the United States either do not engage in formal operational thought, or do so only in their field of expertise (Labinowicz, 1980; Lawson and Wollman, 1976).

On traditional Piagetian tasks requiring application of formal operational thought, Elkind (1975) found that adolescent boys consistently out-perform the girls. However, he found that adolescent girls are more likely to apply their formal operational thinking to interpersonal matters, perhaps for social role reasons. Adolescents of average intellectual ability probably attain formal operations, but do not apply them equally to all aspects of reality (Elkind, 1975). Martorano (1977), in her research, found that mean scores on formal operational tasks completed by girls increased consistently during grades six through twelve. Formal operational thinking begins to emerge between twelve to fifteen years, although not even the oldest age-group tested evidenced formal operational performance across all tasks. Other researchers found no sex differences when formal operational tasks were attempted (Jackson, 1965; Killian, 1979; Kishta, 1979). Overton and Meehan (1982) found that learned helplessness, the perception of a lack of control over response outcomes, combined with feminine sex roles, resulted in inconsistent formal operational deficits; although with most problems, no sex differences were found. Hains and Miller (1980) found steady cognitive growth for normal adolescents, but a lack of such growth in delinquent youth. Older groups of delinquent youth performed no better on concrete or formal operational tasks than their younger counterparts.

Thus, while research on attaining formal operational thought would indicate that most adolescents achieve hypothetico-deductive reasoning in some situations, in a few individuals and in some settings abstract thinking does not occur. Empirical research would indicate that to expect formal operational thought to occur consistently within the adolescent population, across a variety of contexts, is unrealistic. However, an examination of secondary curricula in American schools indicates that formal operational thought is expected of adolescents across all content areas.

Another group of researchers attempted to correlate formal operational thought and spatial ability. Bart, Baxter, and Frey (1980) found spatial ability to be unrelated to formal reasoning task performance. Late maturers tend to have higher spatial ability relative to verbal performance than early maturers, regardless of sex (Waker, 1977). Diamond, Carey, and Back (1983) found that girls who mature earlier are disadvantaged on certain tasks requiring visuo-spatial ability compared with those who mature later. They suggested that the relationship between genetically timed physical and mental growth is a source of constraint on explanations of cognitive development. For example, this study, as well as others (Carey, Diamond, and Woods, 1980; Flin, 1980), observed a disruption of face perception during adolescence. Children, presented with photographs of unfamiliar people to remember, steadily increased their rate of accurate recognition between the ages of two and ten. This is followed by a plateau from ten to fourteen years of age, and usually by an actual decline in performance at age twelve, the average age of puberty in this country for girls. Attainment of the adult level of proficiency occurs by age sixteen. This disruption of development at twelve is not currently understood. Perhaps the disruption is related to pubertal development, but Strauss (1982) has examined other developmental dips (i.e., a behavior appears, disappears, and reappears) where no maturational timing component is implicated.

Higher level language behaviors have had an uncertain relationship with formal operational thought. Piaget's view that the level of cognitive development is not dependent on concurrent language development has been supported by empirical research (Davelaar, 1977; Jones, 1972). Performance on formal operational reasoning tasks, for example, has not been found to be related significantly to subordinate clause use or to tentative statement use such as "it looks like" (Davelaar, 1977). However, Rosenthal (1979) found a relationship between formal operational thought and use of dimensional language. Concrete operational thinkers describe events by using comparatives and superlatives, while formal operational thinkers cite the most general statement possible (e.g., "The most important thing is the length of the string.").

Empirical data for concept development during adolescence is sparse (Elkind, Barocas, and Johnsen, 1969; Peel, 1971). In general, the studies revealed that the adolescent's conceptual ability is more flexible than that of the child's; the adolescent's conceptual orientation can shift back and forth between abstract-categorical and perceptual (Crager and Spriggs, 1969; Elkind et al., 1969; Kagan et al., 1964; Olver and Hornsby, 1966). Olver and Hornsby (1966) concluded that adolescents' thinking becomes increasingly freed from perception. However, there remains the flexibility to classify perceptual characteristics at an analytic level (e.g., both a ruler and a watch have numbers) (Elkind et al., 1969; Kagan et al., 1964). Adolescents have a greater ability than children to classify by homogeneous functions (e.g., a lighter and a match go together because they can start fires) and abstract functions (e.g., a camera and a pencil go together because they can make a record of events) (Crager and Spriggs, 1969).

A Conceptual Learning and Development (CLD) model of concept attainment utilizing four successively higher levels has been proposed (Klausmeier and Allen, 1978):

Concrete Level—an object is recognized as being the same from one encounter to the next.

Identity Level—an object is recognized as being the same from one encounter to the next when observed from a different spatiotemporal perspective or sensed in a different modality.

Classificatory Level—two or more different examples of a given concept are recognized as members of the same class.

Formal Level—hypotheses are formed concerning the relevant attributes of a concept, remembering the hypotheses, and evaluating the validity of them.

Experimental evidence has suggested that adolescents utilize hypothetico-deductive strategy (i.e., formal level) to solve verbal problems (daSilva, 1979; Peel, 1971; Rhys, 1979). Hager (1982) has found that concrete thinkers in grades seven, nine, and eleven attempted solutions in terms of one aspect of the presented data, while formal thinkers combined two or more pieces of evidence relating them through cause and effect or sequence. Only a small percentage sustained arguments resting on assumed hypotheses developed inductively or deduced analytically, even at the eleventh grade level.

It appears that the adolescent has an increasing facility to use words as a means of conceptualizing. Vygotsky (1962) suggested that the ability of the adolescent to use language as a vehicle for the acquisition of new concepts is the major intellectual advancement during this period in the lifespace. He also observed that while the young child thinks by remembering, an adolescent remembers by thinking. Acquisition of concepts becomes increasingly important for the adolescent as the secondary-school curriculum focuses almost exclusively on the acquisition of conceptual knowledge in the content areas (Wiig and Semel, 1980).

The general cognitive developmental changes that occur from childhood to adolescence can be summarized as follows:

1. A growing ability to think about one's own thinking (metacognition)
2. The ability to consider events removed in time or space, real or imagined
3. The ability to consider all possible alternatives to a problem or situation
4. The ability to formulate hypotheses and test them.

COMMUNICATION DEVELOPMENT

Information on the normal development of verbal and nonverbal communication during adolescence is extremely limited. And yet, it is difficult, if not impossible, to determine what is abnormal communication unless professionals have some notion of what is normal development. That the process of normal language acquisition extends into adolescence has been documented by Cromer (1974; 1970), Kramer, Koff, and Luria (1972), and Menyuk (1975). This section presents information that is currently available on the adolescent population regarding verbal and nonverbal communication development. Data have been gleaned from three sources: Surveys and interviews, standardized test data, and empirical research.

Surveys and Interviews

The most recent extensive survey of adolescents was completed by interviewing 160,000 youth between the ages of thirteen to eighteen. The results were published in *The Private Life of the American Teen-ager* (Norman and Harris, 1981), also known as the Norman/Harris Report. During the interview survey, adolescents reported their perceptions of various communication situations. The results indicated that strong beliefs and feelings exist among the majority of adolescents on a variety of issues related to speaking and listening. These adolescents' advice to adults was to be "up-front" and honest with them; to listen to them, and to try to understand them.

In addition to the Norman/Harris Report, exact transcripts of responses to interview questions given by early adolescents have been recorded in *Listen to*

Us! (Kavanaugh, 1978). Professionals who desire to become more familiar with normal syntactic, semantic, and pragmatic aspects of adolescent's language would find considerable data within this resource. The book also provides adults with a perspective on what adolescents think and talk about. The transcripts appear to be actual recorded English, complete with grammatical errors and "verbal mazes" in which the subjects engaged in multiple verbal revisions of content.

Using a field work format, which extended over eight and a half years, Folb (1980) interviewed over three hundred black teen-agers in south-central Los Angeles. Her research is reported in a book entitled *runnin' down some lines* (Folb, 1980), an excellent source for data on black teen-age vernacular. She specifically studied name terms in the black community, forms of manipulation, male-female interactions, the vocabulary of drugs, and the dynamics of vocabulary use.

Standardized Test Data

Standardized test data have been used to compare language performance across instruments, and to describe language development during adolescence. We have serious reservations about whether adolescents' communication development should be described using standardized tests. Prather (1984) examined changes made on subtests of formal language instruments when individuals were between the ages of eleven and eighteen. She found that some language characteristics show no change in development while others show a positive correlation between age and correct responses. For example, Prather examined the *Clinical Evaluation of Language Functions (CELF)* (Semel and Wiig, 1980) and found six subtests that showed no change in the criterion scores from sixth grade through twelfth grade. The greatest change was reflected by a gain of approximately one point a year for the following subtests: "Processing relationships and ambiguities," "Producing word associations," and "Producing model sentences." Prather (1984) concluded that the quality of oral language required during these subtests possibly does continue to improve or emerge during adolescence. We question whether a one point a year gain is significant enough to indicate a quantitative or a qualitative change in oral language. The *CELF* is not alone in reflecting small changes in criterion scores throughout adolescence.

We examined the *Fullerton Language Test for Adolescents* (Thorum, 1980) for similar increases and plateaus in scores across age levels. The data indicated equivalent mean scores for the ages eleven to eighteen and one-half years for the areas of auditory synthesis, morphology competence, oral commands, convergent production, syllabication, and grammatic competency. One interpretation is that little, if any, development occurs in these communication areas after age eleven. One skill, auditory synthesis, actually showed a gradual decline in mean scores between the ages of eleven and eighteen years, perhaps indicative of the lessening practice and emphasis on this oral language behavior as higher grade levels are reached. Two subtests, "Divergent Production" and "Idioms," showed a gradual improvement as adolescents became older. This exercise confirmed our earlier hypothesis that norms on discrete point tests may not provide appropriate quantitative or qualitative changes in adolescents' oral language.

Another concern about the use of standardized test data to describe normal language development during adolescence is that the assessment items selected for inclusion in a given test do not necessarily match those behaviors that show the greatest changes from ages twelve to twenty years. According to Muma (1978), ". . . norms obscure important information about individual differences, strategies of learning, systems and processes, contextual constraints, communicative intent, verbal functions and speech acts, and alternative codes. The result is that they deal with superficial aspects of language: the products of acquisition." (p. 146). A better approach would be to generate empirical research that describes underlying processes of language acquisition.

Empirical Research

Developmental milestones of oral and nonverbal communication have revealed that communication continues to develop during adolescence. These developmental trends are summarized below.

Voice Characteristics One of the most obvious changes in oral communication during puberty is that both boys and girls experience a lowering of the modal pitch. In males, the vocal folds increase in length and thicken, and the pitch drops about a full octave (Zemlin, 1968). In females, the larynx continues to grow at the same rate in adolescence as it did during childhood, resulting in a drop of two to three musical notes (Zemlin, 1968). Males between the ages of nine and thirteen years have a modal pitch of 220 Hz, those between ages fourteen and sixteen years have a modal pitch of 180 Hz, and those between ages seventeen and eighteen years have a modal pitch of 130 Hz before the voice stabilizes at 115 Hz in adulthood (Wilson, 1979). Corresponding modal pitches in females are 240 Hz, then 225 Hz, before the voice stabilizes at 200 Hz in adulthood (Wilson, 1979).

Comprehension of Linguistic Features Subtle changes occur in the adolescent's ability to understand oral communication. Professionals should not expect adolescents to comprehend everything that is spoken to them, since certain linguistic features may not be entirely understood even by adults. For example, it has been found in both children and adults that sentences with relative clauses located in the middle of them are more difficult to comprehend than sentences with clauses at the end (Sheldon, 1977). Also, sentences that violate the minimal distance principal are persistently treated as if they adhered to the principle (Chomsky, 1969; Reed, 1977; Sanders, 1971). A sentence that adheres to the minimal distance principle contains a subject and a verb in reasonably close proximity, thus allowing accurate comprehension. Also, comprehension of the ask/tell distinction is late developing and is never fully resolved by some individuals (Kramer, Koff, and Luria, 1972). Using ninth graders as subjects in a pilot study, Thomas and Walmsley (1976) found that the students made errors in complement sentences with *ask* and *tell*, *promise*, *persuade*, and *threaten*. The investigators reported that errors may have been caused by factors other than linguistic deficiency (i.e., the students' current level of metalinguistic development).

The development of the comprehension of metaphors in normal students between four to fifteen years was investigated (Galda, 1981). Results indicated that metaphoric understanding increased with age. Once students were in the concrete operational period, their metaphoric understanding and linguistic abilities increased, resulting in their ability to comprehend and to explain abstract metaphors.

Production of Linguistic Features One of the most extensive studies to date that explored language production was that of Loban (1976). He completed a thirteen-year longitudinal study on 211 normal subjects from kindergarten through grade twelve. He selected a group high in language ability as reported by teachers, a group low in language ability, and a random group of subjects representative of the total group. The characteristics that teachers used to describe those in the high group included the use of a varied vocabulary, the adjustment of speaking pace to listeners' needs, and the ability to remain in control of ideas expressed. The subjects spoke freely, fluently, and effectively, and listened attentively. The characteristics that teachers used to describe those in the low group included unawareness of listeners' needs and meagerness of vocabulary. Their language rambled without apparent purpose, and projected a hesitant, faltering style.

Each year, Loban (1976) completed an oral interview from all subjects, and from grade three on, he collected one or more written compositions. The purpose of Loban's research was to determine if differences existed between pupils who ranked high in language proficiency compared with those who ranked low. He also wanted to know if growth in language followed a predictable year-by-year sequence.

Using communication units as his basic measurement, Loban (1976) charted the average number of words per unit during oral language. A communication unit was defined as an independent clause with its modifiers. Those students with a high average number of words per communication unit were the same students who were rated high on a checklist of language skills by teachers.

A random group of subjects (i.e., a mixture of students rated high or low on language skills by teachers) was investigated. This investigation revealed that a year of language growth was typically followed by a plateau, then by another year of growth. See Table 2.2 for a comparison of the relative growth of the three groups during grades one through twelve.

In addition to examining the average number of words per communication unit, Loban analyzed the percentage of total words that were in mazes. When a maze is removed from a communication unit, ". . . the remaining material constitutes a straightforward, acceptable communication unit" (Loban, 1976, p. 102). All groups ended grade twelve with virtually the identical percentages of verbal mazes used in grade one, with erratic fluctuations evidenced during the middle years of school. These percentages are summarized in Table 2.3.

The average number of words per maze was also relatively stable throughout all twelve grades. (See Table 2.4.) The high language ability group consistently showed the smallest degree of maze behavior as a percentage of total words, and the lowest average number of words per maze. Although the low language ability group used a lower average number of words, they simultaneously used a larger amount of verbal maze behavior.

In comparing the average number of communication units in oral language with written language, Loban found that his subjects tended to speak *and* write in units that had similar average lengths. He found that those students who were superior in oral language skills in kindergarten and first grade, *before* they learned to read and write, were the same students who excelled in reading and writing by the time they were in sixth grade. The inclusion of longer and more complex adjective clauses was a primary mark of increasing language development, both oral and written. The growth of adjectival clauses was centered mainly in junior high school, grades seven through nine.

In most oral language measurements taken by Loban (1976), the high language ability subjects were approximately four to five years advanced in comparison with low language ability subjects. There was a strong correlation between high socio-economic status and entry into the high language ability group. A similar correlation existed between the low language ability group and low socio-economic status. While subjects from minority ethnic groups (i.e., Oriental, Mexican, Black Americans) comprised a disproportionately high percentage of the low group, and low percentage of the high group, social inequity, not ethnic background, affected language proficiency. As Loban stated, "Minority students who came from securely affluent home backgrounds did not show up in the low proficiency group. The problem is poverty, not ethnic affiliation" (Loban, 1976, p. 23).

Additional research on normal oral communication development of minority groups is limited. Labov (1969) found that black teen-agers used their language to convey the same range of functions that standard English speakers did; but this communication behavior generally occurred away from school. Labov argued that it is not so much a language problem that the child from a minority lower-class background finds in school, but is instead a prob-

TABLE 2.2 AVERAGE NUMBER OF WORDS PER COMMUNICATION UNIT—ORAL LANGUAGE

Grade	Average Number of Words per Communication Unit (mean)			Relative Growth[a] (in percent)			Year-to-Year Velocity[b] (in percent)		
	High Group	*Random Group*	*Low Group*	*High Group*	*Random Group*	*Low Group*	*High Group*	*Random Group*	*Low Group*
1	7.91	6.88	5.91	67.61	58.80	50.51	—	—	—
2	8.10	7.56	6.65	69.23	64.62	56.84	+1.62	+ 5.82	+6.33
3	8.38	7.62	7.08	71.62	65.13	60.51	+2.39	+ 0.51	+3.67
4	9.28	9.00	7.55	79.32	76.92	64.53	+7.70	+11.79	+4.02
5	9.59	8.82	7.90	81.97	75.38	67.52	+2.65	− 1.54	+2.99
6	10.32	9.82	8.57	88.21	83.93	73.25	+6.24	+ 8.55	+5.73
7	11.14	9.75	9.01	95.21	83.33	77.01	+7.00	− 0.60	+3.76
8	11.59	10.71	9.52	99.06	91.54	81.37	+3.85	+ 8.21	+4.36
9	11.73	10.96	9.26	100.26	93.68	79.15	+1.20	+ 2.14	+2.22
10	12.34	10.68	9.41	105.47	91.28	80.43	+5.21	− 2.40	+1.28
11	13.00	11.17	10.18	111.11	95.47	87.01	+5.64	+ 4.19	+6.58
12	12.84	11.70	10.65	109.74	100.00	91.03	−1.37	+ 4.53	+4.02

[a]Relative Growth uses the scores of the Random group at grade twelve to equal 100 percent.
[b]Year-to-Year Velocity is the percentage change in any given group from one year to the following year.

(Reprinted with the permission of the National Council of Teachers of English.)

TABLE 2.3
MAZE WORDS AS A PERCENTAGE OF TOTAL WORDS—ORAL LANGUAGE

Grade	*High Group*	*Random Group*	*Low Group*
1	7.61	7.46	9.04
2	6.21	8.03	8.31
3	4.71	6.39	7.98
4	6.39	8.38	11.06
5	6.41	7.53	9.04
6	6.98	8.29	10.33
7	5.82	7.76	11.08
8	6.08	8.12	9.30
9	5.31	7.29	10.18
10	7.45	7.40	7.51
11	7.32	7.04	9.01
12	7.25	7.04	9.19

(Reprinted with the permission of the National Council of Teachers of English.)

TABLE 2.4
AVERAGE NUMBER OF WORDS PER MAZE—ORAL LANGUAGE

Grade	*High Group*	*Random Group*	*Low Group*
1	1.94	2.09	1.81
2	1.89	1.89	1.90
3	1.88	1.85	1.98
4	1.97	2.06	1.99
5	1.93	2.09	2.07
6	2.15	2.21	2.16
7	1.90	2.06	2.17
8	1.96	2.01	2.11
9	1.78	1.98	2.18
10	1.85	1.92	1.92
11	1.94	1.97	1.97
12	1.77	1.99	2.24

(Reprinted with the permission of the National Council of Teachers of English.)

lem of cultural conflict. These students may not want to be heard saying things that are encouraged at school lest it imply they are accepting the values coded in the language of the middle class. Taylor and Peters (1982) have presented an excellent description of Black English features by reviewing 29 linguistic rules. These twenty-nine linguistic rules (e.g., invariant "be," negation, plurals, questions, and pronouns) have been analyzed to determine where there is overlap between Black English and several other dialects, i.e., Southern English, Southern White Nonstandard English, and Appalachian English. They also briefly reviewed Spanish-influenced English in terms of phonological and syntactic features. A more extensive study by Mendelberg (1984) investigated the language of Mexican-American adolescents of migrant origin. The analysis of the data revealed distinctive language patterns used in different settings. Initially, it would seem that the language patterns chosen are determined as a matter of the subject's personal choice. However, upon further investigation it appears that underlying the choice is the role played by language as a symbol of the group and the position the group occupies in the present social system. There is a relationship between language use and the development of a group identity. These findings concur with Taylor and Peters (1982), who concluded that major social and cultural factors influence language acquisition and behavior.

Discourse: Conversations and Narrations A review of the literature revealed that numerous studies have investigated discourse of adolescents. Data are presented on two types of discourse—conversations and narrations.

Conversations Various researchers have investigated communicative maturity during conversations. For example, Wiig (1982a) found communicative maturity to be developed by age thirteen. At this time, youth can make the transition between an informal language code (i.e., peer register) and a more formal language code (i.e., adult register) of language. Moreover, Wiig found that by age fifteen teen-agers will use the more formal register, not only with adults but also with their own peer group, unless the peers are their very closest friends. Different surface structures of the speech act are appropriate for different situations depending upon the listener, setting, topic, and objectives (Wiig, 1983). Modification of the verb phrase is the most important aspect in making the surface structure changes (e.g., "Close the door" versus "Would you mind closing the door?"). A mature communicator will have many different structural forms to express the same intent.

As communicative maturity increases, inept communication acts should decrease. By third grade, students are able to recognize an inept communication act, but they cannot yet correct it (Johnson, Greenspan, and Brown, 1980). By sixth grade, students improve inept communication acts if those acts attempt to influence others' actions (e.g., "You're studying for a test at school. Lou calls you up and wants to come over to visit. You say, 'You picked a fine time to visit.' How would you correct your statement?"). Not until ninth grade can students correct inept attempts to have others feel better (e.g., "Tom is sad because his dog died. You say, 'Cheer up, it's nothing to be upset about. Pretty soon you'll forget all about it.' How would you correct your statement?").

A possible explanation as to why inept communication acts decrease in late adolescence is that the person is capable of using more sophisticated communication strategies; for example, taking the perspective of the listener. Also, older adolescents have a greater range of interpersonal constructs that they apply to communication situations (Ritter, 1979).

We have completed the second year of a six-year longitudinal study in which we analyzed spontaneous conversational speech of eight normal adolescents, four boys and four girls while they were in the seventh and eighth grades, under two experimental conditions. In one condition, adolescents talked with a familiar peer of their choice, while in the other condition they talked with an unfamiliar adult of the opposite sex. These two conditions were selected to represent bipolar situations.

The results of this study to date revealed that adolescents used more questions when with a peer than with an adult. They also initiated more topics and used more frequently the language functions of describing feelings and of entertaining. With an adult, they used more supportive gestures (e.g., head nodding "yes" while saying "yes"), and the language function of giving information. The study found that boys, more so than girls, used a higher frequency of figurative language, positive verbal interruptions (e.g., saying "uh-huh" while someone is talking), neutral gestures (e.g., no gesture or no new gesture), conversational units, and the language functions of giving information and describing feelings. Although the girls took fewer turns, they used more time per conversational unit than the boys. Seventh graders used more complex sentences and fewer fragments than they did a year later in the eighth grade. We have no explanation as to why this regression occurred in the eighth grade, except that it would illustrate that growth is not a continuous process (Lipsitz, 1979) and that dips occur in development (Strauss, 1982). The eighth graders, more than the seventh graders, used a higher frequency of nonspecific language, verbal mazes, positive verbal interruptions, supportive gestures, conversational units, and indications of readiness for further communication.

Topic maintenance changes have been studied by Dorval (1980), who found significant differences between children and adolescents. The results of the study revealed:

1. Non-elaborated topic related remarks increased in frequency during the elementary years, but started to decrease during high school as more complex topic-related remarks increased.
2. More complex remarks such as factual and perspective oriented evaluations/elaborations/questions were made during ninth grade and increased in frequency thereafter.

3. In ninth grade, but declining thereafter, there was a high proportion of evaluation comments relative to elaboration comments and evaluations, elaborations, and questions that focused on people's perspectives or feelings. Thus, conversational quality (i.e., coordination associated with topic management) changes with age.

Topics of conversation have been indexed and classified using taped transcripts of fifteen-year-old adolescents (Rutherford, Freeth, and Mercer, 1969). While analyzing younger children, two broad topics surfaced—domestic and educational. Rutherford et al. (1969) found these topics to be insufficient when classifying topics of adolescents and they added a third general area called "philosophical." This added category absorbed topics that did not relate to the individual's immediate environment of school and home. Philosophical topics were discussed without immediate personal experience or knowledge, and often reflected facts or opinions derived from television. Although these data were obtained from England, it is probable that the classification of the conversational topics of American youth would also require a philosophical category.

Rutherford (1976) made the astute observation that it is the way in which adolescents talk *about* certain topics, such as pop singers, that causes adults to complain that adolescents "speak another language." The current system of beliefs and attitudes of adolescents can be seen through the medium of their conversations. Adolescents make remarks that allow peer group members to share the feeling expressed, but which intentionally prevent adult onlookers from understanding (e.g., "Well, just . . . [laugh] him" and "Well, not just his voice . . . but himself" [Rutherford, 1976, p. 113]). Such utterances are not analyzable according to Rutherford. Remarks such as the ones quoted above are part of normal adolescent secretiveness, a necessary mechanism that allows the child to grow up and away from parents. Much of the secret nature of their lives is reflected through their language (Rutherford, 1976).

Narrations All of the preceding studies have focused on one aspect of discourse, i.e., conversations. When narration has been studied, normal children have been found to produce true narratives by five to six years of age. Complex stories with multiple embedded narrative structures do not emerge until eleven to twelve years of age (Westby, 1984).

One way that narrations have been studied is through the use of story reformulation tasks. Several researchers have proposed that story schemata are used by listeners to guide comprehension and recall (Mandler and Johnson, 1977; Rumelhart, 1975; Stein and Glenn, 1979). Weaver and Dickinson (1982) summarized the way that efficient listeners maximize verbatim recall by using processes:

1. Recognition of verbal formulae (e.g., "Once upon a time there was . . .")
2. Prediction of sentence structures based upon the constraining power of preceding sentences

3. Recognition and use of conjunctions and prepositions to mark relationships (i.e., temporal, causal, spatial) among propositions during encoding
4. Integration of information gathered from these multiple sources.

Chappell (1980) found that early adolescents were pragmatically aware of what information needed to be retold, and they used appropriate syntactic structures. By adulthood, a story being retold is "filled in" if the original story does not follow a predictable story sequence (Johnston, 1985).

The amount of information recalled during story reformulation tasks showed developmental changes as age increased; however, basic organizational structure did not vary across ages (Mandler and Johnson, 1977). Young children tended to emphasize action sequence outcomes, but older children and adults emphasized the actions themselves or the internal events motivating them (Mandler and Johnson, 1977). Across all age levels, the most important units of a story were recalled most frequently (Brown and Smiley, 1977). Thus, while some aspects of story reformulation differed with age (e.g., amount of information recalled, emphasis during recall), other aspects did not (e.g., organizational structure, judgment of importance of units). As Weaver and Dickinson (1982) pointed out, story grammar taxonomies such as Stein and Glenn's (1979) are relatively insensitive to developmental changes.

Summary of Empirical Research On Oral Communication From the studies encompassed within this section, one can generalize that significant changes occur during adolescence regarding development of communication behaviors. Adolescents become more adept at social communication, more flexible in their language use, and more secretive in their conversations with close peer group members. Their narrations become lengthier and include multiple embedded episodes.

Nonverbal Communication Nonverbal patterns in today's adolescents may be quite different from those in the past (French, 1978). French (1978) has described several nonverbal behaviors now considered normal for adolescents, which in the past would have been signs of hostility and rebellion. One such behavior is the blank stare, or focusing the eyes beyond the listener when engaging in a conversation. Another is the eye roll, once used as an expression of impudence. Now, the eye roll is used so extensively that the message it once conveyed has been weakened (French, 1978). Another behavior is the back turn, or shifting the body slightly, to expose the back to the receiver during the conversation. French believes the back turn has been influenced by the black culture, which views it as signs of trust and of understanding what was said. He also described the "Black Walk," which is slower than the "White Walk." It is more of a stroll, with the head slightly elevated and casually tipped to one side. French (1978) analyzed the nonverbal message conveyed by the White Walk to be, "I am a strong [person], and I'm in a hurry to get somewhere." (p. 544). The nonverbal message conveyed by the Black Walk is, "I am strong. I am 'cool.' I can't be bothered by anything in this world." (p. 544). French has observed that both white and black youth have adopted nonverbal communication patterns of the black culture.

Some of the research in nonverbal communication during adolescence has analyzed recognition of facial expressions. In the 1920s, Gates (1923) conducted a facial expression recognition study and found that laughter was identified by age three, pain by ages five to six, anger by age seven, fear by ages nine to ten, and surprise by age eleven. None of the individuals studied had recognized scorn by age fourteen. The findings of this study have not been seriously challenged since then (Knapp, 1978). According to a report by Blanck and Rosenthal (1982), older children develop some degree of distrust toward facial expressions when accompanied by discrepant vocal cues. The researchers summarized the data on older children as evidence that these children put more weight on facial expressions under normal conditions of communication, and less under conditions of discrepancy.

Age changes in deceiving and detecting deceit have been reported by DePaulo and Jordan (1982). Before adolescence, children's distinction of deception from truth by reading only facial expressions is by chance. When given both verbal and nonverbal cues, adolescents perceive feigned expressions of liking as less positive than sincere expressions of liking, and feigned expressions of disliking as less negative than the honest expressions of disliking. Girls between five to twelve years are increasingly adept at masking their deceptions facially; the reverse tends to occur for boys. The strategy that seventh graders use to deceive a person is to convey the feigned affect with the same degree of intensity as when it occurs naturally when telling the truth, while college students deceive by exaggerating the dissimulated affect. Researchers speculated that students learn and practice deception by playing card games, board games, party games, and sports.

Two studies examining the development of eye contact, or gazing, disagree on whether there is a gradually increasing or decreasing trend in looking behavior, up to adolescence (Ashear and Snortum, 1971; Levine and Sutton-Smith, 1973). Knapp (1978) reported that adolescence represents a low point for eye gazing. Such lack of eye contact noted in normal adolescents is important data for professionals to keep in mind when they are assessing gazing behavior during conversational speech.

Listener feedback, such as head nods and vocalizing "mm-hmm," has been found to be nearly absent through fifth grade (Dittman, 1972). Before junior high school, adults probably cannot expect much overt feedback, such as head nods, to indicate that children are listening to them. Our findings (McKinley and Larson, 1983) concur with Dittman's results. We found eighth grade students provided considerable nonverbal listener feedback during conversations, even more than they did while in seventh grade.

The decoding of nonverbal cues is a gradually increasing skill from kindergarten through ages twenty to thirty, after which time a leveling off occurs (Dimitrovsky, 1964). On tests of nonverbal sensitivity, females consistently outperformed males from grade school through the middle twenties (Knapp, 1978). Nonverbal ability was not found to be significantly related to intelligence quotients, class rank, Scholastic Aptitude Test (SAT) scores, or vocabulary test scores (Knapp, 1978). The findings show that, in general, if persons were good senders of nonverbal communication, they were also good receivers (Knapp, 1978).

The empirical research reported in this section underlines the continuing development of nonverbal communication during adolescence. Developmental changes in both encoding and decoding nonverbal cues occur in normal adolescents.

SUMMARY

This chapter presented information on theories of adolescence, as well as data on normal physical, psychological, and communication development. The four major theoretical positions of adolescence were discussed: biological, anthropological, sociological, and psychological. The reader was presented with a rationale for why knowledge of theories is important, as well as the theoretical framework to which we subscribe. Physical development and psychological development, specifically personality and cognitive development, were considered. Communication development of adolescents was extrapolated from three sources: Surveys and interviews, standardized test data, and empirical research. The empirical evidence reveals that many changes occur in comprehension and production of linguistic features, discourse processes (both conversations and narrations), and nonverbal communication during the adolescent period. These changes include improvement in specific behaviors (e.g., correction of inept communication) or emergence of new ones (e.g., listener nonverbal feedback such as head nods). While the data base is still meager and fragmented, it is our hope that interest in normal adolescent research can be piqued through the review of communication development during adolescence.

DISCUSSION QUESTIONS

1. How does your own comprehensive theory of adolescence interact with your theory(s) of cognition, language, and communication development?

2. What relevance do the physical and psychological data have upon the adolescent's communication behaviors?
3. Critique the data presented on normal cognition and communication development. Describe three research topics that would significantly add to this data base.

SUGGESTED READINGS

Loban, W. *Language Development: Kindergarten Through Grade Twelve.* National Council of Teachers of English, Urbana, IL, 1976.

Muuss, R. *Theories of Adolescence.* Random House, New York, 1975.

Norman, J. and Harris, M. *The Private Life of the American Teen-ager.* Rawson, Wade Publishers, New York, 1981.

CHAPTER 3

Reaching Adolescents: A Service Delivery Model

GOALS:

To report current trends in educating university students about a prototype delivery model

To define the six components of the delivery model

To discuss the first two components of the delivery model:

* Information Dissemination
* Identification

It is one decision to advocate that services for adolescents with communication disorders are needed; it is another to plan and provide such services in the variety of settings in which adolescents are located. Although most adolescents are in public schools, speech-language pathologists cannot ignore other places because youth in settings such as juvenile detention centers and residential institutions have a high incidence of developmental disabilities, which are likely to have associated communication disorders (ASHA, 1984; Lakin et al., 1983; Taylor, 1980; 1969).

Approaches to service delivery are influenced by the professional's university program. We question whether university students are being adequately prepared to meet the challenges of serving the adolescent population. Programs in communication sciences and disorders have traditionally emphasized the study of disability categories (e.g., stuttering, aphasia). Increasingly, programs are organizing coursework by age groupings. It is not unusual to find university programs focused on specific age groups, such as the preschool and geriatric populations, but adolescents rarely benefit from such focus. As awareness of the needs of the adolescent surfaces, some university programs have begun to provide coursework that specifically addresses these needs. A pilot survey in the late 1970s (Boyce, Godwin, and Larson, 1979) revealed that only 50 percent of the university programs in a five state upper-midwest area accredited through the American-Speech-Language-Hearing Association had specific classes or course content that prepared students to work with adolescents. Yet all of the universities expected their students to provide appropriate clinical services to this population.

In an updated survey completed for this book in 1985, all programs in the United States were polled for their current emphasis on educating their students about adolescents with communication disorders. The return rate was 42 percent. The results of this survey are reported in Table 3.1.

University personnel expect their students to interact clinically with adolescents, yet they do not consistently provide them with necessary information on this population. Perhaps this phenomenon is partially explained by the fact that only fifty-two percent of the respondents envisioned an employment market for speech-language pathologists with adolescents with communication disorders. Another explanation is that fifty-eight percent of the programs mentioned insufficient research data, and fifty-two percent mentioned insufficient assessment instruments and intervention strategies. Whatever the explanation, many students majoring in communication sciences and disorders are not receiving the curriculum to prepare them to work with the adolescent population. However, upon graduation, they are working with adolescents in junior and senior high schools, juvenile detention centers, prisons, graduate equivalency degree (GED) programs, and academic skill resource centers for marginal students in vocational-technical institutes, colleges, and universities. Too often, graduates are ill-prepared for these jobs. Furthermore, they are inadequately prepared to create jobs in these settings.

The delivery model that follows is intended to provide a general framework for the development of speech-language programs in settings where adolescents are housed. In some settings, extensive in-roads already lead to delivery of service. In other cases, the in-road is barely a path (e.g., adult basic education facilities). In this chapter and in later chapters, we occasionally illustrate how to apply various components of the delivery model to the primary settings in which adolescents are found: Secondary schools, adult-education facilities, hospitals, juvenile detention centers and prisons, and institutions (i.e., residential placement for persons with hearing impairment, mental retardation, or emotional disturbance).

TABLE 3.1 SURVEY OF UNIVERSITY PROGRAMS IN COMMUNICATION SCIENCES AND DISORDERS: CURRENT EMPHASIS ON SPEECH-LANGUAGE SERVICES FOR ADOLESCENTS

Questions	Responses (In percentages)			
	Yes	No	Other	NR
1. Do you provide specific courses on adolescent development?	16	80	0	4
2. Do you provide specific courses on adolescent communication disorders?	4	93	0	3
3. Do you provide specific course content on adolescent development?	39	54	0	7
4. Do you provide specific course content on adolescent communication disorders?	51	45	0	4
5. Do your students have any opportunity to assess and/or remediate adolescents with communication disorders?	95	2	2	1
6. Does your faculty feel that it is important to train students specifically in assessment and intervention of adolescents?	58	26	4	12
7. Does anyone on your faculty have an interest and/or expertise in the assessment and intervention of adolescents with communication disorders?	66	26	1	7
8. Have students in your training program expressed an interest in being trained to work with communicatively handicapped adolescents?	35	63	0	2
9. Is there an employment market for persons trained to work with communicatively handicapped adolescents?	54	25	3	18
10. Is there a sufficient data base to draw upon for serving the adolescent population with regard to:				
a. Research	28	60	2	10
b. Assessment instruments	33	54	2	11
c. Intervention strategies	31	54	2	13

PROTOTYPE DELIVERY MODEL

The prototype delivery model that is proposed has evolved out of models previously described (Boyce and Larson, 1983; Larson and McKinley, 1985a; McKinley and Larson, 1985). The model consists of six major components: Information dissemination, identification, assessment, program planning, intervention, and follow-up. All six components must be intact to ensure that appropriate services are provided to adolescents with communication disorders. Mutual interdependency exists among components: A missing component, or lack of coordination, will result in disparate services.

Each of the six components of the delivery model includes direct and indirect services. Direct services refer to activities in which speech-language pathologists have actual contact time with adolescents who are, or may be, viable candidates for speech-language services. For example, selectively screening adolescents with suspected communication disorders, assessing the adolescent, and providing intervention sessions are direct services in the sense that the interactions are between the speech-language pathologist and the adolescent. Indirect services refer to activities in which speech-language pathologists do not have actual contact time with adolescents. Rather, they assist, train, and consult with other persons important to the adolescent (e.g., a teacher, a parent, a friend) for the benefit of the adolescent with a communication disorder. For example, training professionals to utilize a referral form to identify adolescents with suspected communication disorders and organizing parent support meetings are indirect services.

Whenever indirect services are discussed hereafter, reference will be to the adolescent's environmental and educational systems. The environmental system refers to family members and peers who interact with the adolescent with a communication disorder. The educational system encompasses the adolescent's structured learning situations and the speech-language pathologist's interactions with professionals and paraprofessionals in those settings. Learning situations may be traditional (e.g., a senior high school) or nontraditional (e.g., homebound instruction for hospitalized youth; instruction at a juvenile delinquency center for incarcerated adolescents). The professionals who may be involved within the educational system are classroom teachers, administrators, special educators, social workers, psychologists, guidance and vocational counselors, nurses, and probation officers. The paraprofessionals who may be involved are teacher aides, communication aides, and peer tutors. Obviously, the educational system is a part of the environmental system. However, since the educational system plays a major role during adolescence, that system is presented as a separate area within indirect services.

A comprehensive delivery model includes both direct and indirect services. While an individual adolescent might receive only direct or only indirect services, it is more common that a combination of direct and indirect services are needed.

Information Dissemination

The first component, information dissemination, refers to educating people about adolescents' communication disorders and varied characteristics. Information dissemination is synonymous with what business calls "marketing the product." Surveys have found limited awareness of speech-language pathology services both in rural (Killarney and Lass, 1981) and large metropolitan areas (Pearlstein, Russell, and Fink, 1977). Van Hattum (1983) wisely asserted:

> "No matter how good, how precise, how dependable our product is, it won't sell without marketing . . . Overall, the person on the street has no more idea what we do than he or she did in 1940 . . . we have maintained our own feelings of professionalism and ethical cleanliness by minimizing our expressions of our importance and of minimizing our public relations effort . . . people must know we are there, must know what and who we are, must be aware of our competence, must know we do better than anyone else can . . ." (pp. 48–49).

This seems especially true as it relates to speech-language services for adolescents: The average person does not know what can be done. Sometimes, even those within the discipline of communication sciences and disorders do not know what can be done or how best to proceed. Normally, jobs are already in existence, but jobs with the adolescent population frequently need to be created. Professionals need to express with clarity and conviction why a school board should add a new speech-language pathologist to work at the secondary level during hard economic times. (After all, they reason, if the communication disorder was not cured during elementary years, why spend more time and money now?) Perpetuating a lack of visibility makes professionals vulnerable to being considered an expendable service. Thus, it puts at risk any guarantee of appropriate services to adolescents with communication disorders.

Visibility of speech-language pathology must be heightened for adolescents (direct services) as well as for persons important to the adolescent (indirect services). As adolescents and the people around them become aware of what constitutes a communication disorder and how they might benefit from a speech-language program, the identification component is activated. Until people know what constitutes a communication disorder during adolescence, what impact such a problem can have on the individual, and what intervention services can be provided, referral for a suspected disorder will not occur.

Identification

The second component in the delivery model is identification, the process of defining which adolescents have a suspected communication disorder that warrants further evaluation by a speech-language pathologist. Many agencies rely on screening for identification. The term "screening" refers to ". . . the use of a systematic procedure to identify provisionally those [individuals] from a population who manifest, or are likely to manifest, an attribute which is judged to require special attention" (Hill, 1970, p. 1). Complete screening programs involve at least three elements: (1) a goal (i.e., for what are we screening?); (2) a screening procedure; (3) a criterion against which the effectiveness of the procedure can be measured (Hill, 1970). Unfortunately, a more common practice has been to begin with an instrument, assume the goal is clearly established, and hope that some criterion may be found that will evaluate effectiveness. Models of screening (Hill, 1970) include:

1. The Illness Model
2. The Developmental Model
3. The Crisis Model
4. The Match-Mismatch Model.

The Illness Model looks for problematic behaviors regarded as symptoms of underlying pathology. The Developmental Model focuses on delays in the onset of behaviors expected to emerge at a given age. This screening instrument yields information that can be compared with developmental norms. The Crisis Model detects individuals who are having difficulty coping with a crisis, (e.g., loss of a parent through death or separation, retention in a class). The Match-Mismatch Model detects students who fail to match the expectations of others who constitute a given social environment (e.g., a high school). This model anchors screening to the social system in which the problematic behavior occurs. We recommend this model as the most appropriate to use with adolescents.

Assessment

Assessment, the third component in the delivery model, is the thorough documentation of speech-language-hearing performance. A primary question to answer during assessment is where is the problem, i.e., within the adolescent, within the educational system, and/or within the environmental system. A thorough assessment considers not only the adolescent's performance, but also the contributing factors from other situations (e.g., school, home).

The adolescent's school experience must be considered, to determine if the problem may be within the educator and/or the curriculum. The educator may lack the ability to teach. The curriculum may not be sequentially organized or at an appropriate developmental level. The educator's inability to teach and inappropriate curriculum should not be misdiagnosed as a language disorder within the adolescent. For example, if many students are struggling to comprehend the content presented by a specific teacher, it would be erroneous to diagnose those students as having language disorders. At the same time, the student with a language disorder within such a classroom is likely to experience extreme frustration. A thorough assessment isolates how much of the academic difficulty can be attributed to the student and how much to flaws within the educational system.

Professionals must consider the environmental system during assessment, to rule out the possibility that a language difference exists. Students with adequate language for their primary linguistic community risk being labeled as disordered if environmental conditions are ignored.

The adolescent's evaluation (direct services) may include obtaining appropriate case history data and administering instruments and informal testing procedures, such as analysis of a representative spontaneous language sample (Boyce and Larson, 1983; Loban, 1976). Indirect assessment services may include analysis of curricula materials for language, surveying teacher attitudes toward communication disorders, and observing how peers with normal language interact.

Assessment should confirm or reject initial impressions of a communication disorder observed during identification and determine if it constitutes a handicapping condition that warrants special services. Assessment should also document the awareness that adolescents have about their communication disorder, and their motivation to modify their communication behaviors. Adolescents with documented communication disorders who acknowledge their problem, and are willing to work to improve their communication, may be better candidates for program planning than adolescents without these traits.

Program Planning

The fourth component, program planning, is the connecting link between assessment and intervention. Before effective intervention can occur, an appropriate individual plan must be drafted. This planning might involve the adolescent directly. For example, adolescents may offer suggestions for their own goals and objectives (e.g., Individualized Educational Plan in the schools). Indirect services related to program planning might include planning with teachers on how to modify curricula or how to modify the learning environment for the benefit of the adolescent.

Program planning occurs both before an adolescent's entrance into intervention as well as during the adolescent's involvement. Ongoing program planning might involve contracting with the adolescent to learn specific behaviors, or earning points toward a quarterly grade for speech and language. These ideas will be discussed in greater detail later in this book.

Intervention

Intervention, the fifth component in the delivery model, refers to any method of ameliorating or reducing the communication disorder within the adolescent. One of the primary goals of intervention during the period of adolescence is acquisition of functional communication for academic, personal-social, and vocational settings. As such, intervention will involve a coordination of efforts among a variety of professionals who may be working with the adolescent in different environments. The *Stage I*—early adolescent will tend to have intervention goals and activities directed toward functional communication for academic and personal-social settings. The *Stage II*—middle adolescent will often have functional communication goals for all three settings: Academic, personal-social, and vocational. By *Stage III*—late adolescence, goals of intervention usually focus upon personal-social and vocational settings.

Intervention for a given adolescent may include direct or indirect services, or a combination. Direct services may be delivered through an itinerant program, a resource room, or a self-contained classroom (Committee on Language, Speech, and Hearing Services in Schools, 1983). Indirect services frequently employ a consultation model. Such a model has become a viable and important alternative to direct services. Frassinelli, Superior, and Meyers (1983) define consultation as ". . . a three person chain of service in which a consultant interacts with a caregiver (consultee) to benefit an individual (client) for whom the caregiver is responsible" (p. 25). Consultation enables a larger population to be served, and it retains a natural environmental setting for communication. Consultation may be combined with some direct services, periodic or ongoing (Frassinelli, Superior, and Meyers, 1983).

While consultation is typically thought of in conjunction with teachers, the families of adolescents cannot be forgotten. The families are an essential link to the generalization of newly acquired functional communication. At the same time, families may need information about the adolescent's communication deficits, and assistance in coping with their feelings.

Intervention will vary in intensity and content, depending upon the individual needs of the adolescent. Ongoing assessment and program planning during intervention, whether it be direct or indirect, is necessary to remain most responsive to the changing needs and abilities of youth with communication disorders.

Follow-up

The last component in the prototype delivery model is follow-up. Follow-up refers to any activity designed to measure the real and perceived benefits of speech-language programs. We believe that the discipline of communication sciences and disorders has not validated its intervention approaches. For a given communication disorder, little evidence exists that approach X is more successful than approach Y.

Current research shows a "continuum of failure" as children grow older, i.e., young children with language deficits often have residual problems during adolescence. (See Chapter 1, page 8). If they do receive intervention during the secondary level, will these youth continue to experience significant communication problems during their post high school years? Only valid follow-up studies will begin to answer this question.

Adolescents who receive speech-language services might be involved in follow-up activities (direct services), or other adults might be used as informants (indirect services). If follow-up activities are used, they should occur both during speech-language services and after services are terminated.

INITIATION AND MAINTENANCE OF THE DELIVERY MODEL

For professionals initiating services in an agency, there is a sequential hierarchy of the six components of the delivery model. First, people need to know what speech-language services are and why they exist, i.e., *information dissemination.* They also need to recognize when adolescents have suspected communication disorders and how to refer such individuals. Only then can complete *identification* of adolescents needing assessment take place. The identified adolescents participate in *assessment.* Next, those determined to need speech-language services require *program planning.* Once planning is completed, *intervention* is commenced. And finally, the *follow-up* component is implemented to determine the short and long-term results of services.

During initiation of the delivery model, one component flows into the next. For example, information dissemination will lead to identification, which leads to assessment. However, just because identification has occurred does not mean that information dissemination stops. Rather, the components add cumulatively to one another: First, information dissemination occurs alone; then in conjunction with identification; and then the two of these components combine with the assessment component. As each new component is added, the preceding ones are expanded by adding new features. For example, when information dissemination is initiated, the process may consist of giving colleagues a brochure about the speech-language program and explaining when speech-language pathologists will be in their building. After identification is added to the model, information dissemination may expand to include an in-service to explain expectations and problems among adolescents. Once assessment is begun, information dissemination may broaden to include lectures to adolescents to encourage self-referrals. Upon adding program planning, information dissemination may be expanded again to include speaking to various parent groups in the community. When the intervention component is initiated, a computerized network system may be established which informs colleagues across the nation about service delivery models, which accesses a data base system to learn how others are providing services to adolescents.

During maintenance of the delivery model, the components interact with one another while at the same time the overlap among the components is constantly changing. Once the speech-language program is at a maintenance phase, the professional might on any given day engage in an information dissemination activity, handle a referral (i.e., identification), assess an adolescent, participate in a staff meeting for the purpose of program planning, and provide actual direct intervention.

The primary thrust of the maintenance model is interactive, while the primary thrust of the initiation model is accumulative. This does not imply that interaction among the components is lacking during initiation of the prototype delivery model. Interaction does occur, but is secondary to the accumulative aspects of adding components and features within components. Similarly, the maintenance model encourages the addition of features within components; however, this is secondary to the interaction among components.

While differences exist between initiation and maintenance of the delivery model, there are many similarities. All six components are present in both levels, although in varying degrees. Coordination of the components is paramount for success in either the initiation or maintenance levels. What is done within each component remains similar whether at the initiation or the maintenance levels. For example, *what* is assessed about the adolescent's communication remains the same whether you are initiating a program or maintaining one. Likewise, *how* each of the components are implemented remains similar. For example, inservice is a common approach to disseminating information whether initiating a program or maintaining one, although the content is likely to vary.

A common error in initiating a program involves jumping to one of the last components, e.g., intervention, too quickly. Successful intervention does not occur without being preceded by the other four components. Another common error is being impatient and giving up too soon. We have known school districts, for example, that have taken two years to progress from the information dissemination component to the identification component. One speech-language pathologist reported that it took him approximately five years to develop his program to the point where it was understood by administrators, teachers, and parents.

The most common error during maintenance of the delivery model is failure to initiate the follow-up component. Yet without evidence that speech-language services at the secondary level produce significant changes that follow students past high school age, these services remain suspect. With the growing use of computers to track administrative duties such as client files, follow-up studies should become less difficult. Another error in the maintenance of programs is the failure to engage in information dissemination activities. Yet without an ongoing marketing of what speech-language programs can do for adolescents with communication disorders, the lack of visibility will continue. The first component of the delivery model, i.e., information dissemination, remains pivotal to the success of the speech-language program whether being initiated or maintained.

INFORMATION DISSEMINATION

Information dissemination can involve the adolescent directly or indirectly. Table 3.2 illustrates who might be receiving the information, what might be disseminated, and how the information could be disseminated.

Direct Services

Information must be disseminated to adolescents for several reasons. First, the likelihood of self-referrals will increase once adolescents understand what kind of problems constitute a communication disorder, and what benefits they can expect from speech-language services. Second, adolescents may be more tolerant of speech-language programs once they become familiar with them. Third, many adolescents have reached a level of metacognitive awareness that allows them to think about their communication and communicate about their thinking. This makes them more receptive to information about how a communication disorder could affect their academic, personal-social, or vocational performance.

Classroom lectures are a good vehicle for disseminating information directly to adolescents. However, lectures should be modified (e.g., level of vocabulary, length of the presentation, types of examples to illustrate a main point, usage of media) to accommodate the various stages of adolescence. During an initial lecture, it may be beneficial to begin with a simulation activity which approximates a language disorder. Raschke and Dedrick (1986), who have provided several specific simulation scripts for use with junior and senior high school students, have found that adolescents reexamine their beliefs regarding students with disorders, following these simulation activities. Adolescents then should be provided the information listed in Table 1.1, Characteristic Problems of Adolescents with Communication Disorders, so that they can begin to identify themselves or peers. The normal developmental data, limited as it is at the adolescent level, should be shared where appropriate. Throughout dissemination of information to adolescents, the benefits of adequate communication for daily living should be stressed. For example, bring in a page of want ads and illustrate how many of the ads require the applicant to possess appropriate language skills.

TABLE 3.2 INFORMATION DISSEMINATION COMPONENT

	Who?	What?	How?
DIRECT	Adolescents Early Middle Late	Expectations and problems Normal developmental data Benefits of adequate communication Self-referral process Prevention	Publications Career days; job fairs Classroom lectures Intake screening
INDIRECT	Educational system members	Expectations and problems Normal developmental data Benefits of adequate communication Referral process How related professionals can help the adolescent Prevention	Inservice Media Telecommunications
	Environmental system members	Expectations and problems Normal developmental data Benefits of adequate communication Referral process How family and friends can help the adolescent Prevention	Media Telecommunications Informational and support meetings

Classroom lectures are generally able to be scheduled through colleagues such as the English teacher or the speech communication specialist. With a little forewarning, most teachers will give up a class session to discuss communication disorders, the benefits of good communication, and so forth. Table 3.3 contains a suggested outline for an initial classroom lecture to adolescents on the topic of communication disorders. Examples of the expectations and problems outlined in Table 3.3 should be developed by the professional delivering the lectures, e.g., what would be some specific difficulties that adolescents might have when organizing information?

During later information dissemination, professionals might discuss with adolescents how to *prevent* certain communication disorders. Prevention is ". . . the elimination of factors which interfere with the normal acquisition and development of communication skills" (Marge, 1984, p. 29). The preventable causes of disabilities within the next generation of children should be discussed (e.g., elimination of drug and alcohol abuse, RH incompatibility, and low birth weight), some of which may include communication disorders. Marge (1984) outlines preventable causes of communication disorders in a way that could be used with adolescents. There are also prevention plans which could eliminate or reduce communication disorders acquired later in life by the adolescents themselves (e.g., reduction of noise levels, such as music or employment equipment, to eliminate hearing deficits).

Additional mediums for information dissemination are publications (e.g., brochures, posters) and participation in school orientation days, career days, and job fairs. Student service handbooks, school catalogs, and campus newspapers should all contain information about the availability of speech-language services. These dissemination vehicles are open primarily to school and adult-education facilities and have less applicability to other settings in which adolescents are located.

Less information would be disseminated by the alternatives cited above, to adolescents housed in juvenile detention centers, prisons, and residential institutions. Rather, a primary means for information dissemination is to take advantage of the adolescent's screening upon entrance, or intake. As part of this initial screening process, speech-language pathologists can disseminate information about communication disorders and self-referrals. Although the intake screening may prove false, these adolescents should be instructed about self-referrals and when they should make such a referral, assuming that the adolescent has the capacity to understand that information.

Indirect Information Dissemination Services

Two primary groups, in addition to adolescents, need to know who speech-language pathologists are, what they can do, and what positive benefits their services can have on the adolescent's academic, or personal-social, or vocational levels. One group includes people who interact with the adolescent

TABLE 3.3 SUGGESTED OUTLINE FOR A CLASSROOM LECTURE TO ADOLESCENTS ON THE TOPIC OF COMMUNICATION DISORDERS

I. **What is a communication disorder?**

   A. Problems in hearing

   B. Problems in speech (stuttering, voice, articulation errors)

   C. Problems in language (difficulty in understanding what others are saying or in expressing yourself)

   D. Simulate problems in language (refer to Raschke and Dedrick [1986] for script)

II. **What is expected of you by parents, teachers, and peers during communication?**

   A. To use thinking abilities that help to understand and express language

      1. To organize information (e.g., If you were in charge of a school dance [a rock band; building a zoo] how would you organize what needs to be done?)

      2. To put information in order (e.g., Federal government is larger than state government, which is larger than county government.)

      3. To identify and solve a problem

      4. To find and select information for assignments (e.g., If you had a paper due that needed three outside resources or references, how would you find them?)

      5. To think about ideas and events that are not "here and now" (e.g., You think about imaginary places and people; you think about how life might be different.)

   B. To have adequate listening abilities

      1. To understand complex sentences, words with more than one meaning, and figurative language

      2. To follow oral directions that are long and have many steps

      3. To understand main ideas and relevant details, especially during lectures

      4. To listen and ask questions during conversations

      5. To listen to speakers and judge what they're saying (e.g., Do you agree or not agree with what they're saying? Are they telling facts or opinions?)

   C. To have adequate speaking skills

      1. To use the right words and sentences that say what you mean

      2. To give directions clearly

      3. To ask and answer questions appropriately

      4. To use language that is organized and understandable to others

TABLE 3.3 CONTINUED

5. To make oral reports, tell or retell stories, or explain something
6. To carry on a conversation
7. To tell opinions, attitudes, moods, and feelings

D. To use appropriate nonverbal communication

1. To interpret and use correct gestures and facial expressions
2. To stand the right distance from others

III. What are characteristics of adolescents with language problems?

A. Thinking abilities that help to understand and express language may be low

1. Difficulty in organizing information
2. Difficulty in putting information in order
3. Difficulty in identifying and solving problems
4. Difficulty in finding and selecting information for assignments
5. Difficulty in thinking about ideas and events that are not "here and now"

B. Listening abilities may be weak

1. Difficulty in understanding complex sentences, words with more than one meaning, figurative language
2. Difficulty in following oral directions that are long and have many steps
3. Difficulty in understanding main ideas and relevent details
4. Difficulty in listening to conversations
5. Difficulty in listening to speakers in order to judge what they're saying

C. Speaking abilities may be weak

1. Difficulty in using sentences that say what you mean
2. Difficulty in finding the right words to express yourself
3. Difficulty in giving directions clearly
4. Difficulty in asking and answering questions appropriately
5. Difficulty in using language that is organized and able to be understood by others
6. Difficulty in making oral reports, telling or retelling stories, or explaining a process
7. Difficulty in carrying on a conversation
8. Difficulty in expressing opinions, attitudes, moods, and feelings

D. Nonverbal communication may be weak

1. Difficulty in interpreting and using correct gestures and facial expressions
2. Difficulty in standing the right distance from others

TABLE 3.3 CONTINUED

IV. What should you do if you suspect a communication disorder?

A. Talk with the speech-language pathologist (The speech-language pathologist should provide a current schedule of available conference times and where to receive messages; schedules should be periodically updated.)

B. Refer yourself for testing

V. What will happen during testing?

A. Tests will be given to you by the speech-language pathologist, and possibly by other professionals (Show and/or demonstrate several representative tests to reduce fear of speech-language "tests.")

B. You will be asked to describe what you think the problem is

C. Test results will be discussed with you

D. Recommendations will be made for how you can be helped

E. You will be encouraged to participate in language intervention if you meet the program's entrance requirements

F. You have a legal right to accept or to refuse the recommendations

G. You have a legal right to obtain a second opinion

VI. What if you are recommended to receive speech-language services?

A. A time for seeing the speech-language pathologist will be determined

B. Services will be planned that specifically address your problem(s)

C. Services may be provided on a one-to-one basis or within a small group (Show a videotape of adolescents in intervention to help eliminate the mystery of what would happen if services are initiated.*)

D. You will receive credit and a grade for your participation**

*Make certain the adolescents on the videotape are unfamiliar to those hearing the classroom lecture; permission to show the videotape must be obtained from the videotaped adolescents.

**Include this information in the lecture, if credits are available for adolescents in your setting.

within the educational system and the second group consists of individuals within the environmental system. Both groups need to understand the expectations during normal adolescence and the resultant problems that occur when these expectations are not met (See Table 1.1 in Chapter 1). Each of these groups needs to have literature on normal communication development and an explanation of the importance of adequate oral communication. Without knowledge of normal adolescent communication, it is difficult to judge when adolescents do not meet developmental norms. Both groups also need to become familiar with the referral process since they will be most involved in identifying adolescents with suspected communication disorders.

In addition to these topics for information dissemination, two others emerge: (1) What can members of the educational and environmental systems do to assist adolescents with communication disorders, and (2) how might preventative measures be taken to avoid additional communication disorders in other adolescents? Adolescents who have already been identified as having communication disorders may be assisted by modifications people make during oral communication (e.g., slowing the rate of oral directions). Chapter 8 contains information on the role of the educational and environmental systems' members who are intervening with adolescents. This same chapter offers suggestions that could be used during dissemination activities.

Preventing additional communication disorders is a critical topic for indirect information dissemination. The national focus on prevention (Committee on Prevention of Speech-Language and Hearing Problems, 1984; McGinnis, 1984) should be emphasized, and a community plan should be encouraged (Marge, 1984). Such a community plan should include strategies for primary prevention (i.e., elimination of the onset of a communication disorder), secondary prevention (i.e., early detection and treatment of the disorder), and tertiary prevention (i.e., reduction of a disability by attempting to restore effective functioning). A long range plan specifying objectives and strategies is needed, as is effective leadership. With the adolescent population, particular attention should be paid to known causes of communication disorders during that period of life. For example, hearing impairments due to loud music (Lipscomb, 1972) and high school shop noise (Roesser, 1980; Woodford, 1980; Woodford and O'Farrell, 1983) have been documented. Vocal abuse in cheerleaders is common (Andrews and Shank, 1983). Drug and alcohol-related motor vehicle accidents during adolescence often result in brain damage for survivors. The initial impetus for a community prevention plan can be provided by speech-language pathologists working with secondary-level students.

Inservice Inservice is one of the most common vehicles for information dissemination to educational system personnel in all of the settings where adolescents are located. While audiences at the inservices may vary, what is emphasized about adolescents remains similar. For example, speech-language pathologists, in schools, must disseminate information to classroom teachers, guidance and vocational counselors, special educators, school administrators, medical personnel, and social workers. In hospitals, the audience might include professionals in related therapies, nurses, and physicians. Regardless of the audience, the focus tends to be on recognizing problems that characterize communication disorders during adolescence, stressing the benefits of good communication, and urging referral when adolescents have difficulties that are suspect. See Table 3.4 for a suggested outline of an inservice about adolescents with communication disorders.

Fafard (1980) stated that inservice is most effective when the local setting is used, and when programs are designed and delivered by local staff members. Inservice, although traditionally defined as occurring within a group setting, can also be effectively delivered in a one-to-one or small group situation. Furthermore, settings such as adult-education facilities may not be suited for assembling large groups. Frequently, professionals maintaining a program find themselves combining information dissemination and program planning. The informal atmosphere offered by a one-to-one inservice may be more conducive to a give-and-take exchange, until the other professional becomes more comfortable with the services provided by the speech-language pathologist for adolescents with communication disorders.

Staff meetings should not be overlooked as a vehicle for inservice and information dissemination. Everyone should remain alert at staff meetings to advocate for adolescents with communication disorders on issues that could potentially affect them.

Media Another means for reaching people in both the educational and the environmental systems is use of the media. Publications such as brochures, posters, and newspaper articles usually promote increased understanding of our role, if done well. Professionals considering the use of publications to disseminate information might consider available resources for how to design a brochure and to write an article (Jewler, 1981; Zinsser, 1985). The American Speech-Language-Hearing Association and many state associations have resources to inform people about the discipline. Some of these publications are specifically for promoting "May is Better Speech and Hearing Month."

Radio and television presentations and interviews, using both public access and local network channels, can also promote speech-language services, if done appropriately. Professionals may wish to consult a source such as *On Television! A Survival Guide for Media Interviews* (Hilton and Knoblauch, 1980) before participating in an interview, since a poorly conducted radio or television appearance could be worse than no appearance at all. After all, speech-language pathologists serve as communication models for other people. If those professionals appear inadequate for the situation, they will have difficulty convincing others that they are able to assist those with disorders.

An aspect of media that is useful for information dissemination is professional publications outside the discipline of communication sciences and disorders. If other professionals are to understand what can be done for adolescents with communication disorders, speech-language pathologists need to make a

TABLE 3.4 SUGGESTED OUTLINE FOR AN INSERVICE TO RELATED PROFESSIONALS ON THE TOPIC OF ADOLESCENTS WITH COMMUNICATION DISORDERS

I. What is a communication disorder?

A. Problems in hearing

B. Problems in speech (stuttering, voice, articulation errors)

C. Problems in language (difficulty in understanding what others are saying or in expressing yourself)

II. What is expected of adolescents by parents, teachers, and peers during communication?

A. To use thinking abilities that help to understand and express language

1. To organize information
2. To sequence information
3. To identify and solve a problem
4. To find and select information for assignments
5. To think about ideas and events that are not "here and now"

B. To have adequate listening abilities

1. To understand complex sentences, multiple meaning words, and figurative language
2. To follow lengthy oral directions
3. To understand main ideas and relevant details, especially during lectures
4. To listen and ask questions during conversations
5. To listen critically to other speakers

C. To have adequate speaking skills

1. To use sentences that express what is intended
2. To find the right words to express ideas
3. To give directions clearly
4. To ask and answer questions appropriately
5. To use language that is organized and intelligible
6. To make oral reports, tell or retell stories, or explain a process
7. To carry on a conversation
8. To express opinions, attitudes, moods, and feelings

D. To use appropriate nonverbal communication

1. To interpret and use correct body movements and facial expressions
2. To follow rules for social distance

TABLE 3.4 CONTINUED

III. What are characteristics of adolescents with language problems?

A. Thinking abilities that help to understand and express language may be low
   1. Difficulty in organizing information
   2. Difficulty in sequencing information
   3. Difficulty in identifying and solving problems
   4. Difficulty in finding and selecting information for assignments
   5. Difficulty in thinking about ideas and events that are not "here and now"

B. Listening abilities may be weak
   1. Difficulty in understanding complex sentences, multiple meaning words, figurative language
   2. Difficulty in following oral directions
   3. Difficulty in understanding main ideas and details
   4. Difficulty in listening to conversations
   5. Difficulty in listening critically to other speakers

C. Speaking abilities may be weak
   1. Difficulty in using sentences that express what is intended
   2. Difficulty in finding the right words to express ideas
   3. Difficulty in giving directions clearly
   4. Difficulty in asking and answering questions appropriately
   5. Difficulty in using language that is organized and intelligible
   6. Difficulty in making oral reports, telling or retelling stories, or explaining a process
   7. Difficulty in carrying on a conversation
   8. Difficulty in expressing opinions, attitudes, moods, and feelings

D. Nonverbal communication may be weak
   1. Difficulty in interpreting and using correct body movements and facial expressions
   2. Difficulty in following rules for social distance

IV. What should you do if you suspect an adolescent in your classroom has a communication disorder?

A. Talk with the speech-language pathologist and/or complete the Secondary-Level Referral Form found in Appendix A (The speech-language pathologist should provide a current schedule of available conference times and where to receive messages; schedules should be periodically updated.)

B. Refer the adolescent for testing

TABLE 3.4 CONTINUED

V. What happens to the adolescent during testing?

A. Tests are administered by the speech-language pathologist and related professionals (Show and/or demonstrate several representative tests given by the speech-language pathologist, and possibly by other professionals.)

B. Test results will be discussed at an interdisciplinary staff meeting

C. Recommendations will be made for how the adolescent can be helped, including changes in the classroom

D. The adolescent will be encouraged to participate in language intervention if the the program's entrance criteria are met

E. The adolescent has a legal right to accept or to refuse the recommendations

F. The adolescent has a legal right to obtain a second opinion

VI. What if the recommendation is that the adolescent receive speech-language services?

A. A time for seeing the speech-language pathologist will be determined

B. Services will be planned that specifically address the documented problem(s) in speech-language

C. You may be asked to make classroom and/or curriculum changes for the benefit of the adolescent

D. Services may be provided on a one-to-one basis or within a small group (Show a representative videotape of adolescents in intervention.*)

E. The adolescent will receive credit and a grade for participation in intervention**

*Make certain the adolescents on the videotape are unfamiliar to those attending the inservice; permission to show the videotape must be obtained from the videotaped adolescents.

**Include this information in the lecture, if credits are available for adolescents in your setting.

concerted effort to publish in journals read by those who need to know about this discipline. To reach related professionals working in prisons and centers for juvenile delinquents, for example, articles should appear in journals such as *Federal Probation*, *Criminal Justice and Behavior*, and *Criminology*. To reach related professionals within vocational-technical schools, information should be published through the Adult Education Association (AEA). Speech-language pathologists should be publishing in medical journals and general education journals, including the *American School Board*. Other professionals will support the development and maintenance of programs for adolescents only when they are aware that speech-language services for adolescents are beneficial.

Telecommunications Telecommunications has become increasingly important for information dissemination. Computer information services such as *SpecialNet*, which is available through the National Association of State Directors of Special Educators, *Compuserve*, which is owned by H & R Block, Inc., and *The Source*, which is owned by Reader's Digest, are valuable informational retrieval sources and dissemination resources.

Technology will play an increasing role in information dissemination. Speech-language pathologists will be able to share or obtain information about a wide array of topics while sitting at their microcomputers. More specifically, a computer network will allow speech-language pathologists: (1) to exchange ideas efficiently about clinical management procedures that appear to be effective with certain types of adolescents, (2) to ask questions in search of new ways to provide services, (3) to obtain the names of speech-language pathologists who have established innovative service delivery models and therefore might be appropriate referral sources, (4) to submit articles for review and reaction to journal editors or to other professionals, and (5) to co-author articles or books with other colleagues who are thousands of miles away.

Technology will provide innovative and creative ways to offer workshops on professional topics. Already, the capacity exists to transmit electronically the image of a person in three dimensions onto a stage thousands of miles away. To the audience present, it will look as though the person who is providing the inservice is physically present, while in fact that person will be in a studio close to home; it will only look like he or she traveled thousands of miles to appear in person.

Technology will continue to simplify the production of brochures and posters. Computer programs such as *The Print Shop* (Balsam, 1984) and *The Newsroom* (Springboard Software, 1984) offer the flexibility to make posters, brochures, and newsletters. The growing use of media in all forms should allow speech-language pathologists to become more visible to people within the educational and environmental systems.

Informational and Support Meetings Speech-language pathologists should reach family members and friends through informational or support meetings. Frequently, vehicles for informational meetings are already in place in the community. For example, many communities have parent visitation night at the school. Community service groups and church groups are often in need of speakers and welcome information to share with their members. Similarly, special interest groups such as the Council for Exceptional Children and Association for Children with Learning Disabilities are often receptive to speech-language information at their meetings. Both community service and special interest groups should receive information on prevention: Possibly, these groups should be the organizations who spearhead a community plan. Informational meetings are particularly necessary within school and hospital settings. Often, less access is available to family members and friends when professionals are working with adolescents in the settings of juvenile detention centers, adult-educational facilities, and residential institutions. Planning suggestions for informational meetings are presented in Chapter 6.

IDENTIFICATION

The identification component relies heavily on the information dissemination component, and may involve the adolescent directly or indirectly. Table 3.5 illustrates main points of the identification component.

TABLE 3.5 IDENTIFICATION COMPONENT

	Who?	What?	How?
DIRECT	Adolescents Early Middle Late	Match-mismatch with expectations for communication	Self-referral Selective screening
INDIRECT	Adults and peers familiar with adolescent	Match-mismatch with expectations for communication	Observational checklist referral forms

Direct Identification Services

In two major ways, adolescents can be directly involved in the identification component. One direct means is self-referral to the speech-language program. However, this does not happen unless appropriate information dissemination has preceded the referral. Self-referrals tend to be more common among late adolescents than early adolescents. Therefore, at the upper ages of adolescence a concerted effort should be made to let adolescents know about speech-language services and how they can benefit from adequate communication. The only setting in which self-referral is not an option is that of the hospital setting. Currently, physicians alone make the referral for speech-language services at the hospital setting. On the other end of the spectrum are adult-education facilities in which nearly all adolescents who come to the attention of the speech-language pathologist do so through a self-referral process. Adolescents located in these facilities tend to be in Stage III—late adolescence.

Another popular method for identification is screening, although available choices for screening potential communication disorders in adolescents are limited at the present time, if published protocols are used. Currently, several screening tests are available for identifying adolescents: *Clinical Evaluation of Language Functions: Advanced Level Screening (CELF)* (Semel and Wiig, 1980), *Screening Tests of Adolescent Language (STAL)* (Prather et al., 1980) and *Adolescent Language Screening Test (ALST)* (Morgan and Guilford, 1984). All of these tests establish norms, measure language comprehension and production, and require students to be screened on a one-to-one basis, i.e., the tests cannot be used simultaneously with a group of students.

Some schools do mass screening of all adolescents within a given grade level. Tibbits (1982) has recommended that ". . . the entire adolescent population should be screened at least twice after they leave the elementary school (6th grade)" (page 26). As an alternative to tests, O'Connor and Eldredge (1981) have described various ways to screen a large number of students. One method they have found to be most effective is to screen all students in English classes at the seventh and ninth or tenth grades. To obtain information about each student, they have divided the screening process into a written task and a three to five minute personal interview. O'Connor and Eldredge (1981) have recommended that the pass/fail criteria be based on what is appropriate to the population being tested. They have also recommended using input from classroom teachers, as well as observations made during the screening process, when deciding who failed the screening.

A 1985 survey (Larson and McKinley, 1985a), found that no secondary-level program surveyed used only mass screening for identification. Sixteen percent of the respondents used both mass screening and a teacher referral system. While we do not advocate mass screening at the secondary level, some speech-language pathologists have observed that the primary benefit from this procedure is increased awareness of communication disorders.

Usually, a more efficient alternative to mass screening is selective screening, particularly in the school setting. The speech-language pathologist would selectively screen those groups of adolescents at high risk for communication disorders, i.e., adolescents in other special programs such as classrooms for the emotionally disturbed or mentally retarded; early adolescents still in remedial reading while in seventh and eighth grades; adolescents about to drop out of high school; and adolescents with academic deficiencies not connected to attitudinal and/or motivational factors. In addition, those adolescents who were seen as young children, but were dismissed from the speech-language caseload at some point in the past, should also be screened. Few adolescents with language disorders surface for the first time, although some do.

In other settings, notably juvenile detention centers, prisons, and residential institutions, intake screening is recommended. Intake screening refers to screening each adolescent upon entry into that setting, either through direct contact or a review of records. Since time spent in these settings may be short, particularly in juvenile delinquent centers, waiting for a teacher referral would be inefficient. By the time a referral is made, the adolescent may soon be returning to the community. Therefore, intake screening would ensure that minimal time is wasted in identifying students with potential communication disorders.

Indirect Identification Services

Referral by a person familiar with the adolescent is a primary method by which adolescents can be identified. The referral might be from personnel such as teachers, social workers, or physicians; or the referral might be made by a family member. Referrals tend to be more frequent and more appropriate if adequate information dissemination has preceded them. The ability of professionals, such as teachers, to make appropriate referrals has been documented. R. Baldes (Personal Communication, 1983) found that teachers, while they may somewhat over-refer, are able to identify students as accurately as speech-language pathologists.

We have found the use of an observational checklist is preferable to direct screening, which is neither efficient nor cost effective. A revised version of the "Secondary Level Referral Form: Communication Disorders" (Boyce and Larson, 1983) has been developed and appears in Appendix A. It is based on Hill's (1970) Match-Mismatch Model of screening. English, speech, math, and special education teachers have completed the checklist more successfully after students have been in their classes for several months. This alternative approach to direct screening accomplishes the following: (1) the speech-language pathologist can educate teachers and parents regarding adolescents' oral communication skills, (2) teachers and parents can listen to and observe tasks requiring daily communication skills, (3) the speech-language pathologist can learn teacher and parental expectations and incorporate them into the observational checklist, and (4) professionals can observe the adolescents' listening and speaking skills in natural communication contexts. Agencies should establish predictive cut-off points, based on their particular population, for students needing comprehensive assessment who were identified through the referral form. This task can be accomplished more readily through computer technology.

SUMMARY

The lack of attention given to adolescents with communication disorders is a result of the way universities have trained, or failed to train, speech-language pathologists. Educational programming at the university level is needed if future professionals are to learn how to provide appropriate speech-language services to adolescents. A comprehensive service delivery model includes the components of information dissemination, identification, assessment, program planning, intervention, and follow-up. If adolescents are to be served appropriately, each component must be operative within the settings that house adolescents: Secondary schools; adult-education facilities; hospitals; juvenile detention centers and prisons; and institutions for those with mental retardation, emotional disturbance, or hearing impairment.

Specific ideas for how to implement the information dissemination and identification components were shared. Within both components, adolescents should be involved directly and indirectly. In addition, adolescents should be given information about communication disorders through mediums such as classroom lectures and publications. Important others in the adolescent's educational and environmental systems should also be given sufficient information about the nature of communication disorders during adolescence, to ensure the appropriate identification of adolescents with suspected disorders. Identification may also occur through self-referrals, referrals by peers, and selective screening.

DISCUSSION QUESTIONS

1. You have just been employed by a public school system that believes all communication disorders should be "cured" by the end of sixth grade. Prepare your argument for secondary-level services.

2. Select a setting in which adolescents are present, and plan an inservice that describes your delivery model to other staff members with whom you work.

3. How might the discipline of communication sciences and disorders be marketed more effectively?

SUGGESTED READINGS

McKinley, N. and Larson, V. Lord. Neglected language-disordered adolescent: A delivery model. *Language, Speech, and Hearing Services in Schools*, 16(1): 2–15, 1985.

Taylor, J. Speech-language services for youthful and adult offenders. *Federal Probation*. 44(6): 37–41, 1980.

Van Hattum, R. Public information: More is not enough. *ASHA*. 25(2): 47–49, 1983.

CHAPTER 4

Assessing the Adolescent's Communication

GOALS:

To present general assessment principles

To describe what to assess within the adolescent's communication

To describe how to assess the adolescent's communication behaviors

To present formal test instruments available for assessing the adolescent's communication

Assessment is a dynamic process in which the speech-language pathologist selects and administers appropriate measurement instruments (formal tests and informal procedures) and observes and records the adolescent's behaviors for the purpose of determining the existence, type, nature, and severity of the communication disorder. This chapter provides assessment procedures for testing the adolescent during an initial speech-language evaluation, or for periodic retesting. Rather than presenting procedures that test isolated behaviors, a wholistic approach is described.

The comprehensive assessment of the adolescent's communication is illustrated in Table 4.1. This chapter focuses on the following specific aspects within the adolescent who is in an early, middle, or late stage of development: History, learning style, cognition, comprehension and production of linguistic features, discourse (conversations and narrations), nonverbal communication, and survival language skills. Assessment of these specific aspects can be accomplished through use of a case history form, and through formal and infor-

TABLE 4.1 ASSESSMENT COMPONENT: DIRECT SERVICES

Who?	What?	How?
Adolescents Early Middle Late	History Learning style Cognition Comprehension and production of linguistic features Discourse Nonverbal communication Survival language skills	Informal assessment (administration, analysis, interpretation) A. Case history form B. Learning style questionnaire C. Discourse samples 1. Conversations 2. Narrations D. Directed tasks Formal assessment instruments (administration, analysis, interpretation)

mal testing procedures. Speech-language pathologists need to review both formal and informal testing procedures in terms of administration, analysis, and interpretation. The speech-language pathologist's assessment of the adolescent should comply with expectations and possible problems cited in Table 1.1 in Chapter 1 of this book. Before describing *how* to assess the adolescent, background information on general assessment principles, along with a description of *what* to evaluate, is presented.

GENERAL ASSESSMENT PRINCIPLES

I. Purpose of Assessment

The exact reason for doing the assessment must be considered before entering the assessment process. For example, is the purpose to determine the existence of a problem; or to establish appropriate intervention goals; or to decide if dismissal is warranted? Questions such as these must be answered to obtain the information needed and to determine the assessment procedures.

II. Perspective of the Adolescent

The examiner should listen to the adolescent's perspective of the problem. Some adolescents may provide insights into their problems that no one else has. However, other adolescents may be oblivious to their own communication disorders. For example, Diedrich (1984) has found the lack of awareness of the disorder to be a major ". . . diagnostic sign that distinguishes adolescent cluttering from other speech disorders" (p. 312). By asking for an explanation of the problem, the examiner can determine whether there are discrepancies among the following: Examination results, the adolescent's perspective, and the perspectives of persons within the educational and environmental systems. If a discrepancy exists among any of these dimensions, it may suggest the need for further evaluation, educational inservices, or environmental counseling.

III. Adolescent's Right to Know

The examiner should explain to the adolescent, before the evaluation procedure, what behaviors are to be assessed, how they are to be assessed, and the reason for the various procedures. By doing this, the examiner will usually find the adolescent is a more cooperative and active participant. The adolescent should be encouraged to challenge and to question what is being done. After all, who should be more interested in what is happening than the person to whom it is happening?

IV. Multi-Dimensional Assessment

The examiner should evaluate the adolescent across natural communication situations (e.g., in the classroom, at home) and with familiar and unfamiliar listeners. Communication styles change as a function of the situation and the listener. These changes must be taken into account during the assessment process.

V. Formal and Informal Assessment

An individual's behaviors are ". . . relative, conditional, complex and dynamic. Accordingly, clinical assessment must be relative, contextual, process oriented and dynamic." (Muma, 1978, p. 211). This type of clinical assessment can best be accomplished using informal assessment procedures that are wholistic, modifiable, and accommodating to the individual within a natural setting rather than conforming the individual to the test methodology. Not only is the test situation artificial, but the language of formal tests is often characteristically different from daily communicative exchanges (Lund and Duchan, 1983).

Frequently, professionals say they cannot use informal procedures because these procedures are not objective, i.e., they provide no quantitative scores. Also, they say it is too time consuming to obtain and to analyze spontaneous communication samples across relevant situations and listeners. Each of these ideas is examined below.

No quantitative scores Objectivity is assumed when formal (i.e., standardized) tests are administered. Assume for a moment that a standardized test is more objective than an informal procedure of obtaining, observing, recording, and analyzing communication behaviors in a natural context. This objectivity should not be construed as more important than relevance (Muma, 1978). A standardized test that is supposedly objective cannot be considered worthwhile and valid if it is not assessing relevant behaviors in relevant situations.

Quantitative scores may not be as advantageous as professionals have been led to believe. Muma (1978) stated that scores may work against both the examiner and student, because when complex dynamic behaviors are reduced to numbers, essential information about the individual is lost, thus making it difficult or impossible to generate appropriate intervention goals and procedures. As Lund and Duchan (1983) have noted, "... scores are of little value for the purposes of describing language and planning therapy, so clinicians must analyze performance on each item" (p. 299).

Too time consuming A second argument for not obtaining and analyzing spontaneous language samples is that they are too time consuming. What has allowed speech-language pathologists to conclude that assessment must be quick and easy? Perhaps it has been large caseloads, or administrators' number games. Whatever the reasons, those variables that force professionals to conclude that language sampling is too time consuming should be changed, and the sampling procedure should be retained. Quick and easy assessment procedures may lose more than is gained by neglecting the responsibility to assess an individual's needs appropriately (Muma, 1978). None of us would want ourselves or our loved ones to be assessed in a "quick and easy" fashion by a physician or psychologist or speech-language pathologist. The consequences may be far too severe.

At some time during the assessment procedure, the examiner must obtain from the adolescent several spontaneous conversational samples, which in turn can be analyzed for phonological, morphological, syntactic, semantic, and pragmatic features. If such samples are not gathered, and only formal tests are administered, isolated aspects of communication may be obtained. These isolated aspects do not constitute the total communication process and could lead to false conclusions.

VI. Critique of Standardized Tests

A standardized test has four aspects that are standardized: (1) test content is fixed, (2) administrative procedures are prescribed, (3) responses are scored using predetermined criteria, and (4) test scores are interpreted by reference to norms or performance criteria (ASHA Ad Hoc Committee on Instrument Evaluation, 1986). When standardized tests are used, examiners need to find answers to the following questions for each test selected (AERA, APA, and NCME, 1985; ASHA Ad Hoc Committee on Instrument Evaluation, 1986; Boyce and Larson, 1983):

1. Is there a clearly stated purpose and definition of the population(s) with whom the test is to be used?
2. Is the test content relevant to the purpose of the test?
3. What stimulus presentation is used to elicit a response?
4. What response mode is used to determine if a response is correct?
5. Is the test valid for the population on which it will be administered? Does it have content validity?
6. Is the test reliable for diagnosing a communication disorder? Does it have intrajudge and interjudge reliability?
7. What is the rationale on which the test is based? Is it based on empirical data, clinical experience, theoretical constructs, or a combination of these?
8. Does the test avoid cultural and sexual stereotyping and biases?
9. Does it assess communication behaviors in a natural context, and in a dynamic ongoing fashion?
10. Are procedures for recording and analyzing responses clearly specified?
11. Are normative data available on the adolescent population being assessed?
12. Is the sample size adequate? Has the representative sample from the population been adequately described?

13. Are the manual instructions to the examiner and to the adolescent clear and concise?
14. Does the test documentation clearly list the qualifications needed (e.g., education, experience, certification) by the examiner to administer the test?

These questions must be answered to ensure that the test is appropriate for the adolescent and is a valid and reliable measure of performance.

VII. Interaction Between Cognition and Language

Professionals recognize cognition, language, and communication as complex, overlapping, and interrelated systems. A variety of professionals (Anglin, 1977; Bowerman, 1976; Feuerstein, 1980; Piaget and Inhelder, 1969; Vygotsky, 1962) have documented that cognition is intricately related to language. However, the nature of this relationship is a point of theoretical difference. Rice (1983) provided a summary of current hypotheses about the relationship between cognition and language:

"1. Strong cognition hypothesis: Cognition precedes and accounts for language acquisition

2. Local homologies hypothesis: Simultaneous emergence of parallel cognitive and linguistic knowledge

3. Interaction hypothesis: Language and cognition mutually influence each other's development

4. Cognition-anchored-in-language hypothesis: Concepts are unstable until anchored with linguistic forms

5. Weak cognition hypothesis: Cognition does not account for all language development

6. Mental processes not rooted in meanings: Language-specific and/or perceptual processes" (pp. 357–359).

These different hypotheses have cited varying levels of linguistic competence and varying kinds of linguistic phenomena to support each hypothesis. The hypotheses that emphasize the strength of cognition focus on the earlier stages of language acquisition. Those hypotheses that emphasize linguistic influence tend to be based on later stages. In essence, the cognition and language relationship may vary as a function of age, type of cognitive task, and linguistic ability (Rice, 1983; Schlesinger, 1977).

The relationship between language and cognition in later developmental periods remains particularly ill-defined. However, we postulate that an interaction does exist. At times, cognition seems to facilitate language, while at other times language appears to facilitate cognition. Certain communication behaviors do not emerge or stabilize until the later stages of cognitive development (e.g., comprehension of abstract metaphors; use of dimensional language, including comparatives and superlatives). Thus, a thorough assessment needs to include evaluation of cognition.

VIII. Importance of Listening

Listening disorders are problematic because of the adolescent's need to understand the spoken English of others. Listening is the basic language skill that is used the highest percentage of the time. Markgraf (1966) determined that high school students were expected to spend forty-six percent of their classroom time listening. Rankin (1926) was one of the first to study how adults spend their verbal communication time. The study revealed that adults spent forty-two percent of their time listening, thirty-two percent speaking, fifteen percent reading, and eleven percent writing. In 1975, Werner conducted an update of the Rankin study. She found that fifty-five percent of the verbal communication time was spent listening, twenty-three percent speaking, thirteen percent reading, and nine percent writing. Clearly, the need for listening spans a lifetime.

According to the Commission on the English Curriculum of the National Council of Teachers of English (1952), people's attitudes and concepts, whether they are economic, political, or ethical, are influenced and perhaps determined by listening. Although listening is essential for survival in our society, it is the basic skill assessed least in the educational system (Wolff et al., 1983; Wolvin and Coakley, 1982). According to Neville (1959) ". . . more failure in academic and [personal] social growth can be traced to the inability to listen than to any other single aspect of the language arts" (p. 226). Therefore, a comprehensive assessment process must include an evaluation of the adolescent's listening abilities.

IX. Description of Behaviors

Examiners should describe rather than judge adolescents' communication behaviors. This description should not be tainted by the dress, posture, or hair style of the adolescent. When appearance and behaviors do not comply with expectations, objectivity and accurate description may be impeded.

X. Discussion of Results

Adolescents should be active participants in the assessment process. We strongly recommend that adolescents, in conjunction with the professionals and parents present, be given the evaluation results and recommendations. If that is too threatening or otherwise undesirable, then separate meetings could be held with adolescents to discuss evaluation performance and its implications for their academic, social, and vocational goals. Adolescents should be told about their strengths as well as their weaknesses. Whenever possible, the examiner should illustrate how they may use strengths to overcome weaknesses. If intervention is not indicated, this interaction will provide insight into the inconsistencies in performance that they have probably been experiencing. If scheduled for intervention, these comments can prepare adolescents for such experiences.

XI. Assessment/Intervention Dichotomy

We concur with Muma (1978) that assessment and intervention procedures are continuous, ongoing, and intimately related. To separate them into two independent procedures is a fallacy. Although this book has separate chapters on assessment and intervention, those chapters are simply a way to organize the data. Please note that Tables 4.1 and 7.1, which illustrate the overview of assessment and intervention, overlap greatly and demonstrate how interrelated these two processes are.

XII. Assessment of Racial Minorities

The Committee on the Status of Racial Minorities (1983) has stated, ". . . no dialectal variety of English is a disorder or a pathological form of speech or language" (p. 23). Thus, some adolescents will have communication differences and not disorders. Communication differences are defined as communication behaviors that meet the norms of the primary linguistic community, but that do not meet the norms of standard English. It is possible, though, for dialectal speakers to have speech and language disorders within the native language. To determine if the adolescent has a dialectal difference or a communication disorder, speech-language pathologists must have the following competencies (Cole, 1983):

"1. Knowledge of the particular dialect as a rule-governed linguistic system

2. Knowledge of nondiscriminatory testing procedures
3. Knowledge of the phonological and grammatical features of the dialect
4. Knowledge of contrastive analysis procedures
5. Knowledge of the effects of attitudes toward dialects
6. Thorough understanding and appreciation for the community and culture of the nonstandard speaker" (p. 25).

Vaughn-Cooke (1983) presented and critiqued a series of alternatives to traditional testing of minority students. One alternative standardizes existing tests on non-mainstream speakers. This is inappropriate, since the new norms would still be derived from tests developed only for mainstream speakers. Another alternative selects a percentage of minorities in the test sample. This is not always a viable alternative, since sample size frequently is too small and nonrepresentative of the large population. A third suggestion modifies or revises existing tests so they are appropriate for non-mainstream English speakers. Nelson (1976) has attempted to do this with *Developmental Sentence Scoring* (Lee, 1974). However, Vaughn-Cooke (1983) questioned Nelson's failure to provide comparable credit for similar language structures used by non-mainstream and standard English speakers. Hemingway, Montague, and Bradley (1981) modified the *Carrow Elicited Language Inventory* (Carrow, 1974), but Vaughn-Cooke (1983) questioned the revisions because they did not reflect a thorough knowledge of the non-mainstream dialects. A fourth consideration utilizes a spontaneous language sample. However, it too has limitations: It may not provide some of the information necessary to make a diagnosis, and results from such analyses must be interpreted within a developmental framework that currently does not exist for non-mainstream speakers. Another alternative uses a criterion-reference measure, but this too lacks normal developmental data for non-mainstream speakers. Another suggestion from researchers and professional organizations declares a moratorium on the use of all standardized tests that have not been corrected for test bias. According to Vaughn-Cooke (1983), the moratorium alternative is not a solution to the testing problem, but rather a means to dramatize the issue.

The last alternative was the one advocated by Vaughn-Cooke (1983), i.e., to begin immediately developing new tests that are valid and reliable with non-mainstream speakers. We maintain that this should include obtaining and analyzing spontaneous language samples on non-mainstream speakers. Sufficient samples should be obtained and analyzed to establish local norms. Until such assessment procedures are devised, speech-language pathologists need to be extremely sensitive to the assessment of the non-mainstream speaker. If professionals are involved with assessing non-mainstream speakers, they should be familiar with the "Resource Guide to Multi-Cultural Tests and Materials" (Cole and Snope, 1981) and "Supplement I" (Cole and Campbell-Calloway, 1983).

WHAT TO ASSESS

Direct evaluation of the adolescent is a major activity when implementing the assessment component of the prototype delivery model. *What* to assess is addressed in the next section of this book, followed by a section on *how* to assess the adolescent.

History

Relevant data on the adolescent's past history, present status, and future goals should be obtained during the initial part of the evaluation process. Only in this way can an accurate assessment battery be planned.

Information should be obtained about the adolescent's environmental, educational, vocational, and health histories. An environmental history should be accumulated on family members and peers. An educational and vocational history should be gathered on specific strengths and weaknesses in the academic subject areas, and on current and future vocational goals. Relevant health data that might affect performance should be collected (e.g., past and present medications, allergies, seizures). Also, any records of past speech, hearing, and language services should be reviewed.

Another critical area to investigate is feelings and attitudes of adolescents toward their current thinking, listening, and speaking abilities, and their willingness to modify these abilities. This investigation will reveal the adolescent's perspective of the suspected communication problem. It will also assist in documenting metacognition, metalinguistic, and metacommunication awareness.

Feelings and Attitudes Toward Thinking Feuerstein (1980) emphasized that adverse affective-motivational factors can result in deficient cognitive functioning. Furthermore, negative attitude may affect general involvement with cognitive tasks that are demanded in academic and real life situations. "Learned helplessness" is a term growing in usage to describe the phenomenon of individuals who, when faced with a problem, act helpless. Adolescents with learned helplessness view outcomes as uncontrollable. Other effects of learned helplessness are passivity, negative beliefs about oneself, severe reduction in persistence, and depression (Greer and Wethered, 1984). Adolescents with learned helplessness have no strategies, or ineffective ones, for solving the problem, and they perceive few alternatives. These adolescents are frequently those who, by high school, have made so many mistakes and have failed so often, that they mistrust their own thinking. Thus, students who *could* have intact cognitive functions, believe they cannot think, and therefore they do not.

Feelings and Attitudes Toward Listening The adolescent's feelings and attitudes toward listening may be influenced by the following barriers: Calling the subject dull; criticizing the speaker's looks, actions, or speaking style; getting overstimulated and emotionally involved; listening for isolated facts; outlining everything; wasting the extra time available between normal speaking speed (175 wpm) and thinking speed (450 wpm); listening to what is easy to understand; allowing personal prejudices and biases to impair understanding; letting emotionally laden words get in the way; and allowing distractions to interfere (Nichols and Stevens, 1957).

In addition to asking adolescents about their listening, the examiner should investigate whether they have any misconceptions about listening that may interfere with their learning to be a better listener. Wolff et al. (1983) summarized ten major misconceptions about listening. These misconceptions are as follows:

1. *Listening is a matter of intelligence.* Intelligence is not a criterion for listening and there appears to be no strong relationship between intelligence and efficient listening. Efficient listening is more a result of training.

2. *Good hearing and good listening are closely related.* Although there is a relationship between hearing and listening, good hearing does not guarantee good listening. Hearing is a physical activity whereas listening is a mental activity.

3. *Listening is an automatic reflex.* Listening is not an innate skill, but one that is learned.

4. *Daily practice eliminates the need for training in listening.* Practice does not necessarily mean a skill becomes better, especially if it is not practiced correctly. Therefore, to be a better listener one must be trained to practice the skill correctly.

5. *Learning to read will automatically improve listening.* This is a false assumption, since the two activities place different demands on the individual. Listening may actually be a more difficult activity because a listener cannot reread a passage and thus cannot control the rate of the message as one can in reading.

6. *Learning to read is more important than learning to listen.* Wolff et al. (1983) argues that this is not true since most people listen three times more than they read.

7. *The speaker is totally responsible for success in oral communication.* Successful communication is a 50/50 proposition. Equal importance must be given to the role of listening, and listeners should not assume that the speaker is 100% responsible for oral communication.

8. *Listening is essentially a passive activity.* This is an erroneous assumption, since the only way successful communication can occur is if the listener is actively engaged in the process.
9. *Listening means agreement.* Good listeners do not necessarily agree with the speaker but they listen first, then agree or disagree as a result of listening to what the speaker has to say.
10. *Consequences of careless listening are minimal.* This is a misconception, since careless listening can be time consuming, costly, and socially destructive.

Professionals must examine the adolescent's listening habits and determine whether the adolescent holds any of these misconceptions about listening. By realizing that these beliefs are erroneous, the adolescent can begin to develop more efficient and effective listening abilities.

Feelings and Attitudes Toward Speaking The feelings and attitudes of adolescents toward their oral language production can reveal their awareness of communication, their ability to take another's perspective, and their motivation to change behaviors. Adolescents may be marginal communicators who have a "defective" attitude toward communication, but who may not qualify for speech-language services (Blue, 1975). Marginal communicators do not initiate conversation, but they respond with minimal, faint but intelligible utterances in a one-to-one situation. For these adolescents, the assessment procedure will need to determine if only their attitude toward communication is defective, or if their communication system is defective, or both are defective. Attitudes and feelings about speaking may differ, contingent upon the listener (e.g., a friend, a group of peers, a teacher) and upon the setting (e.g., school, home). Therefore, both general feelings and attitudes toward their own communication, as well as variations that occur during specific communicative contexts, should be explored.

Learning Style

It is important to obtain data on how adolescents learn certain tasks best. These data can then assist adolescents to use their strengths to overcome their weaknesses and thus be more successful in school or on a job. Some of the factors to investigate that might affect the adolescent's learning a new or difficult subject are:

1. The best time of day to learn a task (e.g., morning, afternoon, evening)

2. The level of noise in the room (e.g., quiet, music, radio or TV on, conversation)
3. The level of light in the room (e.g., dim, moderate, or bright)
4. The degree of the temperature in the room (e.g., cold, warm, or very warm)
5. The presence or absence of food or drink intake
6. The best place to learn (e.g., home, school, office)
7. The best location to learn a task (e.g., desk, floor, sitting, reclining)
8. The reasons that motivate the adolescent to complete a task (e.g., I want to, My parents expect/want me to, I get money)
9. The desire to work alone or with other people.

In addition to these factors, the professional should investigate the adolescent's approach or strategy for learning materials presented via lectures or textbooks, inside the classroom as well as outside the classroom. Collectively, this information can be analyzed to determine how the adolescent learns best in school and home, and should be shared with teachers and parents. Obtaining this information may also provide adolescents with some insight into their own behaviors, and thus increase their awareness levels and their willingness to change their attitudes toward learning new tasks.

Cognition

While literature on teaching cognitive strategies and thinking skills is rapidly expanding (Hallahan, 1980; Hayes, 1981; Lochhead and Clement, 1979; Maxwell, 1983; Parrill-Burnstein, 1981), there has been no corresponding surge in literature addressing the assessment of cognition. Although most speech-language pathologists would agree that it is important to assess cognition, the specific behaviors evaluated remain dictated, in large part, by the few commercial tests available. Therefore, it is important to have a clear idea of *what* to assess about cognition, and then to select a method by which that information can be obtained (e.g., observation, informal assessment, standardized testing). Too often, in cognitive assessment, this procedure has been reversed. In other words, a test is administered and then analyzed for the cognitive functions that were required. This method can result in piecemeal information regarding cognition.

As with any assessment, examiners can look for functions that are present and intact, or they can look for functions that are weak, deficient, or absent. Ideally, both methods are used, and a pattern of strengths and weaknesses surfaces. The cognitive functions in the input, output, and elaboration phases have proven to be an effective guide for what to assess during adolescence

(Feuerstein, 1979). The input phase involves gathering needed information; the elaboration phase involves using the information that was gathered; the output phase involves expressing the solution to a problem.

A cognitive function that is consistently applied across a variety of contexts is a strength for that adolescent. Cognitive functions may be deficient if they do not appear spontaneously, regularly, and predictably in an individual's behavior. Feuerstein's list of deficient cognitive functions can provide a method for profiling weaknesses within adolescents.

Cognitive functions that should be assessed include those listed in Table 4.2 (Feuerstein, 1979). The interaction of language and cognition becomes obvious when the list of cognitive functions is examined. Many language disorders present during adolescence have underlying cognitive deficits. Professionals should be concerned not only with which cognitive functions are intact or deficient during assessment, but also with the adolescent's awareness of these functions (i.e., metacognition). Feuerstein (1980) contends that a greater awareness of cognitive functions produces more control over applying those functions when the situation presents itself.

Comprehension and Production of Linguistic Features

Wiig and Semel (1980; 1976) have discussed comprehension of linguistic features, including these abilities:

1. Identification of morphological structures, such as compound words, prefixes, and suffixes
2. Differentiation of grammatical phrases, clauses, and sentences as incorrect or incomplete
3. Comprehension of various sentence transformations
4. Comprehension of sentences of various length and complexity
5. Comprehension of semantic features, e.g., multiple meaning words, verbal analogies, inclusion-exclusion, and idioms.

In addition to this list of linguistic features, the examiner should assess the adolescent's ability to engage in informational listening tasks (Boyce and Larson, 1983). Informational listening requires the ability to listen for main ideas and significant details, and to listen for oral directions or a sequence of events. This type of listening also assumes the ability to identify and to recall main ideas, and to take notes on orally presented information. A variety of informational listening skills needs to be assessed:

1. Comprehending factual information (e.g., directions and dates)
2. Concentrating attention on the speaker

TABLE 4.2 COGNITIVE FUNCTIONS (FEUERSTEIN, 1979)

Input Phase

1. Clear perception
   Is the adolescent using senses (e.g., hearing, seeing) to gather clear and complete information?

2. Systematic exploration?
   Is a plan being used so that important information is not being skipped or missed?

3. Labeling
   Is the adolescent consistently naming objects and events so that they can be remembered and talked about clearly?

4. Temporal and spatial referents
   Are events and objects being described in terms of where and when they occur?

5. Conservation/object permanency
   Are characteristics of objects and events recognized as the same even when changes take place? (e.g., Is a square tilted onto a corner still recognized as a square?)

6. Using two sources of information
   Can the adolescent organize information by several characteristics simultaneously (e.g., by date and time of day; by size and by shape)?

7. Need for precision
   Does the adolescent know when and how to be precise and accurate (e.g., when reporting data about an emergency to the appropriate authorities)?

Elaboration Phase

1. Analyzing disequilibrium
   Can the adolescent define problems and determine what needs to be done?

2. Relevance
   Is the adolescent using only the information that is relevant to the problem and ignoring the rest?

3. Interiorization
   Does the adolescent form "good pictures in the mind" about what must be done to solve the problem?

TABLE 4.2 CONTINUED

4. Planning behavior
   Is the adolescent making a plan that includes steps needed to reach a goal?

5. Broadening the mental field
   Are the various pieces of information needed to solve the problem being remembered?

6. Projecting relationships
   Is the adolescent looking for relationships by which separate objects, events, and experiences can be tied together? (e.g., A flat tire, a sick child, and an overdrawn checkbook have made my mother very upset today; therefore, this is not the time to ask for a new jacket.)

7. Comparative behavior
   Are objects and experiences being compared to others to determine what is similar and what is different?

8. Categorization
   Is the adolescent finding the class or set to which new objects or experiences belong?

9. Hypothetical thinking
   Is the adolescent thinking about different alternatives and what would happen if one or another were chosen?

10. Logical evidence
    Is logic being used to prove answers and to defend opinions?

Output Phase

1. Overcoming egocentric communication
   Is the adolescent being clear and precise in language so that the listener understands the message?

2. Overcoming trial-and-error
   Is the adolescent thinking through the response instead of immediately trying to answer and making a mistake?

3. Restraining impulsive behavior
   Is restraint being used before saying or doing something that will be regretted later?

4. Overcoming blocking
   Is a strategy being used to help find answers rather than panicking when stuck on a problem?

3. Using advantageously the time differential between thinking and speaking speed (i.e., people think two and one-half times faster than a speaker talks)
4. Understanding main ideas and supportive details
5. Formulating questions of clarification.

Arwood (1983) argued against looking at comprehension of linguistic features in isolation from the speech act, because professionals may end up assessing products rather than processes. To determine, for example, that a student does not understand comparative adjectives tells the examiner nothing about *why* comprehension is absent, or what effect this has on the speech act. While it is important to assess the adolescent's ability to comprehend language features, examiners cannot lose sight of the reason for doing so, i.e., to determine the impact upon communication.

Essential aspects to consider when assessing the adolescent's production of linguistic features include the following:

1. Use of simple and complex sentences
2. Use of appropriate sentence fragments (e.g., a response of "eleven o'clock" to the question, "What time will you be home tonight?")
3. Avoidance of an excessive number of run-on sentences that are strung together with "and," "and then"
4. Use of a variety of question forms, such as wh-questions, tag questions, interrogative reversals, and questions marked by rising intonation
5. Generation of novel questions and sentences
6. Use of figurative language such as slang, jargon, idioms, metaphors, similes, and language for the purpose of entertainment or humor
7. Avoidance of nonspecific language such as low information words (e.g., things, stuff, everybody)
8. Absence of word retrieval problems.

Discourse

During assessment of discourse, specific aspects of conversations and narrations need to be analyzed: Propositions, cohesion devices, critical listening, communication functions, and verbal mazes.

Propositions are defined as idea units consisting of a relational concept plus arguments (Ripich and Griffith, 1985). An argument is a noun that serves the function of agent, object, goal, patient, beneficiary, or instrument. Relational concepts are predicates, modifiers, or connectives that connect arguments. Discourse should be analyzed to determine the number and quality of propositions.

Cohesion devices should be analyzed to determine whether they contribute to or disrupt the continuity of meaning in the conversation or narration. Devices that contribute to continuity are the referent (i.e., meaning of the word is present from the context); the conjunction (i.e., a linking word whose meaning is appropriate to the words being linked); and the ellipsis (i.e., a redundant word or words that are eliminated from the context but can be determined). Disruptive cohesion devices are: Referent error (i.e., using a word to refer to elements that are absent from the context); conjunction errors (i.e., linking words that are inappropriate to the context); and ellipsis error (i.e., elements are eliminated whose referents cannot be determined from the context).

Critical listening is essential to the adolescent's comprehension during discourse. A critical listener must be a critical thinker, i.e., capable of engaging in higher level thought when required by the situation. The critical listening skills that need assessment include:

1. Identification and recognition of the credibility of the source or speaker
2. Recognition and use of inductive and deductive reasoning
3. Detection of false reasoning (e.g., the ability to discriminate between fact and opinion)
4. Recognition of propaganda devices (e.g., loaded words)
5. Drawing of inferences and judgment of statements heard.

Communication functions have been described by a variety of taxonomies (Austin, 1962; Chapman, 1981, 1972; Dore, 1975, 1974; Greenfield and Smith, 1976; Halliday, 1975; Hymes, 1972; Searle, 1965). The system for the adolescent population to which we adhere was extrapolated from the work of Austin (1962), Searle (1965), and Hymes (1972). The taxonomies developed by Austin and Searle were primarily designed to analyze adult speech acts, whereas the taxonomies developed by Halliday (1975) and Dore (1974) were created to analyze child-based speech acts. Searle (1965) refined Austin's (1962) classification system and proposed this taxonomy: Representatives (i.e., statements that convey a belief or disbelief in an idea), directives (i.e., attempts to influence the listener to do something), commissives (i.e., commitments of self to some future course of action), expressives (i.e., expression of a psychological state, such as "thank you"), and declaratives (i.e., statements of facts that presume to alter a state of affairs, such as "I confer upon you").

Our extrapolated taxonomy includes eight functions (Boyce and Larson, 1983):

1. To give information

2. To get information (i.e., question asking)
3. To describe an ongoing event
4. To get the listener to do, believe, or feel something (i.e., persuasion)
5. To express one's own intentions, beliefs, and feelings (i.e., self-disclosure)
6. To indicate a readiness for further communication
7. To solve problems
8. To entertain.

All eight functions should be present within the language of the adolescent. Missing functions limit the communicative intents that can be expressed.

Verbal mazes can impair communicative intent. While all speakers engage in some verbal mazes (i.e., words, or unattached fragments not necessary to the message), the expectation is not to exceed significantly what is normal for a given grade level (Loban, 1976). Some adolescents use verbal mazes with such high frequency that it is impossible to comprehend their spoken message. Along with verbal mazes, the speech-language pathologist should assess the presence of false starts at the beginnings of utterances (e.g., "you know," "guess what?"). Both verbal mazes and false starts during conversations and narrations can be distracting to listeners and can interfere with the clarity of the speaker's message.

Conversations A variety of rules govern conversational exchanges. In conversation, one person selects a topic that is maintained until a topic shift is initiated. When assessing adolescents' use of conversational rules, speech-language pathologists should observe these behaviors:

1. Initiation of conversations in a variety of situations
2. Selection of appropriate topics
3. Maintenance of a topic over a number of speaker-listener exchanges
4. Switching of topics in an appropriate and orderly manner
5. Termination of conversations in a timely manner.

Switching topics can be accomplished abruptly with no warning provided for the listener; or it can be cued directly (e.g., Can I talk with you about something else for a minute?) or indirectly (e.g., That reminds me of . . .). During conversation, the speaker and listener take turns. Turn-taking should occur with a minimum of interruption; repairs and revisions should be made when necessary (Rees and Wollner, 1982).

Grice (1975) proposed four fundamental rules of conversations that summarize expectations held by speakers and listeners. We are hypothesizing that these rules are intact by late adolescence, but may emerge even earlier.

A. Quantity: Informativeness

"1. Make your contribution as informative as is required (for the current purposes of the exchange).
2. Do not make your contribution more informative than is required." (p. 45)

B. Quality: Sincerity

"1. Do not say what you believe to be false.
2. Do not say that for which you lack adequate evidence." (p. 46)

C. Relation: Topic Management

"1. Be relevant." (p. 46)

D. Manner: How to be clear

"1. Avoid obscurity of expression.
2. Avoid ambiguity.
3. Be brief (avoid unnecessary prolixity).
4. Be orderly." (p. 46)

Wiig (1983) has stressed the importance of the adolescent's ability to switch registers, or codes, during conversational speech. While talking with peers, an informal register is acceptable. However, when talking with adults, a more formal register is used. A formal register contains more noun phrase elaborations and verb phrase complexity, and it assumes that the speaker and listener do not share mutual information; thus it necessitates more precise descriptions and explanations. A formal register also uses more polite forms than an informal register. Failure to discriminate which register to use for each communicative situation is a major problem for some adolescents.

Narrations The adolescent's ability to comprehend and to produce narratives should be investigated, because this task demonstrates whether or not the adolescent can integrate information. Also, "narratives are structurally midway between the language of the oral tradition and the language of the essayist literary tradition" (Westby, 1984, p. 124). Thus, knowing the adolescent's ability to generate narratives should allow the examiner to determine if the adolescent is ready to develop a more literary language structure and to learn the written form of language.

When analyzing story grammar units the speech-language pathologist can use either a developmental approach (Applebee, 1978) or a story grammar taxonomy (Roth and Spekman, 1986). With a developmental approach during assessment, the professional should keep in mind the developmental hierarchy leading up to the true narrative (Applebee, 1978):

1. Initially, children use prenarrative structures starting with "heap stories." They talk about whatever attracts their attention, without regard for a relationship among the elements or a macrostructure.
2. A second prenarrative stage is "sequence stories," which have a macrostructure, but the storyteller does not actually have a temporal sequence in mind. Rather, characters, objects, or events are put together because they are perceptually associated with each other.
3. The next stage is "primitive narratives" in which characters, objects, or events are put together because they complement each other in some logical way. These narratives are the students' first use of inference in stories. However, their inferences go in only one direction and they do not perceive the reciprocal causality between thoughts and events.
4. Another developmental stage in story grammars is the "unfocused chain." In unfocused chain stories the elements are logically related to each other but not related to any macrostructure. Thus, the story has no theme or plot.
5. The next stage is the "focused chain," which has all the elements or events sequenced and related to the story's macrostructure. However, the story still lacks reciprocal relationships between characters' attributes and events, and among main events. Thus, the story does not have a strong plot.
6. The last stage of development is the "true narrative" that integrates logical cause-and-effect chaining of the macrostructure elements, which are linked to the macrostructure of the story. This results in the story having a strong, well-developed plot.

Normal children are capable of producing true narratives by five to six years of age. Between seven and eleven years of age, children begin to summarize and to categorize stories both subjectively and objectively. Subjectively, the child may categorize or summarize a story as "funny" or "exciting" or "sad." Objectively, the child may summarize a story as rhyming or long. In either case, the child is capable of considering the entire story and placing it in a more general category. Complex stories with multiple embedded narrative structures do not emerge until eleven to twelve years of age (Westby, 1984). However, mid-school learning-disabled students have been shown to have difficulty with narrative tasks (Westby, 1984).

Analysis of stories begins between thirteen to fifteen years of age. In analysis, "the focus shifts to a consideration of how the work might have been structured as well as how it is structured" (Applebee, 1978, p. 109). Analysis is often integrated with evaluation. During this level, the adolescent is capable of story critiques from a series of dimensions (e.g., What were the motives of a character? How does the story make you feel?).

Individuals between sixteen years to adulthood are capable of generalizing about the meaning of a story, formulating abstract statements about its theme or message, and focusing on how they react to the story. They wish to determine if they agree with the work and how it applies to their situation.

It should be noted that the developmental stages of narration progress in a cumulative fashion. Thus, one level builds onto the next level. For example, "Seventeen-year-olds . . . are typically able not only to generalize, but also to muster the resources of all the earlier stages. They can analyze in support of their generalizations; they can categorize and summarize; and they can retell in whole or in part, depending on their purpose." (Applebee, 1978, p. 125).

The other type of story grammar analysis is that of using a taxonomy that identifies the elements common to stories and specifies a formal set of rules underlying the construction of any story (Mandler and Johnson, 1977; Rummelhart, 1975; Stein and Glenn, 1979; Thorndyke, 1977). All story grammars have a setting in which the main character is introduced, and/or have a description of the social, physical, or temporal context of the story. All story grammars have a goal that is met in an episode system. Episodes have a beginning, which is an initiating event; a reaction of the characters to the initiating event; an action, or attempt by the characters to deal with the initiating event; an outcome, or consequence of the attempt; and an ending. All the elements of a story grammar taxonomy should be present in the adolescents' narrations.

Nonverbal Communication

Nonverbal rules govern kinesic and proxemic behaviors during discourse. French (1978) cautioned adults about recent changes in nonverbal communication among youth; however, there are still expectations for appropriate kinesic and proxemic behaviors. The expected kinesic behaviors include the use of gestures that match the spoken message, avoidance of adaptor behaviors that detract from the message (e.g., constantly pushing hair off one's forehead), communication of emotion through facial expression, and appropriate eye contact. Duncan and Fiske (1977) have discussed nonverbal communication behaviors that occur during conversational speech, particularly kinesics and turn-taking signals, and professionals would benefit from reading this resource. Proxemic behaviors include the maintenance of socially acceptable space or distance while conversing. Hall (1959) delineated acceptable ranges of distance for Americans.

Paralanguage features that should be observed while assessing the adolescent include the rate of speech, tone of voice, use of inflection, and unfilled pause time (i.e., silence) within and between utterances. Also, the presence of filled pauses (e.g., "ah," "um," "er") should be noted. Are pauses occurring so often that the message being communicated is significantly impaired? Abnormal paralanguage features impair communication as much as restricted language features do, and thus they become critical variables to evaluate during assessment.

Survival Language Skills

Adolescents with more severely impaired thinking, listening, and speaking often have accompanying survival language deficits, i.e., difficulty functioning in one or more environments because of their language disorder. Valletutti and Bender (1982) have identified six major environments in which the adolescent must function:

1. At home, as a family member
2. At school, as a student
3. In the community, as a citizen
4. In the marketplace, as a consumer of goods and services
5. In society, as a participant of leisure
6. In the workplace, as a producer of goods or services.

Each of these settings demands appropriate cognitive, language, and communication behaviors. Detailed assessment considerations for each of these roles have been previously outlined (Boyce and Larson, 1983).

Assessment of survival language skills is not always a concern during the speech-language pathologist's initial assessment of an adolescent, but exceptions to this are possible. If an adolescent is in a secondary-school setting, and has only a year or two of programming time remaining, survival language skills may be a primary emphasis for both assessment and intervention. If an adolescent is spending only a few months at a juvenile detention center, assessment of survival language skills necessary for integration and survival in the home community would be an extremely legitimate concern. Speech-language pathologists conducting the assessment of adolescents must use their best clinical judgment in determining whether to evaluate survival language skills, and if so, which ones.

Frequently, survival language skills can be assessed better after beginning speech-language services, as part of an ongoing diagnostic intervention paradigm. For example, within the role of consumer of goods and services, adolescents would be expected to comprehend and produce language needed in a restaurant, e.g., a fast food chain. An initial baseline assessment would determine what vocabulary and communication skills were already in the adolescent's repertoire, and which ones were absent. If sufficient communication skills needed for survival in a fast food restaurant were present, then no further work would be done. However, if deficiencies were noted, then intervention would begin to focus on development of appropriate restaurant language.

In addition to completing the type of situational analysis just described, multi-situational skills can be assessed. For example, the language of money, time, space, warning labels, and signs can be evaluated. The vocabulary for these areas crosses a number of settings and roles in which the adolescent functions.

HOW TO ASSESS

Suggestions in this section will emphasize the integration of the assessment process and how to evaluate *simultaneously* cognitive, language, and communication behaviors. Four informal assessment procedures are proposed: A case history form, learning style questionnaire, discourse samples, and directed tasks. In addition, formal tests are listed. Regardless of whether informal and/or formal testing procedures are used, the examiner must be aware of the variables that affect the administration of procedures, analysis of data, and interpretation of the adolescent's performance.

Informal Assessment

Case History Form A general case history form, for obtaining information on the adolescent's health, education, and environmental history, has already been published (Boyce and Larson, 1983). This form has been revised and is reprinted in Appendix B.

Information can be obtained by interviewing the adolescent or a parent/caregiver. Some of the information may be derived from cumulative records. In most instances, the case history form should not be given to the adolescent to complete, but should be retained by the examiner who asks questions and records responses.

If adolescents have the necessary skills, another alternative would be to have them write or audio tape an autobiography. These options can provide insight into their perspective of the past, present, and future.

A supplemental case history form has been previously published for use during assessment of the adolescent's feelings and attitudes toward thinking, listening, and speaking (McKinley and Larson, 1984). A revised version of this form is reprinted in Appendix B. A questionnaire devised by Schwartz and McKinley (1984) has also been included for assessment of the adolescent's misconceptions about listening.

The general case history form should be reviewed to determine whether the student has had previous speech-language services. If so, is the student ready to receive additional services? Also, the case history should be analyzed to determine a need to refer for additional professional services. The supplemental case history form should be reviewed to see if the students are aware of their own thinking, listening, and speaking abilities. The students who are aware of their abilities may be more motivated to change these behaviors and therefore, may be good candidates for speech-language services.

Learning Style Questionnaire A learning style questionnaire has been developed to determine when, where, what, why, and how the adolescent learns best. (See Appendix C.) The adolescent should not be expected to read the form independently, but should be given a form to follow along with the examiner. The examiner should systematically go through the form, asking the adolescent questions and recording responses. This gives the examiner the opportunity to explain any unfamiliar terms or to ask additional questions to clarify a response.

During field testing, the form has not been useful with all adolescents; but it appears to be most useful with adolescents who already possess a good deal of insight and self-confidence. Students who are less secure are more likely to give answers that they think the examiner wants to hear, or that they think are correct, than they are to report how they actually learn best.

Discourse Samples: Conversations Conversational samples are a critical part of informal assessment of adolescents. These samples have been a major recommended source of information for decades, and they are the preferred method of language elicitation from "toddler to adult" (Atkins and Cartwright, 1982). We concur with this position, despite a recent recommendation to speech-language pathologists that stated: "To be comprehensive, descriptive, and yet meet the time constraints within a school setting, a communication evaluation procedure should have some inherent structure rather than rely upon an unstructured format such as conversations or peer interaction or free play" (Simon, 1984, p. 84). While a disadvantage of spontaneous conversational samples is the risk of not eliciting all the language behaviors in the individual's repertoire, a powerful advantage of conversational samples is the more realistic picture of the adolescent's communication that is gained.

Arwood (1983), who advocates unstructured conversational sampling, commented that to determine level of functioning rapidly, professionals have only to listen to the individual talk. What can be detected about the way the adolescent organizes ideas, expresses communicative intents, and uses a variety of structures? To the recommendation to listen, we would add, "watch the adolescent communicate." What can be noted about eye contact, gestures, body space, and facial expressions?

A partial transcript is reprinted in Table 4.3. This unstructured language sample was obtained by a speech-language clinician evaluating a fourteen-year-old boy. This boy successfully passed tests that measured isolated aspects of language (i.e., discrete point tests), and yet his conversational sample revealed problems in communicating messages to listeners. The excessive number of verbal mazes, lack of message cohesiveness, and high incidence of low information words frequently left his listeners confused.

TABLE 4.3 TRANSCRIPT OF A FOURTEEN-YEAR-OLD BOY

Adolescent: What do we talk on? No. Oh, I got a good one. You should see my...um, Uncle Boos had to move and they're in this really cool house. It's, it's like, it's round. It's sort of li...okay, it's, it's peaked at the top and then it gets round or somethin'...no, it goes...it's...

Clinician: It goes down and then (demonstrates)

Adolescent: Yeah! And then inside they, they have this bedroom...They're going... Okay, there's the living room and their bedroom is...ya go up the, the st...and three stairs, and then you go up there and then they're gonna block it that off from the...so people can't see them in the living room and in the kitchen. They're gonna put a door there and plus they got this neat bar and it's real cool. They have it...um, in the living room. It's real cool. They don't have much furniture though.

Clinician: They should get some.

Adolescent: Uh-hum. They'll have a couch and two chairs. You should see. Oh, it's really awesome. You know, like in a restaurant. They have the table and it's like in the kitchen and it's hitched to the wall. It's real cool.

Clinician: Oh!

Adolescent: And then it goes and then the basement...my older cousins have the basement for the bedroom. It's real cool. They have...they have all these bunch of posters, and feathers, and cowboy hats and...cool!

Clinician: (Laughs)

Adolescent: And then...okay, there's...they have about eight kids and there's one downst in the living room but two down in...Wait a minute! They have six, but counting the parents it's eight. And they...okay, upstairs they have...it's like a closet...like it's about maybe this big. About from this square and that's their bedroom. And it's, okay, from there to there. That's their bedroom. Their mom and dad's bedroom. And there's this kind of like closet thing that closes.

Clinician: How can they get into it?

Administration Procedures for obtaining language samples have changed very little since first recommended by McCarthy (1930). Speech-language pathologists should: (1) establish good rapport with the individual being sampled, (2) keep their remarks to a minimum, and (3) use open-ended questions or comments that will facilitate longer responses. Usually, the adolescent population should select their own topics of conversation.

The goal of obtaining a sample is that it be "representative" of the adolescent's communication. However, "representative" has held different meanings in the literature, including "comprehensive," "idealized," and "typical" (Gallagher, 1983). To be comprehensive, a conversational sample has to be large enough to be reliable, but small enough to be efficient. McCarthy (1930) originally proposed a 50 utterance sample; others have recommended 100 utterances (Crystal, Fletcher, and Garman, 1976; Engler, Hannah, and Longhurst, 1973; Tyack and Gottsleben, 1974). Recently Bloom and Lahey (1978) and Miller (1981) recommended a minimum of 30 minutes of sampling time. Bloom and Lahey (1978) also suggested that 200 or more utterances be obtained within the sampling time.

To be a representative conversational sample in the sense of an "idealized" performance, the sample should evoke the best possible sample of abilities (McLean and Snyder-McLean, 1978). The conversational analysis should neither underestimate nor overestimate the adolescent's communication abilities, since ". . . a language sample is considered unrepresentative if it leads to an analysis that results in either one of these errors" (Gallagher, 1983, p. 3). The notion that an "idealized" sample should be collected is contradictory to the notion that it also be "typical," or representative of daily communication performances. When assessing adolescents, we have been most concerned with collecting samples that represent "usual" language performances, rather than optimal samples.

In addition to considering what is a *representative* sample, speech-language pathologists must consider how language use varies with context (Gallagher, 1983). Many clinicians have responded by obtaining language samples in more than one context, using a variety of stimuli, conversational partners, and settings (McLean and Snyder-McLean, 1978; Miller, 1981; Muma, 1978). The problem is that the ". . . number of possible combinations of stimulus materials, conversational partners, and settings is infinite" (Gallagher, 1983, p. 4). The selection of combinations is either arbitrary or the result of trial and error sampling. Therefore, whether sampling in multiple contexts solves the assessment problems arising from language use variability is questionable (Gallagher, 1983).

There is little available data to describe how adolescents' communication varies as a function of changes in stimuli, conversational partners, or settings. Our own longitudinal study (which utilizes a school setting, and no stimulus materials, to gather data while adolescents converse with peers of their choice and with unfamiliar adults of the opposite sex) is some of the first research that describes how language use varies in these contexts (McKinley and Larson, 1983). Clearly, more information is needed. In the meantime, we recommend, at the minimum, that two ten-minute conversational samples be collected, one while conversing with the speech-language pathologist (usually an unfamiliar adult during initial assessment) and one with a peer of the adolescent's choice. Additional samples might be collected using other partners. The conversational samples should require the adolescent to switch from an informal to a formal register. The speech-language pathologist should keep in mind that after age fifteen adolescents begin to use a more formal register even with their peers, unless they are the best of friends (Wiig, 1982a).

Analysis Both partners' turns should be transcribed in order to analyze certain pragmatic features. Rather than delineating utterances, as would be done for young children, conversational units should be marked when transcribing adolescent language. A conversational unit is defined as "... the utterance(s) of one conversational partner that continue(s) until the other conversational partner initiates an independent utterance" (Boyce and Larson, 1983, p. 221). A phonetic transcription may or may not be necessary. If articulation errors are evident, it may be desirable to complete a phonetic transcription. In all cases, the transcription should reflect what was actually said, and include all false starts, verbal mazes, and filled pauses.

Perhaps the greatest difficulty with conversational samples is how to analyze them once they are transcribed. One reason for the difficulty is that calculation of the mean length of utterance in morphemes (MLU-M) for the purpose of comparing it with Brown's (1973) stages of psycholinguistic development is not appropriate for the adolescent population.

How can professionals determine that an adolescent's language system is different from what might be expected? Loban (1976) has described an analysis procedure that allows the quantification of a variety of linguistic characteristics, e.g., maze words, words per communication unit. (See Tables 2.2, 2.3, and 2.4 in Chapter 2.) This quantification begins to give a sense of the system's functioning, but the focus is on products of communication rather than on processes. Thus, adopting analysis procedures that attempt to quantify developmental changes during adolescence should not be the only method used, since the desired outcome is a *description* of the adolescent's communication, sufficiently detailed to suggest if intervention is needed. When quantitative analysis procedures are used, they should still be combined with descriptive data that discuss how the adolescent's language system differs from the normal.

Several procedures that emphasize descriptive data have been suggested in the literature, and are adaptable for the adolescent population. Arwood (1983) has described her system in detail and has developed appropriate summary forms. Prutting and Kirchner (1983) have developed a "Pragmatic Protocol" organized around the utterance, propositional, illocutionary, and perlocutionary acts. Readers are urged to consult the original sources for more information on these analysis procedures.

We have found that Simon's (1979) chart of competent and incompetent language features provides a useful guide to listening to the adolescent's language. The chart provides a gestalt of the adolescent's communication, not just isolated features. By noting competent features that are present, absent, or inconsistent, and describing typical utterances as evidence, the speech-language pathologist can begin to develop a consensus of the total effectiveness and efficiency of an adolescent's communication.

Drawing from a variety of sources (Duncan and Fiske, 1977; Grice, 1975; Hymes, 1972; Rees and Wollner, 1982; Simon, 1979; Wiig and Semel, 1980), we have constructed a form called "Adolescent Conversational Analysis." This form may be reproduced from Appendix D. It is unique from other analyses in that it examines the adolescent's role both as a listener and a speaker, not simply as a speaker, during conversation.

The microcomputer is an excellent clinical tool for assisting the speech-language pathologist to be more efficient and effective in analyzing language samples. Language assessment software programs, such as *Lingquest 1: Language Sample Analysis*, by Mordecai, Palin, and Palmer (1982); and *Systematic Analysis of Language Transcripts (SALT)*, by Miller and Chapman (1983), allow for the sorting, calculating, and tabulating of data from language samples.

Lingquest 1: Language Sample Analysis (Mordecai, Palin, and Palmer, 1982) uses concepts from Lee (1974), Tyack and Gottsleben (1974), Crystal, Fletcher, and Garman (1976), and Miller (1981). *Lingquest 1* provides for an analysis of lexical items including a type-token ratio (TTR) and eight grammatical forms (i.e., nouns, verbs, modifiers, prepositions, conjunctions, negations, interjections, and wh-question words), mean length of utterance in words and morphemes, and an analysis of eighty-one subcategories of parts of speech.

SALT (Miller and Chapman, 1983) is based on the principles and procedures described by Miller (1981). *SALT* has five major features for analyzing a language sample: Transcript entry, transcript utility, standard analysis, search, and wizard word lists. The standard analysis procedures conducted by the *SALT* are: Number and percentage of complete and incomplete utterances, the type-token ratio, mean length of utterance in morphemes, a distributional analysis of the number of utterances by word or morpheme and speaker turns, the frequency of usage of structures designated by the speech-language pathologist, and an analysis of morpheme usage.

From the brief description of these software programs, it can be seen that they offer a range of analysis features and varying degrees of flexibility. How time-consuming a particular analysis system will be is contingent upon the type of analysis that is chosen, the amount of information processed, and the skills of the speech-language pathologist in coding utterances (Schwartz, 1985). Although these software packages should ultimately allow clinicians to be more efficient, the software should also assist them to become more effective in determining the type and severity of a language disorder, and in establishing appropriate intervention programs. Regardless of the software language analysis system used, the speech-language pathologist must obtain an accurate and representative language sample, transcribe the sample accurately, and code the language structures correctly.

Interpretation Quantitative data may be compared to those presented on existing developmental charts such as Loban's (1976). Caution is advised because Loban's results were obtained in a contrived conversational situation. Quantitative data in the form of TTR should not be compared with existing data for children's utterances, or with adult norms. We recommend that local normative data be obtained on the TTR of adolescents. With the use of the computer, this is a realistic goal.

The "Adolescent Conversational Analysis" that we recommend could be interpreted with the use of the profile summary provided in Appendix D. Conversational behaviors are determined to be either appropriate or inappropriate. Determination of the appropriateness and inappropriateness of a behavior is made by judging whether or not it is penalizing to the adolescent; a behavior perceived by the clinician as penalizing is marked as inappropriate (Prutting and Kirchner, 1983). Our clinical experiences have been that the adolescent probably has conversational deficits in need of intervention if a significant number of conversational behaviors are indicated as inappropriate (i.e., thirty percent or more, disregarding items marked "not observed," which approximates two standard deviations below the mean on standardized tests). Certain items should carry more weight during interpretation because they may carry more negative consequences during communication exchanges than other items do, i.e., main ideas, word retrieval skills, fluency, intelligibility, turn-taking. If consistent problems are evident on any one of these items, then direct or indirect intervention should be considered even if most of the other items are judged to be appropriate.

Discourse Samples: Narrations The use of narratives can be an excellent assessment procedure (Arwood, 1983). Narrative tasks are more structured than conversational speech, but less structured than the directed tasks that will be discussed in the section that follows.

Administration The way that examiners obtain a narrative language sample can result in different types of samples. For example, if adolescents are asked to relate a personal experience, they will produce a more orally structured narrative. If asked to tell a story, adolescents will use a more literary style. However, if they are asked to tell a story like it is written in a book, they will use the most literary style.

When both the examiner and the adolescent can see the stimulus picture and share in the pictorial situation, there is a tendency for some students to resort to a more oral style and to make the narrative less explicit. Also, what is depicted in a picture may make a difference. Pictures that display an action may lead a student to describe only the action, whereas pictures that display a setting often yield a more complex story. Telling a story from a wordless picture book requires that the student recognize the scenarios depicted, whereas telling a story from a single picture requires that the student formulate and organize the story, not simply recognize it. Some students show minimal differences based upon how the instructions are given or how the stimuli are depicted. However, others tend to switch from a more oral to a more literary mode, depending on the task. Perhaps this demonstrates that these latter individuals have a metalinguistic awareness toward story grammars.

Story reformulation has also been used as an assessment procedure (Chappell, 1980; Culatta, Page, and Ellis, 1983). In story reformulation tasks, adolescents have to comprehend, retain and recall information, understand sequences, and express themselves precisely when retelling the story.

We recommend that at least two samples of narration be obtained, one being a formulated and the other a reformulated task. The type of story selected for the reformulation task should be sensitive to the adolescent's social-emotional level and to memory capacity. The specific type of formulated task selected would be contingent upon whether a more oral or more literary sample was desired. Generally, we first choose a formulated task that requires the adolescent to relate a personal experience, since the recounting of a personal story and a story reformulation task are the most distant tasks on the oral-literary style continuum. If relating a personal experience is a much stronger ability for the adolescent than reformulating a story, then additional formulated narration tasks requiring a more literary style, may be necessary to determine where the individual falls on the continuum.

Analysis Once a student has formulated or reformulated a story, the speech-language pathologist should transcribe the story. Recall that there are two primary ways in which narratives can be analyzed once transcribed—through a developmental hierarchy and through a story grammar taxonomy. We advocate analysis through the developmental stage progression (Applebee, 1978) because of its underlying theoretical premises (Piaget, 1959; Vygotsky, 1962). Story grammar taxonomies appear to be independent of theoretical constructs. Using Applebee's (1978) developmental hierarchy, we have developed an analysis form to be used. (See Appendix E.) Applebee (1978) noted that stories do not always fit precisely into one of the first six categories. Thus, judgments will need to be made on the basis of the predominant mode of organization.

Interpretation Once the speech-language pathologist has analyzed the adolescent's story to determine the predominant mode of organization in the developmental hierarchy, then it is possible to interpret these data in terms of the underlying cognitive level and the chronological age at which most students learn this aspect of narration. Adolescents whose narrations are consistently three or more years delayed, compared with their chronological age, may be candidates for language intervention.

Directed Tasks We are defining any structured procedure that requires thinking, listening, and/or speaking as "directed tasks." All of these tasks share commonalities:

1. Focus is directed toward the *process* through which the adolescent goes to perform the directed task: The correct *product* is frequently irrelevant.
2. Each directed task should be followed with appropriate metacognitive, metalinguistic, and/or metacommunication questions. For example, examiners would want to consider questions such as:

a. What did you have to think about to solve that problem? What went on in your mind?
b. How did you figure out what was important to listen to?
c. Was that direction difficult for you to understand? Why? Were there some words that were unfamiliar to you?
d. What made that story (message/direction) difficult to tell?
e. Do you think that was a clear message? Do you think I understood what you meant?
f. Why didn't I understand what you meant?

These types of questions help to determine what the adolescent knows about cognitive functions, language, and communication. An adolescent who has little "meta" awareness is likely to be more impaired than one who has awareness, but inconsistent application.

3. Directed tasks that are difficult for adolescents should be administered again, with slight variations, following metacognitive, metalinguistic, and/or metacommunication questions. This will permit the examiner to comment on the adolescent's prognosis for modification, given a structured learning experience. For example, one of the directed tasks presented later is "Organization." If the adolescent failed to handle the grocery store task suggested in "Organization" (see page 112), the examiner should question the adolescent about knowledge of cognitive functions such as categorization (e.g., "Do you know what some grocery store categories are?") and systematic exploration (e.g., "Do you know how you would systematically look for an item in a grocery store?"). Following these metacognitive questions, once they are successfully discussed, the examiner should present a new problem slightly different from the first. For example, "If I send you to a drug store to buy aspirin, cotton balls, and toothpaste, how would you find those items?" Adolescents who can transfer cognitive functions such as categorization and systematic exploration to this new situation would be viewed as having greater potential for learning, and a more promising prognosis than adolescents who failed to benefit from the metacognitive, metalinguistic, and metacommunication discussions.

Problem Solving 1. Areas assessed: The informal assessment task for problem solving provides information primarily on cognition, but it also provides data on conversational abilities when the problem solving task involves dialogue. Survival language skills may or may not receive focus depending upon the content of the problems solved.

2. Administration: During this task, the examiner would want to ascertain whether the adolescent can apply a problem solving model (e.g., Alley and Deshler's [1979] model). A variety of common problems that relate to academic, social, and/or vocational concerns should be presented to the adolescent. Problems to be solved may range from common daily occurrences (e.g.

Which of four homework assignments should be tackled first?) to novel situations (e.g., How would you find a doctor to go to if you moved to a new city?) A number of excellent computer programs (e.g., see *Solutions Unlimited* [Agency for Instructional Technology, 1984]) focus on the adolescent's ability to apply a problem solving model, and these programs could be adapted for use during informal assessment procedures. Guiding questions may be asked by the examiner to determine application of the problem solving model (e.g., "How do you know if you've made the best decision?").

3. Analysis: The adolescent's responses to the various problems presented should be recorded and analyzed as to whether the adolescent could usually respond to the various steps of the problem solving model (with or without guiding questions) delineated below:

a. Identify the problem
b. Propose alternative solutions
c. Choose the best alternative
d. Make a plan to implement the alternative
e. Evaluate the decision.

The steps of the model that were often problematic to the adolescent should be noted.

4. Interpretation: Adolescents have deficits in the area of problem solving that warrant intervention if they do not identify the problem to be solved, propose only one or two alternative solutions, or choose a solution which is not the best one. (See Table 1.1 in Chapter 1.) When requested to justify the "best alternative," if they provide a weak rationale, or none at all, they may be candidates for intervention. If adolescents have difficulty primarily with Steps d. and e. (i.e., making plans and evaluating decisions), this is generally a less severe deficit.

Organization 1. Areas assessed: The informal assessment task for organization provides information primarily on cognition. However, because the task involves a dialogue between the examiner and the adolescent, the task may also provide discourse data. Depending upon the content of the dialogue, information may be obtained on survival language skills.

2. Administration: During the assessment process, the examiner should obtain information about the adolescent's perceptions of organization. A familiar task should be proposed, such as, "Suppose I sent you into a grocery store to buy celery, milk, and ice cream. You have never been in the store before. What is your strategy for finding these food items?" Adolescents should be able to describe a number of strategies such as asking someone, looking for the signs that hang above the aisles, or walking around the outer perimeter of the store and then the aisles (i.e., systematic exploration). If they

do not describe all of the possible strategies, discuss additional approaches they could use to find the named grocery items. From grocery store organization, the examiner can ask questions that bridge to other situations, such as, "What other stores are organized? How are they organized? What is organized besides stores (e.g., schools, hospitals, houses)? How are they organized? Does everything you can think of have some sort of organization? Why do we organize?"

An alternative task to assess organization is to use a computer program such as *The Factory* (Kosel and Fish, 1984), which requires the adolescent to "manufacture" a model product by subjecting raw material to the correct sequence of production steps. The adolescent must apply consistent organizational strategies to be successful at running *The Factory*. As with the grocery store procedure, the adolescent should verbalize a number of strategies for determining the rules for constructing the model products.

3. Analysis: Record responses to the questions posed during administration. Analyze how many different strategies for finding items (e.g., in the grocery store) the adolescent could report. Determine if any strategies discussed during the grocery store example were generalized to other situations presented. Note whether the adolescent recognized that organization differs among settings (e.g., One way that schools are organized is by grade level. This is not an organizational system used in stores.). Finally, analyze whether the student has any awareness of the importance of organization.

4. Interpretation: An adolescent who has no strategies, or only one or two, for finding an item (person) in an organized setting may need focused intervention for organization (See Table 1.1 in Chapter 1.) This finding should match reports from related professionals and/or family members that the adolescent is disorganized (e.g., frequently loses assignments, forgets to bring requested items). If the adolescent's disorganization is accompanied by lack of awareness of the importance and utility of being organized, it is likely that structured intervention is needed to improve organizational skills.

Giving Directions 1. Areas assessed: The informal assessment task for giving directions provides information on comprehension and production of linguistic features. It is expected that adolescents can give directions (see Table 1.1 in Chapter 1). This task can also provide data on cognition, conversation, and survival language.

2. Administration: Having the adolescent describe how to go from one location to another is an appropriate directed verbalization task (Boyce and Larson, 1983). An agreed-upon referent point (e.g., one's house) is needed from which directives (e.g., left, right) can be given to arrive at an ending destination (e.g., one's school). Locations should be familiar to the student; for example, describing how to get from one's house to the nearest grocery store. If the examiner has prior knowledge of the directions, the task can be restructured

to have adolescents pretend to explain to strangers how they would travel between the two points.

A directed task suggested by Arwood (1983) is that of giving directions for a game or sport. For example, the adolescent might describe how a favorite video game is played, or how the sport of football is played. To complete such a task requires organizing the main ideas, sequencing the description, and communicating messages clearly enough for another person to understand them. During this assessment procedure, it is best that the adult examiner demonstrate little or no prior knowledge of the game or sport. Adolescents will feel little need to communicate the information if they perceive that the adult already knows it.

3. Analysis: The directions given by the adolescent should be analyzed for organization, clarity, and precision. Analysis should determine if a listener could follow the direction or would be left confused. Were essential elements omitted that were necessary in the direction? Directions should neither be contaminated with low information words (e.g., junk, thing, stuff), nor filled with verbal mazes that obscure the intended message.

4. Interpretation: Adolescents who consistently leave their listeners confused when giving directions may have a deficit in this area. Whether the confusion is caused by low information words, verbal mazes, or deletion of essential message elements, the adolescent is at a disadvantage when direction giving is lacking.

Referential Communication Activities 1. Areas assessed: The informal assessment task involving referential communication activities provides information on comprehension and production of linguistic features. This task, like the preceding one ("Giving Directions") can also provide data on cognition, conversation, and survival language (McKinley and Schwartz, 1985).

2. Administration: A related procedure to "Giving Directions" is to immerse the adolescent in referential communication activities, also known as barrier games. A referential communication activity involves a speaker who relays messages to a listener across a barrier, or screen, who, in turn, responds to the message. Activities may range from reproducing three-dimensional patterns to describing how to draw an identical two-dimensional design. Messages may be delivered "step-by-step" from the speaker to the listener, or with a number of steps at the same time. When the examiner is giving directions for the adolescent to follow, rate of speech should be varied to determine its effect upon comprehension. The adolescent undergoing assessment should be observed in both the role of speaker and listener during this activity. Excellent opportunities will be afforded the examiner to observe when and why communication breakdowns occur, and whether repair takes place.

3. Analysis: The adolescent's productions should be analyzed when in the

role of a speaker, as indicated in the preceding task "Giving Directions." Likewise, the adolescent's ability to comprehend messages when in the role of a listener should be analyzed by determining how lengthy, and how rapid, the speaker's message can be before the adolescent has difficulty following it. Any responses to messages that break down because of examiner error should be disqualified.

4. Interpretation: Adolescent speakers who consistently leave their listeners confused may have a deficit in this area. Adolescent listeners who do not comprehend adequate speaker messages, or who follow directions only when delivered one step at a time, or who need directions with an abnormally slow rate of speech have a deficit that warrants intervention.

Informational Listening 1. Areas assessed: The informal assessment task for informational listening provides information on comprehension and production of linguistic features. This task may also assess narration if the task is structured to do so (i.e., retelling of the information is requested).

2. Administration: To determine informational listening ability, a five to ten-minute lecture appropriate to the adolescent's current grade level should be played, preferably on videotape. A substitute activity would have the examiner list main ideas and relevant details about a given topic and present the information informally to the adolescent (i.e., do not read the information). Questions are asked, following listening, to ascertain what factual information was retained, whether the main idea was comprehended, and so forth. The syntactical level of the questions should be simple enough so as not to obstruct comprehension by the adolescent. The adolescent could be asked to reformulate the lecture in lieu of, or in addition to, extensive question asking by the examiner in order to assess narration skills.

A second taped lecture, or topic expounded upon by the examiner, should be presented that is equal in difficulty to the first activity. The second oral presentation should be accompanied by a printed outline that guides the adolescent's listening. This will allow a comparison between listening comprehension ability, with and without accompanying visual input. The majority of adolescents should listen better when following along with a printed outline. Improved performance with a printed outline will be important to document if teachers are to be convinced during indirect intervention that listening guides are important (see Chapter 8).

3. Analysis: Main ideas and relevant details of the information presented to the adolescent should be recorded. This information is compared with the adolescent's responses to questions about main ideas and relevant details. The examiner can then compute the percentage of questions answered accurately, given the total number asked for each of the two listening conditions—with and without listening guides. The two percentages should then be compared.

4. Interpretation: An adolescent who consistently answers questions incorrectly is likely to have difficulty with informational listening in a classroom setting. If the number of questions answered accurately increases when the adolescent is given a listening guide, then teachers who expect classroom listening should be informed of the testing results and should be encouraged to supply such guides to their students.

Critical Listening 1. Areas assessed: The informal assessment task for critical listening provides information on discourse. The task also provides data on cognition, since critical listening strongly parallels critical thinking.

2. Administration: Taped advertisements and political speeches may be good stimuli for assessment of critical listening abilities when selected carefully for length and content. Adolescents should listen and then answer questions posed by the examiner about the detection of false reasoning and prejudice, propaganda, or bias. Questions should also be posed that require the adolescent to draw inferences, judge statements, and apply inductive and deductive reasoning. Multiple questions for each critical listening ability should be asked. Questions should be phrased at appropriate syntactic and semantic levels so as not to interfere with the adolescent's comprehension. In addition to answering questions, adolescents can express what they heard in the advertisement or speech.

An alternative procedure would involve presenting oral information to adolescents, and having them detect whether they were hearing fact or opinion, for example, or having them infer what might happen in a given situation. This approach is different from the critical listening tasks adolescents must engage in during their daily living. However, the approach provides some information about their critical listening skills.

3. Analysis: Systematic recording of the adolescent's responses to the various questions presented is necessary. The examiner should note whether the responses appear to follow a consistent pattern, e.g., correct responses to natural situations and incorrect responses to contrived situations; or correct responses to factual questions but incorrect responses to opinion questions.

4. Interpretation: An adolescent who consistently answers questions incorrectly is likely to have difficulty with critical listening in a classroom setting and in other daily living situations. Professionals should consider providing intervention for the adolescent's deficient critical listening, either through direct intervention or indirect consultative services.

Question Asking and Answering 1. Areas assessed: The informal assessment task for question asking and answering provides information primarily on comprehension and production of linguistic features. Within a conversation, this task can also provide data on discourse. The adolescent's ability to ask and to answer questions appropriately also has strong implications for survival language skills.

2. Administration: The adolescent should be engaged in both asking and answering questions if an insufficient number of questions have been generated during other directed tasks. Specific tasks for asking questions might include the following:

a. Establish a quiz game format in which the response is supplied and the adolescent must generate the question.
b. Direct the adolescent to ask a question, given an imaginary situation (e.g., "How would you ask a stranger sitting next to you on the bus what time it is?"). Request the adolescent to generate two or more alternate ways to ask the same question.
c. Role play situations with the adolescent that require question asking behavior (e.g., You role play the math teacher and the adolescent role plays a student who has been out of school for several days and is missing assignments.).

Tasks for answering questions might include these:

a. Role play interviewing the adolescent for a job.
b. Present questions that request action (e.g., "Would you mind moving over a seat?") or state information (e.g., "Can you believe we're having another test in science?") and determine if the adolescent understands what the appropriate responses would be.
c. Ask questions with the same semantic intent, with increasing syntactical complexity, and determine if the adolescent comprehends the question (e.g., "Who is our president?" "What is the name of the person we call President?" "You know the name of our president, don't you?") These questions should be interspersed throughout the assessment, not presented consecutively.

3. Analysis: The adolescent's spoken questions should be transcribed and analyzed for their syntactic structure and semantic intent. A variety of question forms should be evident, and questions should be stated clearly enough to communicate their intended messages. The questions should also be analyzed for their adherence to pragmatic rules. Adolescents may know how to ask questions, but communication is impaired if they ask in a way that offends their listeners.

Responses to questions asked by the examiner should be recorded and analyzed by determining what question types were comprehended. Comprehension is demonstrated by answering with the appropriate category of response (e.g., answering a "Who" question with a name) although the answer may not always be accurate or "correct."

4. Interpretation: Adolescents who fail to comprehend all question types directed at them are at a severe disadvantage academically, socially, and vocationally, since this is an assumed ability by the middle grades. Interference with test taking in the classroom and with demonstration of informational

listening skills are probable accompanying deficit areas.

Adolescents who fail to produce a variety of question forms have restricted strategies for gaining new information about the world around them. Extreme concern should be expressed if adolescents fail to ask adequate questions during the assessment process, even when they are directed to do so.

Word Retrieval 1. Areas assessed: The informal assessment task for word retrieval provides information on comprehension and production of linguistic features and on discourse. While the administration suggestions provided below are contrived situations, word retrieval problems noted during this task are also likely to be observed within natural discourse samples. This task does not need to be completed if word retrieval skills are not suspect in the adolescent.

2. Administration: The examiner should determine the presence or absence of a semantic deficit by obtaining a baseline measure of receptive vocabulary. The student's ability to define words, to identify likenesses and differences, and to state synonyms and antonyms could be measured (Wiig and Becker-Caplan, 1984); or formal receptive vocabulary tests could be administered. The adolescent's receptive vocabulary performance should be compared to either chronological or mental age in order to confirm or refute the presence of a semantic deficit.

Once the presence or absence of a semantic deficit has been documented, naming accuracy and rate should be measured by a variety of tasks such as sentence completion, naming an item upon description, rapid automatic naming, and word association (Wiig and Becker-Caplan, 1984). If a semantic deficit is determined to be present, the examiner should attempt to restrict words to be retrieved to those words known to be within the adolescent's current vocabulary. If no semantic deficit was found, words commensurate with the documented receptive vocabulary level could be used.

3. Analysis: Data should be examined to determine the presence of a semantic deficit, a word retrieval problem, or a combination of the two. If it is unclear which problem is more pervasive (i.e., low vocabulary or lack of word retrieval), Wiig (1983) has suggested an analysis of the student's response to multiple choices. For example, if an adolescent is pausing to find a word, supply a choice of three or four words; the individual with low vocabulary will not necessarily be assisted by multiple choice, whereas the individual with word retrieval problems will appear to recognize instantly the desired word.

4. Interpretation: Everyone experiences word retrieval problems some of the time. However, if word retrieval problems are consistently present, not only in naming confrontation situations, but also during discourse, then a deficit area is in need of intervention. Adolescents found to have significantly low vocabulary (e.g., two standard deviations below the mean), either with or without the presence of word retrieval problems, should also be considered for intervention.

Formal Assessment Instruments

To this point, this chapter has focused on informal assessment procedures for evaluating cognition, language, and communication behaviors of adolescents. Additionally, an array of formal tests has been published which assesses a multitude of isolated variables. When selecting formal tests to use with the adolescent population, we encourage examiners to refer to the earlier section in this chapter that discusses how to critique standardized assessment instruments. Examiners may also wish to refer to other resources that provide criteria for the evaluation of tests (ASHA Ad Hoc Committee on Instrument Evaluation, 1986). Having done this, examiners can cautiously proceed with selecting one or more standardized tests that are relevant to the adolescent being assessed.

Table 4.4 presents a variety of tests that the examiner might choose when assessing an adolescent's cognition, language, and communication behaviors. Tests whose norms end at age twelve years have been intentionally deleted from the list. A number of variables have been summarized for each test, including age range, primary area(s) assessed, theoretical construct stated, content validity, interjudge reliability, normative data, stimulus presentation (modality and type of auditory input), and response mode. The information cited in the age range column matches what the author(s) of the test reported in the examiner's manual; however, at times the age range cited by the author(s) was discrepant from the age range sampled for the normative data. Likewise, information recorded in the columns labeled "theoretical constructs stated," "content validity," "interjudge reliability," and "normative data" was taken from the perspective of the author(s) of the test. We do not necessarily concur with the conclusions drawn by the writers of the tests. For example, Vallett (1981) stated that his test was based on Piagetian theory, and explained no further. Although a "yes" was recorded in the "theoretical construct stated" column, it is questionable whether this variable warranted credit.

The information in Table 4.4 recorded in the columns "primary area(s) assessed," "stimulus presentation," and "response mode" was taken from our perspective. This information was gathered by carefully reviewing the test materials.

Related Assessment Instruments in Other Disciplines In addition to utilizing formal tests designed to measure cognition, language, and communication of adolescents, speech-language pathologists should be aware of additional data that can be gleaned from tests administered by other professionals. For example, intelligence tests administered by psychologists can be a rich source of information. Tests of reading and writing abilities can provide additional insight into the adolescent's linguistic system, as can annual tests of academic achievement. It is our contention that speech-language pathologists

TABLE 4.4 FORMAL TESTS OF COGNITION, LANGUAGE, AND COMMUNICATION

TESTS	AGE RANGE	PRIMARY AREA(S) ASSESSED			THEORETICAL CONSTRUCT STATED	CONTENT VALIDITY	INTERJUDGE RELIABILITY	NORMATIVE DATA	STIMULUS PRESENTATION		RESPONSE MODE
		Thinking	Listening	Speaking					Modality	Type of Aud. Input	
Clinical Evaluation of Language Functions. Semel, E., and Wiig, E. Charles E. Merrill Publ. Co., Columbus, OH (1980).	Grades K-12		X	X	No	Yes	Yes	Yes (Grades K-12)	A & V	Words Sentences Connected Speech	Oral Pointing
Detroit Tests of Learning Aptitude. Baker, H., and Leland, B. Bobbs-Merrill Co., Inc., Indianapolis, IN (1967).	3-19 yrs.	X	X	X	No	No	Yes	Yes (3.0 to 19.0 yrs.)	A & V	Words Sentences Connected Speech	Oral Performance Pointing Writing (opt)
Detroit Tests of Learning Aptitude (DTLA-2). Hammill, D. Pro-ed, Austin, TX (1985).	6-0 to 17-11 yrs.	X	X	X	Yes	Yes	No	Yes (6-0 to 17-11 yrs.)	A & V	Words Sentences	Oral Performance Pointing Writing
Fullerton Language Test for Adolescents. (Second Ed.) Thorum, A. Consulting Psychologists Press, Inc., Palo Alto, CA (1986).	11-18 yrs.		X	X	No	Yes	Yes	Yes (11.0 to 18.5 yrs.)	A & V	Words Phrases Sentences	Oral Performance
Expressive One-Word Vocabulary Test-Upper Extension. Gardner, M. Academic Therapy Publ., Novato, CA (1983).	12-16 yrs.			X	No	Yes	Yes	Yes (12-0 to 15-11 yrs.)	V		Oral Writing (opt)

TABLE 4.4 CONTINUED

TESTS	AGE RANGE	PRIMARY AREA(S) ASSESSED			THEORETICAL CONSTRUCT STATED	CONTENT VALIDITY	INTERJUDGE RELIABILITY	NORMATIVE DATA	STIMULUS PRESENTATION		RESPONSE MODE
		Thinking	Listening	Speaking					Modality	Tupe of Aud. Input	
Interpersonal Language Skills Assessment. Blagden, C., and McConnell, N. LinguiSystems, Moline, IL (1984).	8-14 yrs.			X	No	No	No	Yes (8-0 to 13-11 yrs.)	A & V	Connected Speech (of peers)	Oral
Inventory of Essential Skills. Brigance, A. Curriculum Associates, Inc., North Billerica, MA (1981).	Secondary Level Students	X	X	X	No	Yes (rating scales only)	No	No (Criterion-referenced)	A & V	Words Sentences Connected Speech	Oral Performance Writing
Let's Talk Inventory for Adolescents. Wiig, E. Charles E. Merrill Publ. Co., Columbus, OH (1982).	9 yrs. - young adulthood			X	No	Yes	Yes	Yes (7 to 14 yrs.)	A & V	Connected Speech	Oral
Peabody Picture Vocabulary Test (Revised). Dunn, L. American Guidance Service, Circle Pines, MN (1980).	2½-40 yrs.		X		No	Yes	Yes	Yes (2½ to 40 yrs.)	A & V	Words	Pointing
Psycho-Educational Battery (Part One: Tests of Cognitive Ability). Woodcock, R., and Johnson, M. Teaching Resources, Highham, MA (1977).	Preschool-geriatric level	X	X	X	No	No	No	Yes (3.0 to 80+ yrs.)	A & V	Words Phrases Sentences	Oral Performance Pointing

TABLE 4.4 CONTINUED

TESTS	AGE RANGE	PRIMARY AREA(S) ASSESSED			THEORETICAL CONSTRUCT STATED	CONTENT VALIDITY	INTERJUDGE RELIABILITY	NORMATIVE DATA	STIMULUS PRESENTATION		RESPONSE MODE
		Thinking	Listening	Speaking					Modality	Type of Aud. Input	
Schools Council Oracy Project Listening Comprehension Tests. Wilkinson, A., Stratta, L., and Dudley, P. Macmillan Educ. Ltd., London (1974). (Distributed in the U.S. by Thinking Publications, Eau Claire, WI)	10; 13; 17 yrs.		X		Yes	Yes	Yes	Yes (10-11; 13-14; 17-18 yrs.—in England)	A	Connected Speech	Oral
Structure of Intellect (SOI) Learning Abilities Test. Meeker, M., and Meeker, R. SOI Institute, El Segundo, CA (1975).	Kinder-garten—adult	X			Yes	Yes	Yes	Yes (K-adult)	A & V	Words Phrases Sentences	Performance Writing
Test of Adolescent Language. Hammill, D., Brown, V., Larsen, S., Weiderholt, J. Pro-ed, Austin, TX (1980).	11-18½ yrs.		X	X	No	Yes	Yes	Yes (11.0 to 18.5 yrs.)	A & V	Words Sentences	Oral Pointing Writing
Test of Concept Utilization. Crager, R. Western Psychological Services, Los Angeles, CA (1972).	5-18 yrs.	X			No	Yes	Yes	Yes (4.5 to 18.5 yrs.)	A & V	Sentences	Oral

TABLE 4.4 CONTINUED

TESTS	AGE RANGE	PRIMARY AREA(S) ASSESSED			THEORETICAL CONSTRUCT STATED	CONTENT VALIDITY	INTERJUDGE RELIABILITY	NORMATIVE DATA	STIMULUS PRESENTATION		RESPONSE MODE
		Thinking	Listening	Speaking					Modality	Type of Aud. Input	
Test of Language Competence. Wiig, E., and Secord, W. Charles E. Merrill Publ. Co., Columbus, OH (1985).	9 yrs. - adult		X	X	Yes	Yes	Yes	Yes (9-0 to 18-11 yrs.)	A & V	Sentences Connected Speech	Oral
Test of Nonverbal Intelligence. Brown, L., Sherbenou, R., and Dollar, S. Pro-ed, Austin, TX (1982).	5-0 to 85-11 yrs.	X			Yes	Yes	No	Yes (5-0 to 85-11 yrs.)	V		Pointing
Test of Syntactic Abilities. Quigley, S. et al. Dormac, Inc., Beaverton, OR (1978).	10-0 to 18-11 yrs.			X (written)	Yes	Yes	Yes	Yes (10-0 to 18-11 yrs.)	V		Writing
Vallett Inventory of Critical Thinking Abilities. Vallett, R. Academic Therapy Publ., Novata, CA (1981).	4-15 yrs.	X			Yes	Yes	No	No (Criterion-referenced)	A & V	Words Phrases Sentences Connected Speech	Oral Performance

should be knowledgeable of other test content being completed with the adolescent, and that these results should be integrated, as appropriate, with data gathered on the parameters discussed in this chapter. Does testing completed by other professionals support or refute findings by the speech-language pathologist? The speech-language pathologist should request that other examiners record oral responses of adolescents verbatim, thus allowing the opportunity for later analysis by the clinician.

An intelligence test like the *Wechsler Intelligence Scale for Children (Revised)* (Wechsler, 1974) will provide both a verbal and a performance quotient. The verbal performance of an individual relies heavily on oral communication skills. So, too, does the performance quotient rely on language when the stimulus presentation utilizes an auditory modality. The most commonly used intelligence tests should be familiar to speech-language pathologists, including the *Leiter International Performance Scale (Revised)* (Leiter, 1979), the *Slosson Intelligence Test for Children and Adults* (Slosson, 1963), the *Stanford-Binet Intelligence Scale* (Terman and Merrill, 1960), the *Wechsler Intelligence Scale for Children (Revised)* (Wechsler, 1974), and the *Wechsler Adult Intelligence Scale* (Wechsler, 1955). The *Hiskey-Nebraska Test of Learning Aptitude* (Hiskey, 1966) has been widely used with adolescents with hearing impairments. Watson (1983) has stressed the importance of using more than one measure of intelligence for this population.

Academic achievement tests with which speech-language pathologists may need to be familiar include the *California Achievement Test* (Tiegs and Clark, 1963), the *Comprehensive Tests of Basic Skills* (1968), the *Iowa Test of Basic Skills* (Lindquist and Hieronymus, 1971), the *Metropolitan Achievement Tests* (Durost et al., 1970), *Peabody Individual Achievement Test* (Dunn and Markwardt, Jr., 1970), the *Science Research Associates (SRA) Achievement Series* (Thorpe, Lefever, and Naslund, 1968), the *Sequential Tests of Educational Progress* (1958), the *Stanford Achievement Tests* (Madden et al., 1973), and the *Wide Range Achievement Test* (Jastak and Jastak, 1978).

Reading and writing tests with which speech-language pathologists may want to be familiar include the *Diagnostic Reading Scales* (Spache, 1963), *Durrell Analysis of Reading Difficulty Test* (Durrell, 1955), the *Gates Reading Surveys* (Gates, 1958), the *Gray Oral Reading Test* (Gray and Robinson, 1967), the *Nelson-Denny Reading Test Vocabulary-Comprehension-Rate* (Nelson, Denny, and Brown, 1960), the *Reading Miscue Inventory* (Goodman and Burke, 1972), the *Test of Syntactic Abilities* (Quigley et al., 1978), and the *Test of Written Language* (Hammill and Larsen, 1978). Readers are encouraged to examine these assessment instruments for the cognitive, language, and communication behaviors they demand in order for the adolescent to respond accurately to test items.

SUMMARY

This chapter presented twelve general assessment principles to consider when testing adolescents: Purpose of assessment, perspective of the adolescent, adolescent's right to know, multi-dimensional assessment, formal and informal assessment, critique of standardized tests, interaction between cognition and language, importance of listening, description of behaviors, discussion of results, assessment/intervention dichotomy, and assessment of racial minorities. An extensive description of what behaviors to assess was provided by category: Cognition, comprehension and production of linguistic features, discourse (conversations and narrations), nonverbal communication, and survival language skills. Emphasis was placed on an integrative assessment process, i.e., evaluating the on-going, interactive dynamics of cognition, language, and communication behaviors. Specific informal methods for how to assess these behaviors were proposed: Case history forms, learning style questionnaire, analysis procedures for conversations and narrations, and directed tasks. Formal tests that might be selected for adolescents were summarized according to a predetermined set of variables. In addition, assessment instruments from related disciplines were listed.

DISCUSSION QUESTIONS

1. Discuss additional general assessment principles under which you would operate during the assessment process with adolescents.
2. Describe several specific informal assessment tasks that would permit the examiner to gather integrated information on cognition, comprehension and production of linguistic features, discourse, nonverbal communication, and/or survival language skills.
3. Select two intelligence tests, two achievement tests, or two reading tests appropriate to administer to adolescents. Summarize and critique the tests for cognitive, language, and communication skills needed to complete items successfully.

SUGGESTED READINGS

Feuerstein, R. *The Dynamic Assessment of Retarded Performers: The Learning Assessment Potential Device, Theory, Instruments, and Techniques.* Scott, Foresman, Inc., Chicago, IL, 1979.

Muma, J. *Language Handbook: Concepts, Assessment, Intervention.* Prentice-Hall, Englewood Cliffs, NJ, 1978.

Prutting, C. and Kirchner, D. Applied pragmatics. In: T. Gallagher and C. Prutting (eds.), *Pragmatic Assessment and Intervention Issues in Language.* College-Hill Press, San Diego, CA, 1983.

Wilkinson, A., Stratta, L., and Dudley, P. *The Quality of Listening.* Macmillan Education Ltd., London, 1974.

CHAPTER 5

Indirect Assessment of the Adolescent

GOALS:

To present what to assess in the educational system

To explain how to assess the educational system

To present what to assess in the environmental system

To explain how to assess the environmental system

A complete assessment of the adolescent includes the investigation of variables in the educational and environmental systems that may be contributing to the suspected communication disorder. Thorough assessment is important for several reasons:

1. The primary problem may not be a language disorder within the adolescent; rather the major problems may be identified within the environmental and/or educational system (e.g., a language difference in the adolescent's home; curricula inappropriate for the student's developmental level).
2. A language disorder may be present within the adolescent with concomitant problems in the educational and/or environmental systems. Difficulties caused by the adolescent's communication disorder may be escalated by these contributing variables.

3. A language disorder may be within the adolescent, but with no accompanying problems in the educational and environmental systems. Difficulties caused by the adolescent's communication disorder may be de-escalated by these supportive systems.

This chapter presents the major variables and procedures for assessing adolescents indirectly, i.e., when assessing their educational and environmental systems. Table 5.1 summarizes our model for indirect assessment of the adolescent. The content of this table will be elaborated in the remainder of this chapter. For both the educational and the environmental systems, what to be assessed will be presented first, and then, how to accomplish the assessment will be explained.

TABLE 5.1 ASSESSMENT COMPONENT: INDIRECT SERVICES

Who?	What?	How?
Educational system members	Structure of system	Structure of educational system checklist
	Teacher's language	Self-evaluation technique
	Teachers' and administrators' attitudes	Attitudinal scale
	Curriculum variables	Curriculum analysis form
Environmental system members	Family members' perceptions of the adolescent Environmental system members' feelings and attitudes Communication styles	Interviews Observation

WHAT TO ASSESS: EDUCATIONAL SYSTEM

Chapter 3 offered a broad definition of "educational system." We acknowledge that a variety of professionals could potentially interact with the adolescent, not all of them from within the discipline of education. For the purposes of this chapter, the assumption is made that teachers comprise the *majority* of professionals with whom adolescents interact in the educational system. Those teachers are located in junior and senior high schools, colleges or universities, vocational-technical schools, jails or juvenile delinquency centers, residential institutions, or homebound programs for hospitalized youth. Therefore, the assessment format presented has primary application for teachers and secondary application for related professionals, e.g., social workers, nurses.

Four major areas of assessment need to be considered: The structure of the educational system, the teacher's language, teachers' and administrators' attitudes toward adolescents with communication disorders, and curriculum variables. *What* to assess within each is described in the next four sections, followed by corresponding sections explaining *how* speech-language pathologists might assess the educational system of the adolescent by using a variety of evaluation forms from the appendices.

Structure of System

The structure of the educational system is important to assess because it indicates how flexible administrators and teachers might be when modifications to the system are proposed. This assessment is important for speech-language pathologists who are initiating a prototype delivery model, since implementation of the model requires system modifications and some flexibility of colleagues. When speech-language pathologists are unfamiliar with the structure of the setting in which they are employed, they may be operating at a disadvantage. It is difficult to advocate for changes if the current structure is an unknown. What to assess concerning the structure of the educational system is summarized below in six key variables. Later, in the "How to Assess: Educational System" section, a suggested assessment procedure will be described.

Response to Educational Reports The first variable to assess is the response of members of the educational system to the reports that are calling for reform of American schools. Publicized reports such as "A Nation At Risk: The Imperative for Educational Reform" (National Commission on Excellence in Education, 1983), "A Study of Schooling" (Goodlad, Sirotnik, and Overman,

1979), and "High School: A Report on Secondary Education in America" (Carnegie Foundation for the Advancement of Teaching, 1983) have heightened concern about the state of American education. These reports share common themes: Education is in trouble; reform is necessary.

From these reports, numerous responses have occurred at the local level. Many local educational agencies have formed their own task forces, introduced curricula changes, and changed their standards in an attempt to educate their youth better. We have found that speech-language programs for adolescents generally fare better when they are located within those educational settings that are committed to excellence in programming for all students. Speech-language pathologists in such settings can appeal to this search for excellence, and to the need for educational reform, when defending their right to be involved with adolescents with communication disorders.

Drop-out Rate A second key variable to assess is the existing drop-out rate of adolescents from the educational system. Historically, the number of high school graduates increased from ten out of every hundred students in the 1900s to a peak of seventy-eight out of a hundred students in the 1970s (Hunt and Clawson, 1975). From 1970 to 1980, the percentage of high school graduates actually declined nationwide (Lambert, Novak, and Dougherty, 1981). Since 1980, the percentage of students graduating from high school has declined from seventy-six percent to seventy-three percent (Hodgkinson, 1985). When this number is analyzed by ethnic groups, forty percent of Hispanic students, twenty-four percent of Black students, and fourteen percent of white students do not finish high school.

From our personal experiences, it is common for speech-language caseloads to include a number of potential school drop-outs. This phenomenon is so common that selective screening should be considered for any student contemplating leaving school. Some youths are leaving with severe deficits in the areas of listening and speaking (R. Comer, Personal Communication, 1981). Others are being "pushed-out" when they fail to meet state-based "reform" legislation graduation requirements (Hodgkinson, 1985). This situation is distressing, because as Hodgkinson (1985) pointed out, "Eliminating low performers from the public schools [is] a way of displacing the problem, not solving it. Out of school, these students present more of a social and economic problem than they do IN school." (p. 12). Yet few states that have passed "reform" legislation have specific plans to provide remediation to those who do not meet the higher standards. These states apparently are willing to have a higher drop-out rate from secondary schools, even though the economic costs of this position will be very high (Hodgkinson, 1985).

There is anecdotal evidence that speech-language intervention with adolescents who are at risk for leaving school may reduce the number of actual school drop-outs (ASHA, 1986). If this evidence can be substantiated through controlled research studies, the discipline of communication sciences and disorders will have a powerful argument for increasing the availability of services for adolescents. We have found that schools that are making a concerted effort to prevent drop-outs and "push-outs" are often more supportive of speech-language services for adolescents.

Minimum Competency Testing A third variable is whether adolescents must pass minimum competency tests to graduate. The establishment of minimum competencies in basic skill areas, and subsequent testing of those identified competencies, is intended to guarantee that all students function at or above a level designated to be sufficient by the educational system. It is assumed that high school students who pass minimum competency tests possess enough basic skills to function as workers and citizens within a community. Basic skills, as identified by the federal government, include reading, writing, mathematics, reasoning, and oral communication (i.e., listening and speaking). Often, minimum competency testing is administered only for reading, writing, and mathematics while oral communication and reasoning are ignored (Backlund et al., 1982a; Backlund et al., 1982b).

If competency tests for listening and speaking have been designed, the content of the test(s) should be checked against the guidelines suggested by the Speech Communication Association of America (1979). To be recommended as a minimal requirement for high school graduation, the speaking or listening skill should meet these criteria: (1) It is functional, i.e., needed by adults to achieve typical purposes in life including occupational, citizenship, and maintenance; (2) it is educational, i.e., appropriate for development by instruction in the schools; and (3) it is general, i.e., needed by graduates from all regions of the United States. Table 5.2 lists suggested speaking and listening skills that could be included in a competency test, according to the Speech Communication Association of America.

Forty-three states have strengthened high school graduation requirements (Hodgkinson, 1985). Most of these states include minimum competency examinations within their requirements. A few states (e.g., Utah, Vermont) test all the basic skills, but the majority test only the traditional three (i.e., reading, writing, mathematics). Many states with minimum competencies administer the test initially when students are freshmen or sophomores in high school. The minimum competencies frequently are designed to reflect approximately a ninth or tenth grade achievement level. Typically, students who fail the test are retested at regular intervals until they pass. These are the students who need provisions for special tutorial help or alternative courses, possibly including those offered by speech-language pathologists when oral communication is interfering with their academic performance. Adolescents whose oral communication is vastly different from the expected minimum competency level may have a higher incidence of language disorders than their peers. This hypothesis needs to be tested by studying those students who fail minimum competency testing in states that assess oral communication.

What is the educational system's response to adolescents who have repeated failures on tests? Graduation from high school may be prevented, de-

TABLE 5.2 MINIMUM COMPETENCIES: SPEAKING AND LISTENING

Communication Codes

A. Listen effectively to spoken English
   1. Use words, pronunciation, and grammar appropriate for the situation
   2. Use nonverbal signs appropriate for the situation
   3. Use voice effectively

Oral Message Evaluation

A. Identify main ideas in messages
B. Distinguish facts from opinions
C. Distinguish between informative and persuasive messages
D. Recognize when another does not understand your message

Basic Speech Communication Skills

A. Express ideas clearly and concisely
B. Express and defend with evidence your point of view
C. Organize (order) messages so that others can understand them
D. Ask questions to obtain information
E. Answer questions effectively
F. Give concise and accurate directions
G. Summarize messages

Human Relations

A. Describe another's viewpoint
B. Describe differences
C. Express feelings to others
D. Perform social rituals

(Reprinted with permission of the Speech Communication Association of America)

pending upon state and local policies, and probably the students will become drop-out statistics (R. Comer, Personal Communication, 1981). These students may have dropped out even without minimum competency test pressure. The reason(s) for dropping out will remain uncertain until the effect of minimum competency testing on borderline academic students and those with disabilities has been fully researched.

Organizational Framework A fourth variable to assess is how the educational system is organized. Sizer (1983) observed that the same organizational framework exists today as in the late 1800s for most U.S. secondary schools. This lack of change persists despite significant evolution in our country from an agricultural society, to an industrial society, and now to an information society.

Goodlad (1983) stated: "a school is a school is a school," meaning teachers teach as they were taught (i.e., lecturing, monitoring, and quizzing), using the same topical arrangement. High schools continue to be horizontally structured by age group (i.e., freshmen, sophomores, juniors, seniors) and vertically organized by program track (e.g., college-bound, vocational education, special education), despite educational literature that has decreed this system as creating inequality among people (Jencks et al., 1972; Rosenbaum, 1976). When identifying which students warrant referral for special education, less than two percent of teachers attribute student problems to inadequate instruction or to "school system" problems (Ysseldyke, 1983). Teachers overwhelmingly view problems as being within students, and fail to see that problems are occasionally within the educational system, despite the current outcry for the need to reform education.

It is important for speech-language pathologists to assess the organizational framework of their secondary schools for several reasons:

1. Horizontal structuring by age group may influence how students are grouped. If horizontal structure is rigid, it may be impossible to group adolescents in one grade with those in another because of conflicting time schedules. This rigidity may prevent efficient organization of peer groups with similar needs. Horizontal structuring can also result in adolescents identifying with only one grade level and preferring not to interact with older or younger peers.
2. Vertical structuring may result in the speech-language pathologist being perceived by other teachers as associated only with those students in the special education track. This perception could result in few or no referrals from the vocational education or college-bound tracks. Also, students functioning primarily within the mainstream often wish to avoid receiving intervention from a professional working mainly in the special education track.

Interdisciplinary Team Process A fifth key variable to assess within the structure of the educational system is the interdisciplinary team process. Especially, speech-language pathologists initiating a service delivery model should determine which adolescents have, in the past, been referred for testing and which professionals have served on the interdisciplinary evaluation teams. This will reveal the past utilization of speech-language pathologists and the placement statistics that have followed referral and testing. Algozzine,

Christenson, and Ysseldyke (1981) have found that seventy-eight percent of those students referred for testing are recommended for special education placement. These data document the effectiveness of a teacher referral system for identification of students. This is the referral method recommended in Chapter 3. Data should be analyzed to determine if any teacher(s) appears to be over-referring, or referring for inappropriate reasons. For example, Ysseldyke (1983) found that teachers often refer students who disturb or bother them.

The case manager(s) who makes decisions about the assignment of team members as specified by P.L. 94–142 should be identified. Does this person know about the discipline of communication sciences and disorders, and know when speech-language pathologists should be assigned to test the adolescent who is referred? If so, has past information been correct? In one prototype secondary-level program, the speech-language pathologist is now serving on approximately seventy percent of the interdisciplinary teams assigned to new referrals (D. Boley, Personal Communication, 1986). This was a direct result of informing the case manager in her school, in this instance a school psychologist, about the profession and the contribution speech-language pathologists can make to those with communication disorders.

Entrance/Exit Criteria The last key variable that speech-language pathologists should assess is whether state or local criteria exist for entrance to or exit from their programs. If criteria exist, are they appropriate for older students? Many criteria appear to have been written for younger children. To say that a two-year delay in language production constitutes a significant problem, for example, may not be valid if the person being assessed is seventeen years old.

Criteria should not be so rigid as to disqualify a student for a program if test scores are discrepant or if test results are marginal to a predetermined cut-off score. Both informal assessment results and formal test scores should be incorporated into the criteria as valid measurements of student performance.

If criteria are in place for adolescents, do you agree with their underlying philosophical premises? For example, a common criterion compares mental age and language age; if the discrepancy between the ages is not significant, then no communication disorder is judged to exist. Another typical criterion compares verbal and performance scores on intelligence tests; if no gap exists, communication is not labeled "disordered." These criteria share the underlying premises that mental ages and intelligence quotients are immutable and that intelligence tests are valid measurements of the language that individuals are capable of learning. We do not concur with these premises and would find operating under such criteria inappropriate.

When criteria are not established for caseload entrance and exit, the speech-language pathologist might assess whether there is administrative concern that they be developed, and if so, by whom and by what date. Speech-language pathologists should be an integral part of the committee establishing criteria.

Teacher's Language

Assessment of teacher language in the classroom is essential to determine if modifications are necessary to meet the needs of students. The language of the classroom teacher directly and indirectly influences students' responses (Gruenewald and Pollak, 1984). Teacher language is comprised of an instructional mode (explanations/directions and questions), a syntactical mode (word order and sentence complexity), and a speaking mode (length, rate, and intonation) (Gruenewald and Pollak, 1984).

Some adolescents may find rapid speech, lengthy directions, or complex questions too difficult to process. Therefore, failure in that teacher's classroom continues until modifications are made. Taking into account the three modes of teacher language described by Gruenewald and Pollak (1984), the following aspects of teacher language should be assessed:

1. Rate of speech
2. Tone of voice
3. Length of directions
4. Complexity of directions
5. Level of vocabulary
6. Organization of ideas
7. Ease of listening (to teacher language by others).

Assessment of these parameters should document where communication breakdowns occur—in the teacher's messages and/or in the adolescent's comprehension of those messages. One speech-language pathologist told us how she has helped several teachers analyze their language. She reported how amazed they were to discover the high level of vocabulary and the complexity of directions they were employing. One of the sixth grade teachers whose language this speech-language pathologist helped to analyze requested on-going analysis of her lessons with her "low track" group. A procedure for analysis of teacher language is provided in the "How to Assess: Educational System" section of this chapter.

Teachers' and Administrators' Attitudes

Assessment of teachers' and administrators' attitudes toward speech-language services, and especially toward adolescents with communication disorders, is important. Specifically, attitudes toward the following topics might be assessed:

1. Speech-language delivery model for secondary students
2. Communication disorders within adolescents
3. Teacher and curriculum modifications for students with disabilities.

When the attitudes of a teacher or an administrator are consistently and resoundingly negative, speech-language pathologists could select from any or all of these alternatives:

1. Attempt to change educators' attitudes through information dissemination activities
2. Advocate to place adolescents with teachers who have expressed positive attitudes
3. Counsel adolescents to cope with educators holding negative attitudes.

Assessment data on attitudes are useful when determining the course of intervention. If the identified problem is within the adolescent, then speech-language pathologists should advocate to schedule the student with teachers who have the best attitudes toward disabilities and toward appropriate modifications that might need to be made in their classrooms. If the identified problem is not within the adolescent, but lies within the educational system, attitudinal data may help to document why the problem has its roots in the system.

Curriculum Variables

Adolescents referred by classroom teachers for evaluation are often struggling with the content of particular courses. To determine whether the struggle is stemming from a communication disorder within the student or from problems inherent in a particular curriculum, several variables should be considered:

1. Comprehension of spoken information—Is the adolescent having difficulty understanding what is said in many different situations or primarily in one course? What is the nature of the comprehension problem?
2. Organization of the course—Is the course organized sequentially (little interaction among units, e.g., one topic is "geology" and the next is "electricity") or in a spiral fashion (major interaction among units, e.g., parts of speech are taught to provide the background for sentence dia-

gramming)? If the course is organized sequentially, have all units been problematic for the adolescent, or only some?

3. Requirements in the course—Does the course demand significantly different requirements than other courses in which the student is not struggling (e.g., excessive reading, lengthy term papers, public speaking)?
4. Textbook and tests in the course—Is the readability of the textbook appropriate for the adolescent? Is it organized like other texts that the adolescent is using? Does the student understand how to use the organizational aids? Are the course tests significantly different from those in other courses that the student is taking (e.g., essay questions; objective questions that demand synthesis of information)?

Examiners should keep in mind that it is plausible for several problems to be identified. The student might be having difficulty in a course because of an underlying language disorder, but at the same time there may be problems in the curriculum (e.g., the readability of the text is not at grade level; the course has spiral organization and the student has been "lost" for months, even years). Negative attitude and poor motivation should also be ruled out as major contributing factors to the adolescent's failure in the course.

HOW TO ASSESS: EDUCATIONAL SYSTEM

Structure of Educational System Checklist

The checklist in Appendix F can be used when assessing the six key variables within the educational system that are of concern at the secondary level:

1. Response to educational reports
2. Drop-out rate
3. Minimum competency testing
4. Organizational framework
5. Interdisciplinary team process
6. Entrance/exit criteria.

When initiating programs with adolescents, speech-language pathologists should attempt to use the checklist in Appendix F to assess as quickly as possible the structure of the system in which they are located. The checklist will help to pinpoint the amount of openness to change. Some systems will be ready for change while others will be resistant.

The checklist in Appendix F will also allow better insight into the history of speech-language programs within the educational system in question; history influences planning for future changes. For example, a speech-language pathologist reported that she secured a high school position and wished to implement our prototype service delivery model. Unfortunately, the speech-language program in her setting was preceded by a dozen years of traditional programming by inadequately prepared professionals. She has found the past difficult to combat, but this knowledge has helped her to plan for future change. She realizes that information dissemination efforts will need to be intensified for an extended period of time until her colleagues are reeducated about the role of a speech-language pathologist at the secondary level. She also recognizes that she needs to train her colleagues to identify language disorders within adolescents.

Those speech-language pathologists who have initiated programs in the past, and who are now in the maintenance phase, may use the checklist as a summary of the current status of the educational system. Responses to the checklist questions should be analyzed to determine what variables within the educational system might be changed (e.g., modification of criteria for entrance and exit; increment in the number of interdisciplinary teams to which speech-language pathologists are assigned). When armed with this information, speech-language pathologists are better able to engage in program planning (see Chapter 6) and to initiate modifications in the educational system that are beneficial to adolescents.

Teacher's Language: Self-Evaluation Technique

While teacher language might be analyzed best by speech-language pathologists, we have found that teachers who welcome speech-language pathologists into their classrooms for the purpose of evaluating their language during instruction are rare. More common reactions have been feelings of anxiety, fear, and invasion of privacy or academic freedom. And yet, most teachers are interested in improving their classroom instruction and many are receptive to self-evaluating their language if data remain confidential.

A self-evaluation technique has been designed to be used by a teacher within a classroom situation. (See Appendix G.) Speech-language pathologists should train teachers in this technique. Each student is given the evaluation form in Appendix G immediately following a ten to fifteen-minute lecture or some detailed classroom instructions. Teachers may also wish to complete the form from their perspective. Students should be assured that there are no "wrong" answers and that their answers will not influence their grade(s) for the course. The request for the student's name on the form is to encourage taking the test seriously and to discourage "silly" responses. The requirement of names is, however, at the discretion of the teacher. If there are a number of poor readers in the classroom, the teacher should read aloud the response form for all students before, or during, their completion of the form. Explanations of the characteristics of the teacher's language to be rated should be provided, whether or not students ask for them. Honesty of answers should be stressed.

Teachers should collect the forms and compute means for each item on the response form. Forms containing responses that are on the extreme low end of the rating scale should be analyzed carefully. For example, is only one student evaluating level of vocabulary as too difficult or are a number of students reacting negatively to the difficulty level? Teachers who notice a number of students assessing various aspects of their language of instruction negatively might wish to consider modifications in their language.

It is particularly helpful for teachers to use the self-evaluation technique when a student in their classrooms has been referred for testing for a suspected communication disorder. This self-evaluation will allow a comparison of that student's perception of the teacher's language with the perceptions of peers in the classroom. Is the referred student unique in responses on the form? Were the responses primarily negative? If they were, the teacher's language within that particular course may be problematic for the adolescent.

Attitudinal Scale

Measurement of teachers' and administrators' attitudes toward adolescents with communication disorders may be accomplished through an attitudinal scale. Several attitudinal scales toward disabilities have been developed previously, particularly at the university faculty level (Fonosch and Schwab, 1981; Morris, Leuenberger, and Aksamit, 1985). We have gleaned concepts from these attitudinal scales and from "Attitudes Toward Disabled Persons Measurements" (Yuker, Block, and Younng, 1970) to develop an assessment tool for teachers and administrators. (See Appendix H.) The tool, called the ACDA Scale (Adolescents with Communication Disorders—Attitudinal Scale), measures attitudes toward these variables: Speech-language services, adolescents with communication disorders, and modification of curriculum for students with disabilities. The attitudinal scale should be completed voluntarily and anonymously.

Data obtained from the attitudinal scale identify teachers who are most receptive to working with students with disabilities. These teachers are determined by observing who chooses to complete the sign-up section called "Mainstreaming List" at the end of the ACDA Scale. (See Appendix H.) The other major use of the data is to document on a regular basis (e.g., annually) the predominant attitude toward speech-language services, adolescents with communication disorders, and curriculum modifications. If the general attitude of educational personnel is negative, it may be indicative that the "problem" within the student who is undergoing assessment has all or some of its roots in the educational system itself.

Curriculum Analysis Form

We previously published the CALI: Curriculum Analysis of the Language of Instruction (Boyce and Larson, 1983) as a procedure for assessment. A revised version of CALI is presented in Appendix I and its name has been abbreviated to "Curriculum Analysis." The intent of the Curriculum Analysis form is not that it be completed for every student undergoing assessment for every content area. Rather, the form should be completed whenever one or two subject or content areas are particularly troublesome to the student undergoing an initial assessment. Completion of the Curriculum Analysis form would help to locate the problem (i.e., within the adolescent and/or educational system). This is necessary for appropriate program planning.

The Curriculum Analysis form may be especially helpful once adolescents with language disorders begin intervention. The form then serves as an organized, coherent approach to studying the adolescent's abilities within existing curricula. The form may also serve as a referent for needed modifications in the classroom if a consultation model is used.

An alternative procedure for curriculum assessment is proposed by Gall (1981). In her *Handbook for Evaluating and Selecting Curricula Materials*, she suggested establishing an inventory of evaluative criteria (e.g., cognitive level) stated as bipolar adjectives (e.g., concrete-abstract), with an accompanying rating scale (e.g., a "1" means a very concrete curriculum; a "10" means a very abstract curriculum; numbers between 1 and 10 mean a combination of concrete and abstract features). This method for evaluating curriculum materials could be adapted by the speech-language pathologist when assessing the cognitive and language levels of curriculum materials. Other evaluative criteria and bipolar adjectives (noted in parentheses) to be rated might include these: Vocabulary (basic—advanced), sentence structure (simple—complex), and main ideas (obvious—obscure). Examiners desiring to use Gall's complete (1981) procedure should consult her handbook.

Another option is to use the detailed procedures offered by Gruenewald and Pollak (1984) for analyzing the language required for classroom learning. Their basic premise is that there is continuous language interaction among the triad of teacher, student, and language content/concepts in the teaching and learning process. All components of this triad must be considered when analyzing their interaction. Gruenewald and Pollak's (1984) strategies for analysis include: (1) identification of the interacting language components and their effect in instruction, (2) description of developmental information related to the language components, (3) hypotheses formulation which attempts to stimulate thinking about possible solutions to why a student might have had problems during instruction, and (4) identification of possible intervention strategies.

WHAT TO ASSESS: ENVIRONMENTAL SYSTEM

Assessment of the environmental system includes an examination of relevant variables within peers and family members that affect the adolescent with a suspected communication disorder. Before presenting what to assess, it is important to consider some basic definitions.

Peers are defined as people who are equal in age, rank, or ability. During adolescence, acceptance by peers and membership in a group become important for the development of a positive self-concept. Adolescents with communication disorders may lack the necessary socialization skills for group membership (Donahue and Bryan, 1984). Thus, it becomes important to assess interactions and reactions of the adolescent with a communication disorder to peer group members, and vice versa.

Family can be defined ". . . as a small, interdependent social system within which may be found smaller subsystems, depending upon the family size and defined roles" (Buscaglia, 1975). Traditionally, the parents, father and mother, form the central unit as head of the household. However, intrafamily relationships are also present (e.g., father-daughter, mother-son, brother-sister) (Buscaglia, 1975). Most family units have defined family roles. Their agreed-upon norms and values change whenever there is an alteration in the composition of the family unit, such as an addition (birth of a child) or a removal of a family member (divorce of the parents or an older child leaves the family). The family, although a social unit unto itself, does not exist in a social vacuum, but is part of other social units such as the community.

Examiners who are assessing the environmental system should realize that the American "family" has changed dramatically over the past decades. Before the nineteenth century, most activities revolved around the family, and parents were responsible for educating their own children. The economy was agrarian, and all family members (which usually included extended family members) worked to sustain the unit. The Industrial Revolution brought profound changes, such as families moving from farms to cities, and women entering the work force (Simpson, 1982). As a result of these two changes, urban families, unlike rural families, decreased their contacts with extended family members; and attitudes, values, and beliefs about the family unit changed. Also, with women in the workforce, less of their time was spent with family members. As a result, children began to spend more time without parental supervision; thus, the peer group and the educational system began to assume a stronger role in attitude and value formation.

Since World War II, monumental changes in the American family have occurred. For example, family units today rarely include grandparents and extended family members such as aunts and uncles; frequent moves from one geographical location to another are common; single parent and reconstituted families are increasing in frequency; families where both parents are working outside the home have become the norm, and some parents expect the schools to fulfill roles traditionally assumed by the family (Simpson, 1982). The "average traditional" American family, more than ever, does not exist (Simpson, 1982).

It is important for examiners to know about the adolescent's environmental system because it provides the foundation for language and communication. Major purposes for assessing variables within the environmental system include these:

1. To understand the family's perspective of the adolescent's communication disorder, or suspected disorder, including past history and future goals
2. To gather information on feelings and attitudes of family members toward adolescents with communication disorders and toward the educational system; this may indicate how supportive and tolerant the environment is of disabilities and how amiable the relationship has been between the environmental and educational systems.
3. To obtain information about the family's and peers' communication styles; this permits speech-language pathologists to determine if a language difference exists.

Following is a summary of variables to assess to determine whether a problem exists within the environmental system. In the last section of this chapter, how to assess these variables will be explained.

Family Members' Perceptions of the Adolescent

During direct assessment of the adolescent, examiners are encouraged to gather data on the student's perceptions of the problem, the previous speech-language services, and the need to improve speaking, listening, and thinking. These data may also be gathered from the family and compared with the adolescent's responses for agreement. The family's answers may provide insight into the adolescent's diagnosis and prognosis. Consider information gathered on past speech-language services, for example. Five years of articulation intervention on the /s/ will not remediate a continuing syntactic, semantic, or pragmatic problem. However, ten years of intensive speech and language intervention, working on all aspects of phonology, syntax, semantics, and pragmatics, but resulting in minimal intelligible oral communication, reveals something quite different. While this information would not necessarily deny the reinstatement of speech-language services, any prognosis should be guarded.

Data should also be gathered from families to address these issues:

1. Do the family members feel that a problem exists, or do they feel that the school or someone else is fabricating the problem?
2. If a communication disorder exists, is it a primary concern or a secondary concern?
3. If they feel that a problem exists, are they frustrated, embarrassed, guilty, and ashamed; or are they accepting of the adolescent's communication?
4. How does or doesn't the family attempt to cope with the adolescent with a communication disorder? (e.g., Is it done by talking for the adolescent; by excluding the adolescent from the mainstream of family life and decision making; or by ignoring the disorder?)
5. What are the goals and expectations of the family for the adolescent with a communication disorder, or a suspected disorder? Are they realistic?

Environmental System Members' Feelings and Attitudes

The examiner should investigate the family's attitudes toward adolescents with communication disorders, and toward educational services and professionals providing services. By evaluating the parents' attitudes toward issues such as the value of good communication, the examiner can determine if there is a mismatch between familial or cultural expectations and professional or educational system expectations.

Attitudes and feelings of families may change over time. Family members of adolescents being assessed may have experienced many years of professionals trying to help, and still the adolescent may have problems. As adolescents grow older, parental involvement usually lessens, but not parental concern. For example, parental pressures may not result in the adolescent's willingness to be evaluated, even though the parents are concerned about their child's progress. Parents may become frustrated, anxious, guilty, exhausted, and more negative toward the adolescent and/or the educational system.

Parents/caregivers may need to sort through their feelings toward the educational system or professionals with whom they have interacted. Particularly, if the interaction has not been pleasant, family members should be given the opportunity to express their feelings and attitudes during the assessment process, without value judgments from involved professionals. Families may be resentful of the educational system if they have experienced frustration in getting necessary services, or if professionals have not followed through with their commitments. These feelings should be freely expressed, and in addition, families should be assured that the educational system's goal is to provide the most appropriate services for their child.

Peers' feelings and attitudes toward the adolescent's communication should also be evaluated. If they feel a problem exists, are they teasing, rejecting, or accepting the person as a friend or a member of the group? Do they avoid talking or listening to the adolescent with a communication disorder? What is most disturbing to them about their peer's communication? Answers to these questions will help to document the amount of social isolation the adolescent being assessed may or may not be experiencing.

Communication Styles

To determine whether the adolescent has a communication disorder or difference, the speech-language pathologist must be aware of the family members' communication behaviors. If the adolescent's communication style is similar to other family members', probably a communication difference is present and not a disorder. This decision is complicated when English is not the primary language spoken in the adolescent's home. The adolescent's communication style must be assessed from the perspective of the first language in the family, even if that language is not English. Through the use of an interpreter, the examiner should determine whether the adolescent understands and produces the primary language similarly to other family members who are approximately the same age or older.

Since there is a paucity of data on normal adolescent communication development, an assessment of the peers' language system is also important for determining normal communication behaviors for this age group. By analyzing the peers' communication styles, the examiner can determine how the peers may be requiring the adolescent being assessed to comprehend or produce social-interactive language (e.g., idiomatic expressions, slang).

HOW TO ASSESS: ENVIRONMENTAL SYSTEM

Interviews

According to Emerick (1969), an interview ". . . is a purposeful exchange of meanings between two persons, a directed conversation that proceeds in an orderly fashion to obtain data, to convey certain information, and to provide release and support" (p. 3). Ivey (1971) distinguished interviewing from counseling and therapy. Interviewing is ". . . a process of information seeking," counseling is ". . . seeking to understand another person more fully," and therapy is ". . . helping another person change pathological behavior" (p. 5). The kind of interview needed for gathering the information suggested in the "What to Assess" section (i.e., family members' perceptions of the adolescent, environmental system members' feelings and attitudes, and communication styles) is a combination of the behaviors that Ivey (1971) labels interviewing and counseling.

Eriksen (1979) observed that people conducting helpful interviews consider six interactive dimensions: People, place, problem, purpose, process, and outcome. These six dimensions can be used as a guide when determining how to interview members within the environmental system for their perceptions, feelings, and attitudes.

People In an interview, at least two people are engaged in a helping relationship, e.g., the examiner and a family member or a peer of the adolescent. The person being interviewed should feel confident that the examiner is competent and empathic. Mutual respect is necessary for the interview to be productive.

Sue (1981) has discussed in depth what may happen when the people involved in the interview have different cultural backgrounds and values. Most white middle-class Americans fall into a world view that he labels "internal locus of control—internal locus of responsibility," i.e., a high value is placed on using personal resources for solving problems and on control over other people, things, and forces of nature. An examiner perseverating on this world view will generally have a difficult time being perceived as competent and empathic when interacting with persons from minority and Third World cultures who have other world views. Examiners who desire to understand and to interact with other cultures, need flexibility with other world views. How to develop this flexibility is discussed in Sue (1981), and readers are urged to consult this source.

When the primary language spoken in the home is not English, the examiner should either converse in the other language or use the assistance of an interpreter. Speech-language pathologists should keep lists of capable interpreters. When selecting an interpreter to assist with an interview, care should be exercised not to insult the family members or peers by selecting an individual who represents strong political or religious conflicts, e.g., a family from South Vietnam should probably not be interviewed by an interpreter from North Vietnam; an Arab family who is Moslem should probably not be interviewed by a Jewish interpreter. People involved in the interview go through a period of testing each other's values to decide if the relationship suits them (Eriksen, 1979). When values of the participants conflict sharply, the interview may fail.

Place Location and accessibility to the interview site are important. If family members or peers are expected to travel some distance at their own expense, they may choose not to do so. This should not be interpreted as a lack of concern, but perhaps as a lack of available resources. Examiners should ensure that the necessary resources to travel to the place of the interview are provided; or should allow the family members or peers to be stationary and travel to them or should interview them by telephone.

When the examiner provides the site of the interview, physical setting needs to be considered. Expensive furnishings do not usually encourage rapport with persons from economically depressed areas. Probably, moderate, comfortable furnishings are best in a room free from clutter, ornamentation, or music. Interviews are best conducted when persons are seated relatively close to each other, at comfortable angles, and without a large desk between them. Proxemics may need to be altered for different cultures if interviews are to be successful (Sue, 1981).

Timing during the interview is significant. The examiner needs to be flexible in gauging how long an interview should last. Flexibility may also be needed for the starting time; people in lower socio-economic classes may operate under "minority standard time" (Schindler-Rainman, 1967). So often have these people waited hours for a ten-minute appointment that arriving on time is perceived as doing little good. Examiners often fail to understand this aspect of the interviewees' lives and misinterpret their lateness as a sign of indifference or hostility (Sue, 1981).

Problem The people involved in the interview have met to deal with a specific problem, i.e., the adolescent with a communication disorder, or a suspected disorder. If the interview is the first contact between the examiner and the family member or peer, then it is beneficial to explain how the testing is done, what tests have been or will be given, and how results will be interpreted. This information should be presented clearly and concisely, without professional jargon (Emerick, 1969). Examiners should explain how the family member or peer contributes to the evaluation of the adolescent and why their perspective of the problem is important. We have also found it helpful to give family members and peers some background information on who speech-language pathologists are, and how professionals might help the adolescent in question, before requesting information from them.

Family members and peers should be asked what they think and how they feel about the adolescent's communication (Eriksen, 1979). The case history form (see Appendix B) used with adolescents has many appropriate questions. The form may be used during the interview with the family and peers; however, questions on the form should be modified to eliminate the pronoun "you" (e.g., ask "How well is [*name of adolescent*] understood by others?" rather than "Are you understood when you speak?"). Questions should be presented orally, with the examiner recording responses. The examiner should also develop a specific list of questions that address the issues mentioned under "What to Assess: Environmental System," particularly those suggested within the first two subsections, i.e., Family Members' Perceptions of the Adolescent; Environmental System Members' Feelings and Attitudes.

Asking less personal questions first (e.g., "What has been done for the adolescent's communication problem in the past?", "Describe a typical day for [*name*]."), and more intimate questions about feelings and attitudes last, may be a technique that is successful most of the time. This approach allows time to develop trust and mutual respect. Many people who are culturally different stress friendship as a precondition to self-disclosure (Sue, 1981). These people may be too uncomfortable to discuss frustrations and fears during the initial interview; thus, more than one contact may be needed with the examiner before feelings are expressed.

Purpose The common goal of the interview is to bring about positive change. Family members and peers should be encouraged to state whether they believe the adolescent undergoing evaluation needs to change to improve communication and if so, how. If a number of problems within the adolescent have been identified, family members and peers should be encouraged to express what they think and feel is most or least important to change.

If the need for change is expressed during the interview, examiners should determine how receptive the family members and peers are: (1) toward assisting the adolescent to change to meet the demands of the environment, or (2) toward modifying the environment to meet the needs of the adolescent. Is there a sibling, for example, who is willing to focus on study skills with the adolescent at home? Are peers willing to speak more slowly when communicating with the adolescent?

If the need for change in the adolescent's communication is not expressed during the interview, examiners should make special note. In some cases, this may be additional evidence that a communication disorder is not present within the adolescent. In other cases, the communication disorder is present, but members of the environmental system do not perceive it, or fail to consider it important. Unless members of the system can be convinced otherwise, little support may be provided for the adolescent, and the offer of speech-language services may be refused.

Process The interview process has three discrete phases: Beginning, middle, and end (Eriksen, 1979). The beginning phase explores the problem's size and shape. The person being interviewed is probably testing the examiner for trustworthiness and for values. For many minority groups, these judgments by the interviewee(s) are based more strongly on the examiner's nonverbal communication than on oral language (Sue, 1981). For example, Anglos prefer more distance during face-to-face interactions than do Latin Americans, Africans, Black Americans, and Indonesians. White middle-class examiners who maintain the preferred distance of the Anglo culture may be interpreted as aloof and noncommunicative by members of the cultural groups listed above. Readers should consult Sue (1981) for additional modifications that might need to be made in their nonverbal communication during interviews.

The middle of the interview analyzes the problem in depth (i.e., the communication disorder of the adolescent referred for an evaluation). This analysis determines the relationship between the environmental system and the adolescent's communication. Any necessary note-taking should be done in an undistracting manner. An open invitation to talk should evolve from asking open-ended questions (e.g., "Could you tell me more about your child's past speech-language program?" rather than "Did your child's past speech-language program help?") and from encouraging exploration of thoughts and feelings.

The final phase of the interview process summarizes the information shared with and gathered from family members and peers. Before the interview is terminated, there should be an understanding of "what happens next" in the evaluation of the adolescent. In particular, members of the environmental system should be aware of the staffing about the adolescent that occurs at the end of the evaluation process, and of how they may become involved in the program planning and intervention components.

Outcome Once the interview is completed, the speech-language pathologist should analyze the information obtained. This analysis might summarize major themes in the family's and peers' perceptions of the problem, and attitudes toward the adolescent. Examiners should document inconsistencies in data and note possible omissions of information. From this analysis, examiners must interpret the relationship between variables in the environmental system and the adolescent's communication.

Eriksen (1979) emphasizes the importance of reflecting on an interview for another reason: Analyzing strengths and weaknesses of the interview may help the examiner to conduct better interviews in the future. The difficulty of interviewing people who are culturally different from the examiner makes evaluation of the outcome particularly necessary.

Observation

Observation is the other major assessment procedure to use for gathering information about the adolescent's environmental system. Examiners are most efficient when they use both procedures simultaneously, i.e., close observation is made during the interview(s). Observation should document communication styles of family members and peers. Typical communication of family members and peers should be observed and used as the referent point for comparing the adolescent's language system. For example, examiners may be tempted to mislabel some popular adolescent behaviors as disorders (e.g., the lack of precision of language in Valspeak, a type of teen-age vernacular prevalent in the early 1980s). Adolescents probably cannot be labeled as communicatively disordered if their language is similar to their peers and they continue to function in the mainstream academically, socially, and vocationally.

Observation of the peer group should occur with and without the adolescent referred for evaluation. When the adolescent being tested is present, observations should be made regarding these behaviors:

1. Do the interactions seem primarily positive, negative, or neutral?
2. Did communication breakdowns occur? Why?
3. Was current slang/jargon understood and produced by the adolescent being tested? How much facility with slang/jargon was the peer demanding?

These observations can be made directly (e.g., structure the adolescent being evaluated and the peer to play a board, card, or computer game that requires oral communication while you observe) or indirectly (e.g., tell the adolescent and the peer to have a conversation, which you will tape record while you are out of the room).

When the adolescent referred for assessment is not present, observation of peers will allow the documentation of communication behaviors currently in vogue among adolescents. These observations can be made within more formal communication situations (e.g., volunteer to assist with the high school newspaper or to coach a sport) or within less formal communication situations (e.g., listen to adolescents conversing between classes or during lunch time). Both formal and informal interactions with the adolescent's peers will help to maintain the examiner's perceptions of normal versus disordered communication in older students.

Observation of the family may also occur with the adolescent present or absent. Comparison of the adolescent's communication style with that of the family members may be easier when everyone is interacting, e.g., during an interview situation. However, the constant presence of the adolescent during the family's interview and observation time could curtail the sharing of information and the expression of feelings.

SUMMARY

Too often, when a student is referred for assessment, professionals have assumed the problem to be evaluated is within that student. This assumption may be erroneous. Thorough assessment determines whether the problem being assessed lies within the adolescent, the educational system, the environmental system, or a combination thereof. This chapter examined assessment of the educational and environmental systems. Variables to assess within the educational system are structure of the system, teacher's language, teachers' and administrators' attitudes, and curriculum variables. Procedures for assessing these variables were delineated. Each procedure has a form that was developed for investigating these variables. Within the environmental system, variables to assess include the family members' perceptions of the adolescent, the environmental system members' feelings and attitudes, and communication styles. This assessment is accomplished by interviews and observation.

Once indirect assessment data are gathered, they must be combined with data from direct evaluation of the adolescent. The presence or absence of contributing problems within the educational and environmental systems has major implications for determining the locus (loci) of the disorder and the direction of program planning.

DISCUSSION QUESTIONS

1. Propose additional options for assessing one of the following factors: Teacher's language, teachers' and administrators' attitudes, or curriculum variables.
2. State the criteria you would use to determine whether an adolescent has both a language disorder and a language difference.
3. Discuss strategies that you could use to counter resistance of educational and environmental system members to the proposed indirect assessment procedures.

SUGGESTED READINGS

Eriksen, K. *Communication Skills for the Human Services.* Reston Publishing Co., Inc., Reston, VA, 1979.

National Commission on Excellence in Education. An open letter to the American people. A nation at risk: The imperative for educational reform. *Education Week.* April 27, 1983, pp. 12–16.

Sue, D. *Counseling the Culturally Different: Theory and Practice.* John Wiley and Sons, New York, 1981.

CHAPTER 6

Direct and Indirect Program Planning

GOALS:

To present what to consider and how to engage in direct program planning for the adolescent

To present what to consider and how to engage in indirect program planning for the educational system

To present what to consider and how to engage in indirect program planning for the environmental system

Program planning as defined in Chapter 3 is the connecting link between assessment and intervention. Before intervention commences, and after interpreting the assessment data regarding the adolescent's communication performance, professionals must allow a significant amount of time for program planning. This planning time is essential to establish a comprehensive intervention plan. Such planning may involve the adolescent (direct program planning) and may also include consulting with teachers or family members (indirect program planning). Usually, the greatest amount of program planning time is needed before an adolescent enters an intervention program; however, reevaluation and modification of the program plan often are necessary during the adolescent's involvement in intervention. Some elements of program planning (e.g., educational policies and procedures) may take several years to establish and to implement. A comprehensive model for direct and indirect program planning is illustrated in Table 6.1.

TABLE 6.1 PROGRAM PLANNING COMPONENT

	Who?	What?	How?
DIRECT	Adolescents Early Middle Late	Adolescent's involvement	Writing goals and objectives
		Adolescent's attitude	Motivational procedures
		Group versus individual sessions	Group characteristics
		Program selection	Selecting programs
INDIRECT	Educational system members	Educational policies and procedures	Administrator's involvement
		Consultation	Collaborative approach
		Peer involvement and attitude modification	Peer tutoring
	Environmental system members	Alteration or maintenance of parents' attitudes and behaviors Awareness of referral agencies	Informational and support meetings Newsletters, phone campaigns, home visits
		Sibling acceptance and involvement	Sibling tutoring

Early in the program planning component, a clinical decision must be reached concerning whether the adolescent would benefit from direct and/or indirect program planning. The combinations of possible program planning outcomes are summarized in Table 6.2. The outcomes are labeled by numbers for ease of reference. The first four outcomes include an identified problem (i.e., communication disorder) within the adolescent. Each of these outcomes results in direct program planning for the adolescent; some also include indirect program planning to effect change within the educational and/or environmental systems. Outcomes 5, 6, and 7 result in no direct program planning for the adolescent, since a communication disorder does not exist; however, indirect program planning may be appropriate for the educational and/or environmental systems. Outcome 8 eliminates the need for program planning, because no problems are identified either directly or indirectly.

DIRECT PROGRAM PLANNING

What To Consider: Program Planning for the Adolescent

Adolescent's Involvement When adolescents have been determined to need direct intervention, they need to be included in the program planning component. This is a continuation of the involvement begun during the assessment component, as discussed in Chapter 4. If adolescents resist involvement in program planning, refuse to take responsibility for modifying their disorder, deny the existence of a problem, or remain unmotivated to change, we would recommend that these adolescents not be forced into the intervention component, if indeed force is even possible with this age group. Adolescents will benefit most from intervention if they are willing to take responsibility for their communication disorders and to be involved in the planning of the program.

Adolescent's Attitude It is critical to determine the adolescents' attitudes toward modifying their communication behaviors. Adolescents may be reluctant to work on their communication behaviors for a variety of reasons. Among these reasons are fears that they will be ostracized and laughed at by their peers at a time when peer acceptance may be extremely important to them. Because many of these adolescents have repeatedly failed, they have lowered self-esteem and feel they cannot learn (Brown, 1978). They may have received services previously and felt negatively about them. It may be that other activities such as sports are more important to them than working on their speech-language behaviors. All of these reasons for reluctance may be

TABLE 6.2 EIGHT POSSIBLE PROGRAM PLANNING OUTCOMES FOLLOWING DIRECT AND INDIRECT ASSESSMENT

	1	2	3	4	5	6	7	8
Direct Assessment of Adolescent	Identified problem	Identified problem	Identified problem	Identified problem	No identified problem	No identified problem	No identified problem	No identified problem
Indirect Assessment of Educational System	Identified problem	No identified problem	Identified problem	No identified problem	Identified problem	No identified problem	Identified problem	No identified problem
Indirect Assessment of Environmental System	Identified problem	Identified problem	No identified problem	No identified problem	Identified problem	Identified problem	No identified problem	No identified problem
PROGRAM PLANNING OUTCOMES	Direct and indirect	Direct and indirect	Direct and indirect	Direct	Indirect	Indirect	Indirect	None

operating in an adolescent, or perhaps just one reason is prevailing.

McFarlane, Fujiki, and Brinton (1984) cited four specific types of reluctant clients: (1) the "tardy or absent" type who has a poor attendance record; even when attending intervention sessions, this client type does not work to capacity; (2) the "yes-but" type who attends sessions, but resists the intervention process; (3) the "pleaser" type who attends sessions consistently, praises the clinician's skills and efforts, but never communicates any better; (4) the "semi-success" type who makes significant gains very quickly and then wants to discontinue therapy or direct the course of therapy differently from the course prescribed by the speech-language pathologist. When providing examples of the various reluctant client types, the following observation was made: "If any single age group tends to show this type profile [of a tardy or absent type] to a large degree, it is the junior and senior high school age group." (McFarlane, Fujiki, and Brinton, 1984, p. 91). Planning for the tardy or absent client might include shifting the assigned time, changing the composition of the group, and involving the adolescent in setting the rules for attendance and the consequences for nonattendance (McFarlane, Fujiki, and Brinton, 1984). While the other three types of reluctant clients also exist among the high school age group, they are not as predominant.

Regardless of the number or the nature of the reasons, the end result is a lower motivational level. It is important during program planning to determine the adolescent's attitudes so that procedures can be selected that would increase or maintain the adolescent's motivation toward working on speech-language behaviors. Likewise, a decision may need to be made that if the adolescent's negative attitudes toward intervention cannot be changed, then direct services should not be provided at this time.

Group versus Individual Sessions The speech-language pathologist needs to decide whether adolescents can best accomplish their goals during group or individual intervention. Most adolescents with language disorders would benefit from group intervention, although there are some exceptions to this principle: (1) The adolescent does not have the most basic communication behaviors, and therefore could not interact effectively in a group; (2) The adolescent's communication level is incompatible with existing groups; (3) The adolescent's feelings or attitudes about participation in a group may be so fearful or negative that it may be detrimental to the adolescent or to the entire group.

Our contention that the majority of adolescents with language disorders will benefit most from group sessions is based on several clinical observations. Group sessions help adolescents to derive emotional support from fellow group members and to realize that others may have similar communication disorders. In group situations, conversational skills and pragmatic communication behaviors can be practiced in a naturalistic context; ideas can be exchanged and compared. Many adolescents with language disorders have poor listening skills. An effective way to assist adolescents in developing their assertive and active listening skills is in group interaction with peers (Larson and McKinley, 1985b).

Program Selection As part of direct program planning, the professional will need to select from among a number of programs and then choose what best meets adolescents' needs. In selecting programs to implement with adolescents, the professional will need to consider: (1) the theoretical constructs that undergird the intervention program, (2) the environment that is best for learning, i.e., natural or contrived, (3) the method of intervention that should be used, i.e., traditional or contemporary, (4) the degree of counseling to incorporate into the intervention process, (5) the use of the interaction of language modalities, (6) the general program type adhered to, i.e., basic skills, functional curriculum, tutorial, learning strategies. All these issues should be considered when selecting programs.

How to Engage in Direct Program Planning for the Adolescent

Writing Goals and Objectives One of the best ways to involve the adolescent in the program planning process is simply to continue what should have been started during the assessment process, i.e., to have no "hidden agenda." The professional should communicate to the adolescent openly and honestly what needs to be accomplished during program planning, how it is to be accomplished, and why it is to be done. If the adolescent is willing to modify communication behaviors, then the adolescent should be included in the writing of the individualized goals and objectives. The adolescent should help to identify major goals and objectives for communication and to assist in ranking them according to basic academic, personal-social, and vocational goals. This inclusion of the adolescent in the writing and ranking of the goals and objectives may help to establish that they are responsible for improving their own communication performance.

Motivational Procedures Motivation can sometimes be enhanced by using contracts, offering speech-language intervention as a course for credit, providing grades for speech-language intervention, scheduling speech-language services within existing time modules, developing and using supportive titles for speech-language services, considering carefully the area of the school where services are provided, and encouraging an intrinsic desire to improve communication. Each of these motivational procedures is described below.

Contracting Some adolescents seem to be motivated to work when they sign a contract that specifies goals for communication performance and the time line in which the goals are to be accomplished. When using contingency contracts with adolescents, the professional should make the contract appear adult-like and official (Larson and McKinley, 1985b). The contract should specify the consequences for positive performance or lack of performance. The professional should be flexible when discussing the contract and should allow sufficient time for the student either to agree with the content of the contract or to suggest revisions. A model contract for adolescents containing all essential elements is provided in Appendix J.

Course for Credit Another motivational consideration is recognition of the student's effort by offering speech-language intervention as a course at the junior high level and as a course for credit (e.g., one-fourth credit per semester) at the senior high level. Students invest at least as much time and energy working on their communication skills as they do on other skills taught as courses for credit. How to convince administrators of the need for speech-language courses will be discussed under indirect program planning for the educational system. If a decision is made to offer speech-language intervention as a course for credit, then it should be determined if this is to be an elective course or if a required course can be waived for speech-language intervention (i.e., credit for speech-language intervention substitutes for the required course credit).

Assume for a minute that speech-language courses have been established, and that they may be taken either as electives or as waivers for required classes. During program planning, the speech-language pathologist and the adolescent need to determine which option is most suitable (i.e., elective or substitute). Major considerations when making this decision include these:

1. Is the student attempting to function in required mainstream courses but failing, or nearly failing, one or more? If so, is the failure resulting from poor comprehension of vocabulary and concepts, or from the high cognitive demands of the curriculum? When one or both factors are contributing significantly to failure in a required course, a rationale can be built for the student to receive a waiver from that course on the grounds that insufficient language and cognitive skills inevitably prevent success in the course. When the speech-language course replaces the class being failed, prerequisite language and cognitive abilities become goals and objectives in the student's individualized plan.

2. What other electives are in competition with the speech-language course? Students with language disorders, who need intervention at the secondary level, frequently wish to take vocationally oriented classes which usually are offered as electives. These students need flexibility to take these electives because the courses are important for their future vocational success. Also, adolescents are often more motivated to partici-

pate in elective courses than in required courses. Since these same students may be at risk for dropping out of school, they must be kept in courses that spark their interest. If there are many electives in which the student is interested, it might be best to build a rationale for substitute credit. However, if a rationale for substitute credit is not appropriate, then the adolescent should be counseled to take speech-language intervention as an elective course.

Grading Offering speech-language courses entails giving grades for student performance. There are several options for grading. Giving a letter grade or using a satisfactory/fail system, as other courses would, is appropriate. If the speech-language course is substituting for a required course, a letter grade may be mandatory when this is the grading policy for other required courses. Another option is to grade by progress, resulting in a description of performance and not a letter grade. An example of this type of grading report can be found in Appendix K. Grading by progress most accurately reflects performance on individual goals and objectives, and could possibly be combined with other mandatory grades.

Even when speech-language intervention is not organized as a course for adolescents, grading should be explored as an option. As much as grades appear to be aversive to students, they are inherent in the adolescent's educational experience. Grades are a way to give clout and credibility to speech-language intervention. Several options exist regarding their use:

1. Have the student's performance in speech-language intervention contribute to a percentage of the student's grade in another course. For example, if the adolescent is being removed from part of English class for speech-language services, propose to the English teacher that a portion of the student's grade be determined by speech-language performance.
2. Request a space on the student's regular report card for speech-language performance and record a letter grade or satisfactory/fail.
3. Include a progress report card (see Appendix K) with the student's regular report card.

The option(s) for grading that is chosen should be clarified with the adolescent during program planning. The student needs to understand that grading will occur, and realize when and how grades will be reported. Deriving a grade to evaluate the student's performance may be accomplished in several ways. One alternative is to assign a percentage to each course requirement, e.g., twenty-five percent for class discussion, twenty-five percent for projects, twenty-five percent for examinations, and twenty-five percent for daily assignments. Another way to derive a letter grade is to assign points for participation and work completed and to remove points for inappropriate behaviors. At the end of a grading period a minimum number of points is needed for each letter grade.

Scheduling Another topic to consider during program planning is scheduling the speech-language course so that the student receives appropriate intervention and not token services. Meeting twice a week for twenty or thirty minutes may not be sufficient time to help the adolescent make significant progress in communication behaviors. What may happen during these short time blocks is that the student may taste success but become frustrated further when the intervention time cannot be extended.

A more viable means to schedule intervention is to use existing time modules and to have the administrator incorporate the course into the class schedule like all other subject areas. Meeting for full time modules will allow more time for intervention and will eliminate the problems in junior and senior high schools caused by students entering a class after twenty minutes of speech-language intervention, or leaving a class midway to go to intervention. This obvious entering and leaving causes disruptions within the classes and is one more way adolescents with communication disorders look different from their peer group.

While an obvious solution to scheduling might appear to be removing adolescents from study halls, we would urge caution. Some students offer such extreme resistance to intervention during study time that they refuse to participate, much like elementary children may resist intervention during recess time. Others disrupt sessions so severely that they need to be removed. From the perspective of the professional, these adolescents may be using study hall time inefficiently for academic activities, but students may insist on study hall for social reasons or for relaxation. On the contrary, some adolescents, particularly those in early adolescence, often willingly accept being removed from a study time for speech-language intervention. They would rather work on structured objectives and activities with the speech-language pathologist than work on homework assignments for which they lack basic skills. Also, they may have few friends with whom to relate socially during study hall, and they may possess few acceptable relaxation outlets (e.g., reading a book, writing a letter).

When scheduling options during the regular school day fail, the speech-language pathologist might consider requesting an extended contract day. Some students would prefer not to use school time for speech-language intervention, or have no flexibility in their schedules to do so. However, they would agree to intervention before or after regular school hours. Some secondary level speech-language pathologists now work an extended schedule four days a week, rather than a regular five day week, to accommodate the needs of these students.

Supportive Titles During the program planning phase, the speech-language pathologist must consider and select supportive titles for courses. "Speech therapy" and "language therapy" may be unsupportive titles for adolescents with communication disorders trying to appear similar to their peers. Better titles might be "Individualized Language Skills" or "Oral Communication Strategies." Speech-language pathologists should determine optimal titles for their courses, since preferences will vary according to geographical location.

The title selected is also important because it will appear on the student's report cards and transcript. If speech-language intervention is offered as a substitute course, then professionals may have fewer options for course titles; the substitution may need to be reflected in the title (e.g., Alternative English; Functional Science). If intervention is an elective course, then there is usually more flexibility in titles.

Area of the School Providing speech-language services out of the mainstream areas of the school is frequently viewed negatively by adolescents. A room located in a part of the school that is perceived as part of the mainstream is less likely to carry a negative image.

Many times, because of overcrowded conditions, the speech-language pathologist cannot have a private classroom throughout the day that is large enough for groups of adolescents to meet. However, a classroom somewhere in the building is generally open because secondary-level teachers have staggered preparation periods. Given a willingness to be flexible and to tote their materials from classroom to classroom, speech-language pathologists can meet in areas of the school viewed positively by adolescents. As a toehold is gained for the profession of communication sciences and disorders at the secondary level, buildings being constructed or remodeled should take the speech-language pathologist's space needs into account.

Intrinsic Motivation Note that motivational procedures mentioned thus far are appropriate extrinsic forms of reinforcement for adolescents. Adolescents should be assisted to realize that increasingly successful communicative acts are their own rewards. When extrinsic motivational systems such as points for appropriate communication behaviors have been established, adolescents should eventually be weaned from such a system. Often this weaning process occurs naturally over a long break time from programming (e.g., summer vacation). Students arrive after the break and no longer ask for points (D. Boley, Personal Communication, 1986). They seem to be more willing to participate in speech-language intervention because they realize they are becoming more successful in communicating. We have noted that this change from extrinsic to intrinsic motivational forces often occurs between eighth and ninth grades.

Group Characteristics As stated earlier, planning includes deciding whether adolescents will best accomplish their goals in a group or in an individual intervention situation. Assuming that the group situation is the most advantageous, it is essential to plan for how to establish and to maintain workable groups. When establishing groups several variables need to be considered: Size, grade, gender, and relationships among group members.

The size of the group will vary as a function of the adolescent's needs. Unfortunately, it will also vary as a function of scheduling, particularly in school settings. Group size may vary as a function of availability of other adolescents in hospital settings, and as a function of security considerations in prisons and juvenile detention centers. Groups will not always be homogeneous in their needs; nor is this necessary: Adolescents who are working on a variety of objectives can still be grouped successfully. Groups of as many as ten or twelve adolescents can be considered in an intervention session. In a team teaching situation even more could be grouped.

A one to two grade diversity in the group has been found to be compatible, but usually not greater than that (e.g., a seventh grader and a sophomore would generally not be grouped together). When speech-language intervention is substituted for a required course at a particular grade level, homogeneity is usually necessary. When intervention is an elective course, more flexibility in grouping students from different grades is available.

When general cognition, language, and communication strategies are being taught, we have not experienced problems grouping opposite genders at any stage within adolescence. Wiig (1983) has cautioned that boys and girls should not be mixed in groups during early adolescence. She has also suggested that genders may need to be grouped separately if social communication skills are being taught that would be embarrassing to practice in view of the opposite sex. In our clinical experiences, we have not found this gender separation to be necessary if supportive group dynamics have been established.

A fourth consideration when grouping adolescents, in addition to the age of the group, the grade of the group members, and the genders involved, is the relationship among group members. Group members should perceive one another as equal in status if they are going to work cooperatively with one another, rather than competitively. At other times, groups do not work because the individuals involved simply do not like one another. The presence of a "gang leader" perceived by peers as having more power has dramatically changed the nature of group relationships in settings such as juvenile delinquent centers (S. Robertson, Personal Communication, 1983). Recognition by speech-language pathologists of the social dynamics occurring among adolescents is basic to knowing how to organize peers into cohesive groups.

Wiig (1983) recommended that in public school settings adolescents be seen in a group setting early in the day, followed by individual sessions later. While this may reflect ideal scheduling, it is not realistic in many settings. We would argue that one well-planned, well-executed group session will meet the needs of most adolescents having deficits in cognition, language, and communication. In our clinical experiences, ". . . most adolescents seem to work well and can benefit from being in groups of five to seven students of both sexes, similar chronological ages (i.e., early adolescence versus late adolescence), and compatible communication abilities (i.e., similar but not necessarily identical syntactic, semantic and pragmatic skills" (Larson and McKinley, 1985b, pp. 76–77).

Selecting Programs Six aspects of selecting programs were delineated under the "What to Consider" section. How to engage in program planning for these variables is indicated in the next six subsections.

Theoretical Constructs As emphasized in Chapter 2, our strong recommendation is that every speech-language intervention program be girded with theoretical constructs that provide a framework, rationale, and guideline for the selection of objectives and activities. Lee and Shapero-Fine (1984) stated, "The starting point of any aspect of programming is in its theoretical underpinnings" (p. 339). Johnston (1983) proposed that the question, " 'What is language intervention?' . . . can only be answered within a theoretical model that addresses the nature of language, the nature of change, the nature of language disorders, and by extension, the role of the interventionist" (p. 53).

Consistency and compatibility must exist among and between theoretical constructs and intervention strategies. When the speech-language pathologist extracts from incompatible theoretical constructs, the end result may be an adolescent who becomes confused about the goals and expectations during communication intervention sessions. For example, if a highly structured communication program with a rigid behavior modification paradigm is being used, then a discovery approach to learning would be incompatible. While professionals may perceive this combination of theoretical constructs as being eclectic, the student may instead view the professional's actions as inconsistent and unpredictable.

Natural versus Contrived Learning When planning for an intervention program, it is important to consider whether the learning environment will be natural or contrived. Muma (1978) stressed the importance of utilizing natural, active learning. In most cases, this is not accomplished by using highly structured intervention programs which predetermine the content and sequence of objectives. Exceptions to this can exist. For example, some individuals benefit from a highly structured program when initially establishing a communication behavior in their repertoire. However, most of the time, the contrived learning that results from using these structured programs has a low probability of offering relevance to individual needs.

The content and objectives within natural learning are derived from everyday contexts in which the individual functions. Focus is upon what the adolescent *needs* to learn, not what the speech-language pathologist *wants* the person to learn.

Natural learning is also sensitive to pacing (Muma, 1978). Often speech-language pathologists will have students practice until an objective is at a ninety or one hundred percent correct criterion level; published programs require this also. Repetitive trials may be harmful rather than beneficial for some individuals (Muma, 1978). Perhaps more important than repetition is variation, so that an adolescent sees how a label or a concept or a pragmatic skill applies to many different situations. The number of trials and the variations required for learning to occur are best determined on a case-by-case basis.

Traditional versus Contemporary Intervention The traditional intervention approach has emphasized phonology, then syntax, semantics, and last, pragmatics, if time permitted. A more contemporary approach advocated in current literature is to place pragmatics at the top of the hierarchy with phonology, syntax, and semantics encompassed beneath (Boyce and Larson, 1983). Figure 6.1 illustrates these two intervention approaches.

Why is the contemporary approach a more viable one to use with adolescents? Because the speech-language pathologist should be concerned with whether adolescents can communicate in daily living situations. Can they convey their messages to listeners in an acceptable manner, despite problems in phonology, syntax, and/or semantics? If not, and communication breakdowns are occurring, objectives for phonology, syntax, and/or semantics should be formulated based upon a strong pragmatic rationale.

The contemporary intervention hierarchy never loses sight of the purpose of communication—the meeting of meaning between two or more people. A sentence may have perfect phonological, syntactic, and semantic parameters, yet convey the wrong message because it was said at an inappropriate time, or to the wrong person. Rather than leaving pragmatics until the end of intervention, or never addressing it at all, we would place it at the peak of the hierarchy, the umbrella under which all other parameters fall.

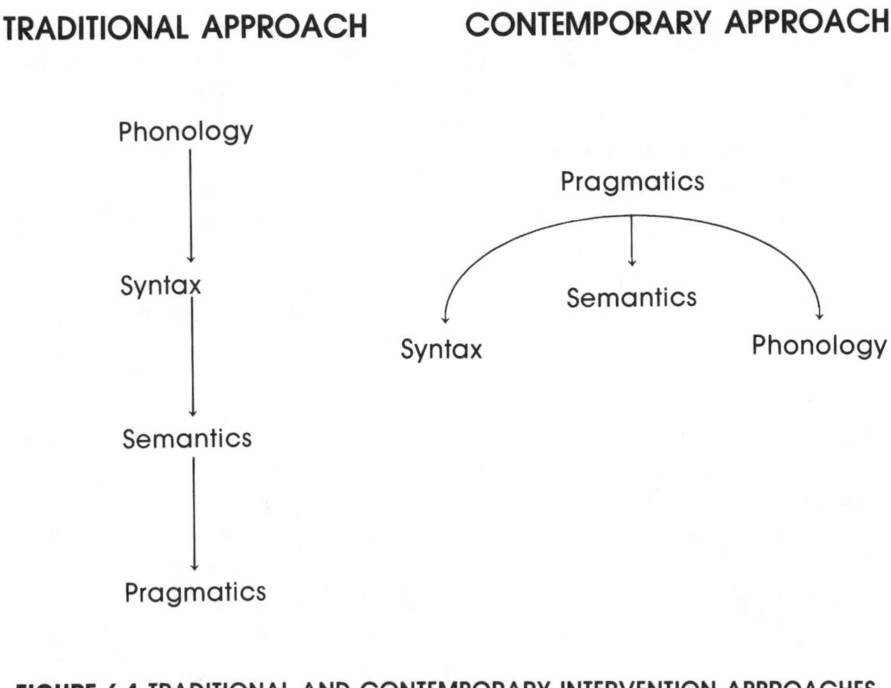

FIGURE 6.1 TRADITIONAL AND CONTEMPORARY INTERVENTION APPROACHES

Counseling When selecting an intervention program to implement with an adolescent, it is important to plan to what degree and when counseling will be incorporated into the intervention program. Simon (1981) commented that as much as fifty percent of intervention with adolescents may involve counseling with them about their communication disorders. It might include giving information, obtaining information, and providing for the release and support of feelings.

Giving information to adolescents might involve telling them about the impact of their communication disorders on listeners, describing appropriate objectives, and explaining strategies that could possibly remediate their problems. They might be given information on how their communication disorder could affect their academic, personal-social, and vocational goals. Information may be given to adolescents on how to monitor their own communication if they choose to terminate intervention, and what options are available to them if they decide to commence speech-language services at a later date.

Obtaining information from adolescents involves gathering their ongoing perspective of the communication disorder, inquiring about their priority needs, and involving them in establishing the best intervention content for their unique strengths and weaknesses. Adolescents might provide information about natural contexts in which they function. Speech-language pathologists might obtain information from them about the effectiveness of assessment and intervention strategies, and about the modifications in objectives and activities that are warranted.

Providing release and support for feelings associated with the communication disorder might involve discussing frustration, anger, and rejection that adolescents have felt. Hartzell (1984) has pointed out that adolescents' feelings run high because ". . . the stigma of a handicap or special need is hard to bear" (p. 3). On the positive end, triumphs and successes might be shared.

Baggett (1969) has offered a number of constructive suggestions for how adults should counsel adolescents. In surveys of youth from rural environments, high socio-economic communities, and correctional schools, these behaviors were found to communicate understanding to adolescents: Suggesting ways to solve a problem, taking time to sit down and talk, spending time to discuss a problem, listening to what the adolescent has to say, asking questions about the problem, and sticking to the problem about which the adolescent wants to talk.

Also, professionals should be aware of the barriers to counseling culturally different populations (DeBlassie, 1978). These barriers are: The counselor's lack of understanding of the socio-psychological background of the adolescent; the counselor's inability to penetrate the language differences of the culturally different adolescent; the culturally different adolescent's lack of familiarity with counseling; the adolescent's hesitation to self-disclose; and the conflict of values between counselor and adolescent.

Interaction of Language Modalities When professionals consider what program to select, they must realize the interaction among the language modalities of speaking, listening, reading, and writing. Speaking and listening have been called the primary language system, and reading and writing the secondary language system (Phelps-Terasaki, Phelps-Gunn, and Stetson, 1983). Myklebust (1960) proposed that writing was the most difficult of the language modalities, and depended on underlying competence in listening, speaking, and reading. Since 1960, many other researchers have emphasized the interrelationship of the four language modes and have documented problems in oral language preceding problems in reading and writing (Aram and Nation, 1980; King, Jones, and Lasky, 1982; Lassman et al., 1980). While normal developmental data suggest listening precedes speaking, which precedes reading, which precedes writing, those who continue to be impaired in all modalities during adolescence do not necessarily acquire language skills according to the developmental model (Johnson, 1982). In some individuals, oral language skills are facilitated by improving written language; in other individuals, written language is facilitated by improving oral language (Johnson, 1982). Phelps-Terasaki et al. (1983) proposed that ". . . oral language activities should accompany writing to get the student involved and thinking about the topic" (p. 362). These authors also emphasized that for some individuals working on oral language, accompanying written activities may be desirable.

Speech-language pathologists working with adolescents on speaking or listening skills should be cognizant of the interrelationship among the language modalities, and should remain open to utilizing writing and reading activities when they assist in the acquisition of oral language skills. While we hold the opinion that the expertise of speech-language pathologists may not lie in teaching reading and writing per se, these modalities should be used when they positively affect the attainment of oral communication goals. It is appropriate and necessary for those in the discipline of communication sciences and disorders working with adolescents to be knowledgeable of the areas of reading and writing (Dagenais and Beadle, 1984).

General Program Types Intervention with adolescents by speech-language pathologists has evolved around either a medical model, a developmental model, or an educational model. Neither of the first two models is appropriate for many adolescents. The medical model is often inappropriate because knowing about the underlying etiology of a language disorder that was identified during the preschool years may be irrelevant by adolescence. The developmental model is often inappropriate because there is no longer time to remediate the gaps in development; instead the adolescent may need assistance in coping with the disorder. The educational model is usually the one selected for adolescents. Four program types based on the educational model have been described by Alley and Deshler (1979). Their critique of the various program types is summarized below.

One general program type to use with adolescents is basic skills remediation. Skills are taught at the level that approximates the student's achievement level. For example, if the adolescent has third-grade listening skills, then intervention tasks will be designed to teach listening skills typically taught at that grade level. The goal is to improve sequentially the youth's performance in the basic skill areas. This program type makes the assumption that identifying and sequencing of prerequisite skills are possible; that past instruction has been inappropriately or incompetently delivered; and that students will benefit in spite of a history of not benefiting from similar intervention in the elementary grades. The strengths of this program type include: (1) the increased competence in basic skills that enables adolescents to perform better, and (2) the relevance that instruction in basic skills has for those youth who have received no intervention or poor remediation previously. However, there are some potential weaknesses as well. For those adolescents in a school setting, there is limited time available, thus making it unlikely that enough progress can be made to reduce the gap between grade level placement and level of functioning. Interest and motivation also may be hampered when adolescents are overexposed to intervention activities and materials identical to those used during the elementary years.

The functional curriculum program type emphasizes equipping adolescents to function in society. The assumption is that survival skills are identifiable and stable over time. This program type has merit in that, at least over the short term, students are equipped to function independently in society. The problem is that survival skills become outdated. A functional curriculum program type also risks ignoring strengths of adolescents and denying them the opportunity to develop normal basic skills.

The tutorial program type "... emphasizes provision of instruction in academic content areas" (Alley and Deshler, 1979, p. 52). A speech-language pathologist using this general program is concerned primarily with assisting adolescents in their academic curriculum. While at first glance it might appear that the discipline of communication sciences and disorders could easily dismiss this tutorial program, it is not unusual in school settings for classroom teachers to request assistance on academic assignments for students on the caseload. Providing tutorial assistance meets the immediate needs of adolescents, and is readily accepted by other teachers, but it is a short-term solution. When the primary goal is to respond to classroom assignments, there is little time to intervene with the actual, underlying problems. We strongly urge speech-language pathologists to resist any temptations to engage in the tutorial program type.

The learning strategies program type, as described and promoted by Alley and Deshler (1979), is advocated as the most appropriate type with the majority of adolescents needing speech-language intervention; we concur. "Learning strategies are defined as techniques, principles, or rules that will facilitate the acquisition, manipulation, integration, storage, and retrieval of information across situations and settings." (Alley and Deshler, 1979, p. 13). Emphasis in a learning strategies program is on *how* to learn (i.e., process) rather than *what* to learn (i.e., product). Advantages of this program type are numerous. Learning strategies allow adolescents to make changes in response to immediate concerns, but the youth also generalize to other situations. The emphasis on how to continue learning is better suited than other program types to the ongoing adaptation adolescents will be facing in their lifetimes, living in a technologically oriented culture. Strategies that allow adolescents to continue learning may be imposed by the adult providing intervention, but they are often most effective if they are generated by the individuals themselves (Levin, 1976).

Initiation of the learning strategies program type is most appropriate and effective as adolescence emerges. Rowher (1971) argued that instruction in learning and thinking skills should begin in early adolescence, and even questioned whether early childhood and elementary years might be relatively inefficient periods in which to teach skills that are learned quickly during the teen years. In addition to the adolescent age range, Alley and Deshler (1979) described the following characteristics of youth who can most benefit from a learning strategies program type. First, it is helpful if those participating in the learning strategies program read at or above the third grade level. Second, students should be able to learn from both symbolic and concrete tasks. And third, average intellectual ability as defined by IQ scores should be present. While a learning strategies program can be used with adolescents who do not possess all three of these attributes, it is likely to be more effective with those who do.

Several major drawbacks to the learning strategies program type exist: (1) heavy reliance on cooperative planning, something not conducive to the structure of many secondary-level schools; (2) failure to address the basic skill and tutorial needs of adolescents; and (3) failure to consider functional life skills. Moreover, limited data are currently available on the efficacy of the learning strategies program type and whether the program accomplishes the major goal of generalization of strategies to other situations. Data are lacking because of the small number of people currently implementing this general program type (Alley and Deshler, 1979).

After considering the four general program types within the educational model, we would recommend adherence to learning strategies that emphasize how to become a more competent communicator. Strategies are taught that should have utility beyond the intervention sessions, yet in this program type adolescents also learn communication behaviors necessary for the immediate environment. This approach is particularly beneficial with adolescents who possess the characteristics that Alley and Deshler (1979) described. When adolescents do not possess these characteristics, and are within the early stage of adolescence, it may be more appropriate to select the basic skills program type in an attempt to prepare them for a learning strategies program. The basic skills program type also relates to one of the primary goals of intervention during early adolescence as presented in Chapter 3, i.e., communication for academic settings. No later than the end of middle adolescence, the basic skills program type should be replaced with a learning strategies program, if students possess the recommended characteristics. If students have not gained prerequisite basic skills, then a functional curriculum program type should be used.

INDIRECT PROGRAM PLANNING

Indirect program planning can be conducted for the benefit of the adolescent in the educational and environmental systems. What to consider when planning for these systems and how to engage in program planning was summarized in Table 6.1, and is detailed below.

What to Consider: Program Planning for the Educational System

Educational Policies and Procedures The speech-language pathologist should plan with school administrators for changes in the speech-language program, such as offering intervention as a course for credit and deciding whether the course should be an elective or a substitute course. Together, they should investigate whether or not an option exists to offer speech-language intervention as a substitute course, since some educational agencies will not allow anyone who does not have an English degree, for example, to teach a course that is replacing the required English credit. If this is true of your educational setting, then you may wish to consider team teaching with someone who has the required credentials.

Speech-language pathologists and administrators need to plan jointly how offering a course for credit will fit into existing educational policies and procedures. Issues to consider include these:

1. How many units of time are required to constitute a course for credit?
2. How many credits can be obtained in special courses that are being used to substitute for required courses?
3. What type of prior approval process has been established to assure a student that the course is an acceptable course substitution?
4. How will speech-language courses be reflected on the transcript?
5. How will the grades earned for speech-language courses be calculated for purposes of determining class rank or honor roll status?
6. Will an individually designed course of study (e.g., an IEP) be acceptable as a substitute if a written curriculum is required?
7. What are the various types of diploma options available to students with language disorders and related disabilities?
8. How will speech-language courses affect the current graduation policy?

Consultation The speech-language pathologist needs to plan for the implementation of a consultation model for indirect intervention. The consultation model is a viable and important alternative service delivery model for adolescents. As noted in Chapter 3, Frassinelli, Superior, and Meyers (1983) defined consultation as "... a three person chain of service in which a consultant interacts with a caregiver (consultee) to benefit an individual (client) for whom the caregiver is responsible" (p. 25). Consultation may enable a larger population to be served, and it retains the natural environmental setting (i.e., classroom) for communication. Along with these benefits to the adolescent, there are other advantages to using a consultation model. It provides us with a medium for inservicing teachers regarding normal expectations about and problems of the adolescent's communication system. Speech-language pathologists utilizing a consultation model may assist teachers to change attitudes about adolescents with communication disorders and to adapt materials and methods to meet the needs of these adolescents.

Peer Involvement and Attitude Modification There is a dual advantage to involving peers with adolescents who are enrolled for speech-language intervention: It will help adolescents with disorders to learn necessary communication behaviors and it will assist in altering the attitudes and perceptions that peers have toward those adolescents who have problems learning (Slavin, 1986). Furthermore, the social benefits and increased self-esteem of all students working together are considerable (Slavin, 1986). However, there may be a disadvantage to including normal peers: Adolescents with language disorders may view the presence of a normal adolescent as an invasion of their privacy. The adolescent with a language disorder should be informed about and consent to having normal adolescents participate in the clinical process.

How to Engage in Indirect Program Planning for the Educational System

Administrators' Involvement Administrative involvement is crucial to making changes in educational policies and procedures. Administrators are the people in the educational system most knowledgeable about educational laws and state and federal guidelines. Sometimes there are no laws prohibiting the modification of existing policies and procedures, only guidelines open to interpretation. It is essential that the administrators approve of the concept behind a change of policy in order for them to accept it and, more importantly, for them to persuade others. Typically, this will require a series of planning meetings between the speech-language pathologist and administrators.

The speech-language pathologist and administrators should decide the written documents that are needed to offer intervention as a course, and a realistic time line for writing the required documents. Also, the person responsible for writing the documents should be designated. For example, if a written curriculum guide needs to be created, what types of information does it need to contain (e.g., scope and sequence of objectives, sample activities)? Who will write the curriculum and when does it need to be completed?

A decision needs to be made about the report card procedure, i.e., will a progress report card be sent home (see Appendix K), will course performance be reflected on the agency's existing report card, or both? Plans must be made either to develop a written graduation policy or to incorporate speech-language courses within an existing policy. A written graduation policy from one school district is reprinted with permission in Appendix L. This policy illustrates the careful program planning and implementation that an educational agency accomplished following the cooperative efforts of a speech-language pathologist, a learning disabilities specialist, and administrators.

Collaborative Approach Consultation may be carried out in the absence of any contact time with the adolescent; or it may be combined with some direct services, periodic or ongoing (Frassinelli, Superior, and Meyers, 1983). Regardless of whether the consultation model is used alone or in conjunction with direct services to adolescents, a collaborative approach rather than an authoritarian approach should be used. In a collaborative approach, the speech-language pathologist does not simply give teachers information, but actively listens to the teacher's viewpoint and then negotiates who is responsible for what in the teaching of the adolescent. The speech-language pathologist should listen to the teacher's viewpoint and withhold providing specific solutions to problems. Solutions are mutually developed and negotiated in a collaborative consultation approach.

When planning a collaborative consultation approach, actions that may be taken, as adapted from Frassinelli, Superior, and Meyers (1983), include these:

1. Select teachers who are willing to devote time and energy to consultation sessions; some teachers are more suitable than others for initial consultation endeavors.

2. Educate teachers about the benefits of and their role in indirect intervention.

3. Assist teachers to change their attitudes about the traditional role of direct intervention by the speech-language pathologist; some teachers believe that the only way to modify behaviors is through direct intervention.

4. Select adolescents who are appropriate candidates for the consultation approach, e.g., those who need to practice newly acquired communication behaviors that were learned during direct intervention in the classroom; those who need to use appropriately the behaviors already within their repertoire, but not being applied.

When establishing a collaborative consultation approach, it is essential to consider when to meet with teachers and for how long. Meetings should be arranged as part of the school day during teachers' preparation times, and not during lunch hour or after school unless it is mutually agreeable. Time for consultation meetings is essential to the success of this approach.

Peer Tutoring One of the major mechanisms for involving peers and changing their attitudes toward adolescents with communication disorders is through a system of peer tutoring. Professionals typically think that the major advantage of peer tutoring is to the recipient. However, peer tutoring may be as important to the tutor, i.e., for changing attitudes. Also, helping another person to learn usually results in all people having a greater understanding of the behaviors being modified.

The peer tutoring system planned by the speech-language pathologist should emphasize teaching tutors how to assist adolescents who have language disorders to improve communication performance. When using a peer tutoring system, the speech-language pathologist must spend a considerable amount of time and energy planning the tutorial program. If a peer tutorial system already exists in the educational agency, then speech-language pathologists should collaborate with those persons implementing that system to determine if it meets existing needs of adolescents with communication disorders. If a peer tutorial system does not exist, then some of the issues to consider when planning such a program are:

1. <u>Gaining Educators' Support</u> Administrators can "make or break" tutoring programs. To gain the administrators' supportive enthusiasm, it is necessary to explain the program to them, the benefits derived from such a program, and the resources needed for the establishment and maintenance of the program. Teachers should be consulted about the program to determine if they are willing to have their students participate and which students might be best in the role of the tutor.

2. <u>Recruiting and Selecting Tutors</u> Obviously, supportive teachers can be instrumental in recruiting and selecting tutors for the program. In addition to the teachers' assistance, the program can be advertised through posters, brochures, newsletters, media, and personal solicitations. Once the tutors have been identified, a structured selection process must be followed. This would entail interviewing the tutors and having them complete an application form (see Appendix M) that reveals their strengths and weaknesses. Using the data submitted on the form and gleaned from the interview, it should be feasible to select good tutors. Some of the characteristics of a good tutor would include: Ability to relate to adolescents with language disorders; knowledge of the behaviors to be taught; patience; ability to teach someone else; positive attitude toward education; available time to participate; and ability to

prepare, to implement, and to evaluate lesson plans and activities.

3. Training, Supervising, and Supporting Tutors It is essential to orient the tutors about the tutoring program. Tutors should be trained to develop interesting activities and lessons; to implement time management techniques; to help tutees feel good about themselves; to respect confidential information about students; to establish and to maintain tutoring logs. Answers to questions such as the following should be provided to the tutor during the training session: Who am I going to tutor? What will I be doing during the session? When will I tutor the tutee? How do I encourage effort and reinforce success? Where am I going to do the tutoring? What type of records must I keep?

   During the training session, it is important to discuss tutoring strategies that make a difference. Some tutoring strategies that have been found to be successful (Koskinen and Wilson, 1982a) are: (1) focusing on the student's strengths, (2) working with the student's interests, (3) listening to students, (4) accepting students at their level, (5) helping students to learn how to pay attention, (6) helping students complete assignments independently, (7) creating a challenging situation for the students, (8) encouraging appropriate risk-taking, and (9) developing and maintaining a learning environment where the tutee feels comfortable to ask questions. In addition, we would recommend that each tutor be required to read about tutoring. For example, *Tutoring: A Guide for Success* (Koskinen and Wilson, 1982b) would be appropriate reading for tutors who are late adolescents or young adults, such as those who are in vocational-technical institutes or colleges and universities. *A Guide for Student Tutors* (Koskinen and Wilson, 1982c) and *Tutoring Can be Fun* (Klausmeier, Jetter, and Nelson, 1972) would be appropriate reading for those who are in early or middle adolescence. These are pertinent resources for helping the tutor to better understand peer tutoring, and the role, responsibilities, and guidelines for being a peer tutor.

   Once the tutor has been trained, it is critical to have weekly or biweekly contacts to evaluate progress and to detect and to prevent problems. The tutor should be supervised and should be encouraged to discuss all issues with the speech-language pathologist as they occur.

4. Selecting the Tutee Not all adolescents with language disorders will benefit from having a tutor. Therefore, it is equally important that careful planning be given to the selection of the tutee. The tutee should be someone who needs to learn tasks that can be taught by a tutor; who is not embarrassed to work with a peer; who has time available to participate in the program. The peer tutoring program is conducted independent of the time spent in speech-language intervention and other courses, and therefore must be incorporated into the students' schedules. Quite frequently, peer tutoring is feasible during study hall hours when both tutors and tutees are available.

What to Consider: Program Planning for the Environmental System

Alteration or Maintenance of Parents' Attitudes and Behaviors Program planning is necessary for two types of parents: Those who need to *modify* their attitudes about and expectations for their son or daughter; those who need to *maintain* their constructive attitudes about and expectations for their son or daughter. Some parents have expectations that are too high, while others have given up on their son or daughter after years of frustration and a variety of "special services."

Awareness of Referral Agencies Parents frequently are unaware of the variety of agencies and services within their immediate geographical area or state. Parents should be informed of available agencies so that they can make knowledgeable decisions about available alternative resources that may assist their son or daughter who has a communication disorder.

Sibling Acceptance and Involvement Siblings may have a variety of negative reactions to the adolescent with a communication disorder. It is important to consider the siblings' reactions and, when necessary, to plan a program that involves the siblings with the adolescent who has the communication disorder in a way that increases their acceptance.

How to Engage in Indirect Program Planning for the Environmental System

Informational and Support Meetings One of the ways to increase parental involvement and to change or maintain attitudes toward the adolescent is to plan informational and support meetings. It is essential to obtain the administrators' support and suggestions for conducting these meetings. The meetings should be scheduled at a time and frequency when the majority of parents can attend. Planning should take into account the schedules of various life styles, such as families where both parents work. An agenda should be created before the meeting to ensure that specific topics are covered in a well-organized manner. Flexibility needs to be built into the agenda so that parents feel comfortable to interject comments and opinions. Also, sufficient time should be planned for parents to talk with each other, since they may learn as much from each other as from a professional.

Before conducting meetings, the speech-language pathologist must develop active listening skills. Also, skills to function as a group discussion leader are essential for successful meetings.

Newsletters, Phone Campaigns, Home Visits Some viable alternatives to keeping parents informed about their son or daughter, besides informational and support meetings, are newsletters, phone campaigns, or home visits. In some families, these alternatives may better meet the needs of the family than meeting in groups.

First, the speech-language pathologist should determine the frequency that a newsletter should be disseminated to parents. At least twice a year appears to be necessary to have a mechanism to disseminate relatively current information. The newsletter should contain information of interest that also meets the needs of the greatest number of parents being served. Likewise, the content of the newsletter should be free of professional jargon, and be written in such a style that the majority of parents can easily read the newsletter. Attractive newsletters can now be published quite efficiently with computer hardware and software packages designed for this purpose. These software programs were listed in Chapter 3. Using a program like *Mailmerge* (MicroPro International Corp., 1983), the speech-language pathologist can effectively and efficiently produce mailing labels for the newsletter, which should be mailed home rather than entrusted to the adolescent for delivery.

Planning a phone campaign in which parents are contacted at predetermined, regular intervals leads not only to disseminating current information but also to obtaining information about parents and answering questions. A phone call will probably not take a considerable amount of time, and yet the returns may be great in that all parties are being kept informed and concerns are being accommodated immediately. It also demonstrates to parents that you are interested in and concerned about keeping them informed; not simply when they must come to the school for a parent conference, orientation session, or open house.

Home visits are another means for keeping some parents informed. Home visits may need to be planned to accommodate parents who do not have work schedules that permit them to attend informational and support meetings, or parents who do not feel comfortable in a school environment. The home visit may provide a relaxing, comfortable, flexible atmosphere in which to converse, assuming that there are not too many distractions or interruptions. It may be necessary to arrange home visits at a time when other children are not home, or are playing, so that privacy of information about the adolescent with the communication disorder is maintained.

At some time during home visits, phone campaigns, or informational and support meetings, every speech-language pathologist will be expected to provide information as to the location of alternative agencies and services that might assist in meeting the needs of a particular adolescent. Therefore, it is essential that the speech-language pathologist establish a data base of appropriate agencies by categories and geographical locations. With computer technology, the establishment and maintenance of such a data base are easily within reach.

Sibling Tutoring To this point, we have discussed ways to engage in program planning primarily for the parents. Siblings, too, may need to be involved actively with the adolescent who has a communication disorder, in order to accept and to understand their brother or sister better. One of the ways to involve the siblings is as tutors, in much the same way as peers have been involved. It should be noted that not all siblings are viable candidates for being in a sibling tutor program. To decide the viability of the sibling to be a tutor, determine the answers to the following questions:

1. Is the sibling someone who has the necessary skills and patience to work with the adolescent who has a communication disorder?
2. Does the sibling desire to participate?
3. Is the sibling willing to be trained and supervised in carrying out assignments?
4. Is the sibling willing to spend the necessary time and energy to teach behaviors to the adolescent?
5. Is there a workable age difference between the siblings to maximize potentials?

The speech-language pathologist should plan to train and supervise the sibling tutor similarly to the peer tutor. The sibling tutor also should be counseled about the important role he or she is playing in the life of the adolescent with a communication disorder.

SUMMARY

Program planning, the connecting link between assessment and intervention, should not be glossed over, because it is essential to establishing a comprehensive intervention program. Program planning includes working with the adolescent (direct) or interacting with people in the educational and environmental systems who are involved with the adolescent (indirect). Direct program planning data were provided on what to consider, i.e., the adolescent's involvement and attitudes, group versus individual sessions, and program selection. In addition, how to engage in the direct program planning process was presented, i.e., writing goals and objectives, determining motivational procedures, considering group characteristics, and selecting programs. Indirect program planning data were presented on what to consider in the educational system, i.e., educational policies and procedures, consultation, and peer involvement and attitude modification. Also, data were presented on what to consider in the environmental system, i.e., alteration or maintenance of parents' attitudes and behaviors, awareness of referral agencies, and sibling acceptance and involvement. Each aspect of what to consider in indirect program planning was discussed from the perspective of how to engage in that aspect of program planning. How to engage in program planning for the educational system was presented as utilizing administrators' involvement, a collaborative consultation approach, and peer tutoring. How to engage in program planning for the environmental system was discussed as developing: Informational and support meetings, newsletters, phone campaigns, home visits, and sibling tutoring.

DISCUSSION QUESTIONS

1. Create a goal and an objective for an adolescent with a language disorder. Then, do the following tasks based upon this goal and objective:
   a. Develop a written contract that incorporates your selected goal and objective.
   b. Decide if you would work with the adolescent in an individual or a group setting; provide your rationale.
   c. Select a general program type (i.e., basic skills, functional curriculum, tutorial, learning strategies) that would support the adolescent's attainment of the goal and objective.
2. Outline your approach for establishing speech-language intervention as a course within the school curriculum. Assume that you have an administrator who is skeptical of the idea.
3. Compare and contrast how you would establish and implement a program to train peers versus siblings to tutor adolescents with language disorders.

SUGGESTED READINGS

Alley, G. and Deshler, D. *Teaching the Learning Disabled Adolescent: Strategies and Methods.* Love Publishing Co., Denver, CO, 1979.

Koskinen, P. and Wilson, R. *Developing a Successful Tutoring Program.* Teachers College Press, Columbia University, New York, 1982.

Larson, V. Lord and McKinley, N. General intervention principles with language impaired adolescents. *Topics in Language Disorders,* 5(3): 70–77, 1985.

CHAPTER 7

Direct Intervention with the Adolescent

GOALS:

To delineate what to modify:

* Thinking
* Listening
* Speaking
* Nonverbal communication
* Survival language

To present general intervention procedures

To illustrate selected specific intervention methods

To summarize commercial resources appropriate for adolescents

Intervention with the adolescent commences once adequate program planning has been completed. The primary purpose of this intervention is to assist the adolescent in the acquisition of appropriate and effective communication for academic, personal-social, and vocational settings (i.e., functional communication). The adolescent's functional communication acquisition should be in the forefront whenever intervention procedures are planned and implemented.

Many suggestions have been presented in preceding chapters concerning how to organize the speech-language program for adolescents. This chapter will focus specifically on what behaviors to modify within the adolescent's communication and on which methods (i.e., procedures and materials) to employ during intervention. The generic term "methods" is being used to describe what speech-language pathologists do during intervention, whereas the term "strategies" is being used to describe what adolescents develop during intervention.

Table 7.1 summarizes the information that will be presented in this chapter. It can be noted from Table 7.1 that reference is made to general procedures and to specific methods. General procedures are those that should be used throughout intervention, regardless of what is being modified or the program type (see Chapter 6) being emphasized. Specific methods are those that are limited to some areas of modification (e.g., the procedure would be used when intervening with listening, but not with nonverbal communication). Specific methods may also be limited to certain general program types (e.g., the procedure might be used during a learning strategies program, but not during a tutorial program).

TABLE 7.1 INTERVENTION COMPONENT: DIRECT SERVICES

Who?	What?	How?
Adolescents Early Middle Late	Thinking Listening Speaking Nonverbal communication Survival language	General procedures A. Mediation B. Bridging C. Discussion Selected specific methods A. Referential communication activities B. Simulation and role playing activities C. Narrative skill building activities Commercial resources

WHAT TO MODIFY

When determining what to modify within the adolescent's communication, several considerations need to be made:

1. What are the behaviors being modified?
2. How should professionals label the behaviors being modified during intervention for adolescents?

3. How should professionals determine what to modify first?

Behaviors Being Modified

Behaviors to modify within the adolescent's communication system closely parallel those assessed informally. (See Chapter 4.) These behaviors have been reorganized into Tables 7.2, 7.3, 7.4, 7.5, and 7.6 to correspond to the labels thinking, listening, speaking, nonverbal communication, and survival language. This reorganization has been completed for ease of use with adolescents. The behaviors listed in these five tables are not intended to be exhaustive. Neither are they intended to translate directly into individualized objectives. Tables 7.2 through 7.6 list behaviors to select from, during intervention with adolescents. No developmental sequence of behaviors is implied within or across tables. Professionals should select those behaviors that most support the adolescent's acquisition of functional communication.

Behaviors within Tables 7.2 through 7.6 are amenable to being taught through a learning strategies approach. For example, the first listening behavior listed in Table 7.3 is "Identifying morphological structures." To accomplish this, adolescents should be taught strategies to identify words and word endings; to use prefixes and suffixes to help them derive meanings of words; and to find the meaning of a word if they do not know the meaning of the root, prefix, and/or suffix (i.e., where this information is located). Similarly, strategies can be emphasized for all other behaviors recorded in the tables.

Behaviors within Tables 7.2 through 7.4 may be selected for a basic skills approach. Nonverbal communication and survival language are not considered within the realm of basic skills. Because a basic skills approach implies that a regimented skill sequence is followed, prerequisite behaviors may need to be taught before behaviors from Tables 7.2, 7.3, or 7.4 are selected.

The behaviors listed in Table 7.6 Survival Language are essential within a functional curriculum program. However, behaviors from the other tables may also be selected depending upon the survival skills a particular adolescent most needs to develop. In a general sense, all of the behaviors on all of the tables could be considered survival language. Remember, the division of behaviors into categories is arbitrary and made for the convenience of organization; the behaviors were first listed as expectations in Table 1.1 (p. 16).

Labels for Behaviors

Recall that in Chapter 4 the adolescent's feelings and attitudes toward the improvement of thinking, listening, and speaking were assessed. During intervention it is important to use these terms when referring to the communica-

TABLE 7.2 THINKING BEHAVIORS (Adapted from Feuerstein, 1979)

Input Phase

1. Using senses to gather clear and complete information
2. Exploring a situation systematically
3. Naming objects and events consistently
4. Describing when and where events and objects occur
5. Recognizing events and objects as the same even when changes occur
6. Organizing information by several characteristics simultaneously
7. Knowing when and how to be precise and accurate

Elaboration Phase

1. Defining problems and determining what needs to be done
2. Using relevant information to a problem and ignoring irrelevant information
3. Forming a "good picture in the mind" about what must be done to solve a problem
4. Making a plan with needed steps to reach a goal
5. Remembering the pieces of information needed to solve a problem
6. Looking for relationships among separate objects, events, and experiences
7. Comparing objects, events, and experiences for similarities and differences
8. Finding the category to which new objects, events, and experiences belong
9. Considering different alternatives
10. Using logic to prove answers and to defend opinions

Output Phase

1. Being clear and precise in language so the listener understands
2. Taking sufficient time to think through a response
3. Restraining saying or doing something that will be regretted later
4. Using a strategy to help find answers

TABLE 7.3 LISTENING BEHAVIORS

Comprehension of Linguistic Features

1. Identifying morphological structures
2. Differentiating syntactical structures as incorrect
3. Comprehending sentence transformations
4. Comprehending sentences of various length and complexity
5. Comprehending semantic features
6. Applying informational listening skills
   a. Comprehending factual information and following directions
   b. Concentrating attention on the speaker
   c. Utilizing the time differential between thinking and speaking speeds
   d. Understanding main ideas and supportive details
   e. Formulating questions for clarification
7. Comprehending adolescent slang

Discourse

1. Applying critical listening skills
   a. Identifying the credibility of the source and/or speaker
   b. Recognizing inductive and deductive reasoning of the speaker
   c. Detecting false reasoning
   d. Recognizing propaganda devices
   e. Drawing inferences
   f. Judging statements
2. Listening to retell a story
3. Utilizing appropriate informational and critical listening skills during conversations

TABLE 7.4 SPEAKING BEHAVIORS

Production of Linguistic Features

1. Using simple and complex sentences to express ideas clearly and concisely
2. Using sentence fragments appropriately
3. Using figurative language
4. Using specific language and applying strategies when struggling to retrieve a word

Discourse

1. Using propositions and cohesion devices appropriately while telling or retelling a story, making a report, explaining a process, or conversing
2. Producing language that fulfills eight functions of communication: To give information, to get information, to describe, to persuade, to self-disclose, to indicate a readiness for further communication, to solve problems, to entertain
3. Applying rules of conversation
    a. Initiating and closing conversations appropriately
    b. Selecting appropriate topics
    c. Maintaining topics
    d. Switching topics orderly
    e. Making contributions to the conversation informative
    f. Making contributions to the conversation truthful
    g. Making contributions to the conversation relevant
    h. Making contributions to the conversation clear, brief, and orderly
    i. Switching to formal and informal registers as appropriate
4. Engaging in narration skills during story telling and retelling
    a. Summarizing/categorizing stories subjectively and objectively
    b. Analyzing and critiquing the story
    c. Generalizing the story's meaning

TABLE 7.5 NONVERBAL COMMUNICATION BEHAVIORS

1. Matching oral and nonverbal messages
2. Determining whether oral and nonverbal messages of others match or mismatch
3. Detecting emotion through facial expression
4. Displaying emotion through facial expression
5. Recognizing the impact of distance (i.e., proxemic behavior) on the message
6. Maintaining socially acceptable distance
7. Maintaining appropriate eye contact

TABLE 7.6 SURVIVAL LANGUAGE

1. Comprehending language for specific situations (e.g., school classroom, restaurant, grocery store)
2. Comprehending language for multi-situational settings (e.g., money, signs)
3. Producing language for specific situations
4. Producing language for multi-situational settings

tion behaviors being modified. Adolescents seem more willing to participate in activities, and more understanding of the activities' purposes, if they can relate them to improving thinking, listening, and speaking in daily living situations.

Thinking, listening, and speaking are artificial divisions that provide a means to organize intervention for the adolescent. The divisions are helpful when it becomes desirable to emphasize one area of modification to the exclusion of others (e.g., when first establishing a behavior in the adolescent's repertoire). However, before the termination of intervention, adolescents should be guided to see the integration of thinking, listening, and speaking during communication. How to accomplish this integration is illustrated later in the "How to Intervene" section of this chapter.

The other two major areas of intervention, i.e., nonverbal communication and survival language, may be labeled as such for adolescents. This labeling presumes that the professional(s) involved in intervention with these areas defines and explains these terms to the adolescent. Definitions for both terms appeared in Chapter 1, although they should be modified as necessary to accommodate the student's level of comprehension.

First Behaviors to Modify

Adolescents who are in the early or middle stage of development when commencing intervention are often operating in a school setting and they are feeling extreme academic pressure. These students may feel burdened by the overwhelming amount and complexity of the curricula material they are expected to assimilate. For these adolescents, a beginning point for what to modify during intervention may be listening and thinking behaviors that will relieve the immediate pressure of academic demands (e.g., informational listening in the classroom; strategies for remembering). Once the academic pressure has been at least partially diminished, adolescents seem more aware of the relevance of language intervention and less resistant to subsequent activities.

When academic pressure is not the primary concern upon commencement of intervention, adolescents at any stage could begin with objectives that assist them to use their existing oral communication system in the most appropriate way possible during personal-social interactions. Most adolescents receiving language intervention have some oral communication system, albeit an inappropriate or ineffectual one that impairs personal-social relationships. Goals and objectives might focus initially on those communication behaviors that are interfering most with personal-social interactions (e.g., maintaining topics of conversation, maintaining socially acceptable distance).

Adolescents in middle or late stages might begin with objectives that focus on adequate communication behaviors for vocational situations that will extend beyond high school, including post-secondary education. For example, goals may emphasize comprehension and production of language needed to secure a job, or improvement of listening skills needed to understand lectures at a vocational-technical institute, college, or university. Goals and objectives should result in a positive influence on the adolescent's future performance in post-secondary experiences.

HOW TO INTERVENE

This section is divided into three major subsections: General Procedures, Selected Specific Methods, and Commercial Resources. When intervention with adolescents occurs, speech-language pathologists may draw upon information from each of these sections.

General Procedures

Three general procedures are described: Mediation, bridging, and discussion. Each of these procedures will have an important role to play during implementation of selected specific methods and when using commercial resources.

Mediation Mediated learning experience (Feuerstein, 1980), also called mediation, was defined in Chapter 2. During mediation, there is purposeful focusing on objects, events, or experiences to anchor them in time, space, or affect. Mediation takes advantage of natural learning by focusing on everyday occurrences surrounding the adolescent. The focusing may frame the whole object, event, or experience, or it may filter out segments; focusing may be accomplished verbally or nonverbally by the professional providing intervention.

During mediation, the adult transmits the meaning underlying an object, event, or experience (i.e., interprets *why* something exists, happens, or may occur), and guides the adolescent to comprehend this meaning. Transmittal of meaning is intentional on the part of the adult. During language intervention, transmittal of meaning through mediation provides adolescents with a strong rationale for the session's objectives and activities. The inclusion of a statement regarding *why* an adolescent is being asked to do something is a key factor in that person's participation in behavioral changes. Adolescents also tend to be less resistant to intervention when they receive an explanation of the relevance of planned activities. It is particularly helpful to anchor the explanation to academic, personal-social, and vocational areas appropriate to the various stages of adolescence. Table 7.7 illustrates examples of mediated learning experiences, as contrasted with nonmediated learning experiences during intervention.

Mediation assists adolescents to become more and more capable of modifying their own communication behaviors as intervention progresses and after it terminates, without the need for the professional's focusing. This is in line with Feuerstein's (1980) theory of cognitive modifiability; the more mediated learning experience an adolescent has, the more capable that individual becomes to learn independently through direct exposure to stimuli. Since the end goal of a learning strategies approach is having the adolescent know *how* to learn, mediation is a particularly important general procedure when using that program type. However, it is a procedure we strongly recommend across the other program types as well.

Mediation for adolescents occurs most obviously at the beginning of an intervention session. At this time, the professional is first introducing the day's activity. Failure to establish the activity's meaning for the adolescent could result in the demise of the session before it begins. This is crucial for professionals to remember when working with older youth since younger chil-

TABLE 7.7 EXAMPLES OF MEDIATED AND NONMEDIATED LEARNING EXPERIENCES FOR ADOLESCENTS

Object, Event, Experience	Mediated Learning Experience	Nonmediated Learning Experience
Open classroom door into a noisy hallway	Please close the door because it's so noisy in the hallway. Maybe we can block the noise until class is over.	Please, close the door now.
A set of photographs for use during intervention placed on the table	Today we're going to tell about these pictures because it's important to describe details clearly to another person. For example, if you were going to buy a new pillow for the sofa, it might be important to describe the color of the sofa, other colors in the room, who might use the pillow, and so forth. Tell me a time when it is important for you to describe something clearly to a salesperson in a store. (Wait for response.) Now we'll talk about when it might be important to describe these pictures clearly.	Tell me what you see in these pictures.
The adolescent has made an off-topic contribution to the conversation	Think about what you said in response to (*previous comment*). What you said is off-topic because it didn't add to what (*name*) just said. When you make off-topic remarks, it's difficult for the listener to follow the conversation. Staying on topic will help you to communicate better with your peers.	Stop! Get back on the topic.

dren do not necessarily need or want the underlying rationale and purpose for the session's activity(s), nor would they necessarily benefit from this mediation. Professionals should keep in mind that opportunities for mediation also occur during and after the session's activity.

When the professional is mediating an object, event, or experience for the adolescent, precise language in context should be used. Feuerstein (1980) has maintained that professionals keep adolescents functioning at a lower level by failing to teach them precise language. In an attempt not to overload adolescents with large words, smaller words are used in a multitude of ways. The end result may be confusion caused by multiple meaning words, plus a continued lack of differentiated vocabulary. Many adolescents with language disorders could become adept at using academic, vocational, and survival vocabulary, if mediated, just as many of them have become adept in using language to describe a current topic of interest (e.g., race cars, sports, popular music groups). The professional needs to focus on the precision of the adolescents' vocabulary that is evident for any topics of interest, and to mediate the importance of being equally precise in language needed for academic and/or vocational success.

Bridging While the professional providing intervention engages in mediation, the adolescent engages in bridging. Bridging is synonymous with the terms "transferring" and "generalizing." We have found bridging to be a preferable term because it tends to be more graphic for adolescents. Without the strong inclusion of bridging in intervention, adolescents will make minimal gains in using their new communication behaviors in other settings.

During bridging, adolescents apply new behaviors and strategies learned within intervention sessions to novel academic, personal-social, or vocational situations. Professionals may guide adolescents to do this bridging, but only the adolescents themselves can make a meaningful application. The application should be specific enough to demonstrate that the adolescent understands how to apply the new behavior or strategy in other relevant situations. Table 7.8 provides examples of strong bridges, in contrast with weak bridges, for a variety of behaviors and strategies.

Within Table 7.8 only one guide question for each new behavior or strategy is indicated. This is not to imply that only one probing question would be used. Rather, the professional should generate many ongoing questions about each behavior or strategy that will trigger bridging responses from adolescents throughout the intervention process. When weak bridges are given (e.g., the first response in Table 7.8 "In math class"), professionals should ask follow-up questions that encourage expansion (e.g., "*When,* in math class, might you switch topics of conversation with the teacher?").

It is a common pattern for adolescents to generate no bridges, or weak bridges, initially. The act of realizing an application for what is being learned in an educational situation appears foreign to many adolescents. However, with guidance from the adult mediator(s), adolescents gradually improve the quantity and quality of their bridges. The improvement is facilitated by the provision of a partial bridge by the speech-language pathologist and the encouragement of its completion by the adolescent. The following transcript, taken from a group session, illustrates this facilitation of bridging which may occur, i.e., when adolescents are reluctant or unable to bridge:

TABLE 7.8 STRONG AND WEAK BRIDGING BY ADOLESCENTS

New Behavior or Strategy	Professional's Guide Question	Strong Bridge	Weak Bridge
Switching topics (of conversation) appropriately	When might you have to switch topics when talking with the teacher at school? (academic bridge)	When I have two things to ask, like what assignments I'm missing and what's on the test.	In math class
Formulating questions for clarification	Are there times when you want to ask qustions for clarification, but it's not appropriate? (personal-social bridge)	I want to ask my mom something, but she's on the telephone; I want to ask my friend something, but he's taking a make-up exam.	At school; at home
Making a plan to reach a goal	Who earns a living by making plans? (vocational bridge)	City planners; architects; air traffic controllers	Adults; everybody

PROFESSIONAL: We have been practicing giving clear messages. We made it a rule to use the fewest words possible, but still to communicate the message. Think for a minute. Where else is it important to give clear messages using the fewest words possible?

ADOLESCENTS: (No response after waiting five to ten seconds)

PROFESSIONAL: Suppose you are at a pay phone. You need a ride home. You put your money in the phone and discover it is a long distance call home. The operator tells you to deposit another coin. You now have no more money. When you call from a pay phone, you can only talk for three minutes before depositing more money. How would giving a clear message be important in this situation?

ADOLESCENT 1: Better tell Mom to pick you up. Tell how to get there fast.

PROFESSIONAL: Good idea! You'd really want to get right to the point of your message when you're stranded at a pay phone. Now think for a minute about telegrams. You've been studying about telegrams and the Morse code in history. Why is it important to send short messages when wiring a telegram?

ADOLESCENTS: (No response after waiting five to ten seconds)

PROFESSIONAL: Does anyone know, is it free to send a telegram or does it cost money?

ADOLESCENT 2: Don't know.

PROFESSIONAL: Let's think about sending messages to other people when we can't see them. It costs to mail a letter. It costs to make a phone call. Do you think a telegram will be free?

ADOLESCENT 2: No, people gotta pay.

PROFESSIONAL: All right. When people send a telegram, they have to pay so much for each word. So why would it be important to send a telegram using the fewest words possible?

ADOLESCENT 2: So it don't cost much.

PROFESSIONAL: Good thinking! So it *doesn't* cost as much. Sometimes sending a clear message may save us money. Let's think of another situation. You are in the middle of study hall and you need to tell your friend something. How will clear messages help now?

ADOLESCENT 3: You better tell your friend fast. O' else the teacher may catch you and put name on the board.

PROFESSIONAL: In our school, that's true. In this case, sending a clear message could help you to avoid trouble. You've done a fine job of bridging when it is important to give clear messages using the fewest words possible.

From the transcript, notice how the professional assisted the adolescents to think about a particular communication behavior as it affected their lives. Sometimes this process is facilitated by the use of a hands-on activity, rather than relying on adolescents answering questions (e.g., bring in a telegraph key to use; practice formulating actual telegrams). With frequent exposure to the general procedure of bridging, adolescents gradually begin to generate spontaneous responses that result in positive transfers in daily communication.

Discussion The transcript included in the "Bridging" section above is a segment of a larger discussion on precise language use. Discussion with adolescents contains these elements:

1. A statement of topic (what is to be discussed)
2. Mediation by the adult providing intervention, and occasionally by one adolescent interacting with another
3. Bridging by the adolescents in response to guiding questions

4. A summation (what was discussed).

The statement of topic and summary statements are usually made by the professional. However, they may also be made by the adolescent, particularly when counseling issues are selected for discussion. Counseling discussions will be described later in this section.

From the transcript in the last section, observe that not all of the discussion's mediation is provided at one time, followed by all of the bridging. Rather, there is a fluid exchange between mediation by the adult and bridging by the adolescent. The discussion most often serves one of two major purposes:

1. To analyze communication behaviors and processes that elude adolescents with language disorders
2. To provide counseling about the communication disorder.

These purposes may also co-exist during a discussion.

Analysis of communication behaviors relies upon metacognition, metalinguistic, and metacommunication abilities, the "meta-abilities." Recall from Chapter 2 that normal adolescents are different from younger children in that they have the capacity to reflect upon and to talk about their thinking, speaking, and listening. They can also discuss the overall effectiveness of communication. The capability to engage in these meta-abilities assists adolescents to analyze their current communication behaviors and to incorporate new behaviors consciously.

Adolescents with language disorders may have deficient or absent meta-abilities. This deficiency impairs analysis of the communication behaviors that are interfering with their academic, personal-social, or vocational success. Through mediation and guided bridging, adolescents can be assisted to develop the ability to analyze their communication and to develop new behaviors.

The discussion segment in the last section illustrates adolescents who have little capacity to engage in meta-abilities independently. The opening bridging question (i.e., "Where else is it important to give clear messages using the fewest words possible?") required meta-abilities to answer. When the adolescents failed to answer this question, the professional assisted the analysis by presenting specific bridging questions related to concrete interactions. Gradually, adolescents with deficient meta-abilities begin to acquire the ability to analyze communication behaviors as demonstrated by their answering of bridging questions. Acquisition of this ability will not be immediate, and adolescents may initially be outright resistant to discussion. However, meta-abilities do begin to emerge and to solidify after several weeks to several years, depending upon: (1) the severity of the adolescent's language disorder, (2) the number of opportunities provided during discussion for bridging, and (3) the quantity and quality of the professional's mediation.

Counseling is the other primary purpose of discussion. The focus of counseling, as mentioned in Chapter 5, is to give information to adolescents about their communication disorder, to obtain information from them about their perceptions of the disorder, and to provide release and support for feelings associated with the disorder. The counseling is specific to problems associated with the communication disorder, not to topics for which speech-language pathologists are unqualified to intervene (e.g., domestic violence, suicide proneness). Adolescents with problems that extend beyond their communication disorders need more help than empathic responses from speech-language pathologists; they need emphatic referrals to trained counselors. It is unethical and impossible to try to handle all of the problems associated with adolescence within the confines of the speech-language program.

Counseling about the communication disorder should not be a segregated part of intervention, but an integral part of the process. Opening each session with a "class meeting" is a recommended way to integrate counseling. The class meeting contains three parts:

1. Adolescents' self-report on how successfully they have transferred two or three communication behaviors outside of the intervention setting
2. Issues or problems that are of primary concern to the adolescent, particularly as they relate to communication disorders
3. Opportunities for adolescents to compliment themselves or one another.

The self-report part of the class meeting targets two or three behaviors that the adolescent is trying to incorporate into daily living situations. These are selected mutually by the speech-language pathologist and the adolescent. Once the adolescent reports appropriate use of the behavior for ten consecutive sessions (the number is arbitrarily selected), it is replaced with a different behavior. The reporting relies on the honesty of the adolescent. While adolescents might occasionally misrepresent the truth, their peers in the intervention session tend to challenge these misrepresentations. Honesty is certainly desirable, but dishonesty does not destroy the value of self-reporting on communication behaviors outside of intervention. Whether honesty or dishonesty prevails, the value of adolescents' analyzing their communication (i.e., metacommunication) is retained.

The issues part of the class meeting affords a routine mechanism for uncovering significant problems in the lives of adolescents. Some days there are no issues, and the class meeting proceeds quickly to the third part (compliments). Other days, problems surface that require referral to other professionals. When speech-language pathologists are open recipients to the adolescents' feelings and attitudes, they often absorb the brunt of listening to significant problems and determining the necessary referral course. On other days, problems surface that are appropriate to discuss within the speech-language program. These problems tend to be paramount to the adolescents at that moment in time. Failure to address the problems would be detrimental to the remainder of the session. The best planned lesson is doomed if adolescents arrive at a session preoccupied with a burning issue or problem and it is dismissed as irrelevant. The best lessons with adolescents use topics of deep interest to them, such as those which surface during the issues section of the class meeting, and weave these topics into existing goals for thinking, speaking, and listening.

When problems are addressed during issues time, it is often helpful to have adolescents refer to a problem solving model chart. An example of such a chart (Thinking Publications, 1983) is illustrated in Figure 7.1. Whether this particular chart is used, or an adaptation, the logical flow of the steps within the model tends to guide the adolescents' discussion of the problem effectively. The professional monitoring the discussion should also mediate how a problem solving model can assist in analyzing and resolving other difficult issues throughout the adolescent's daily life.

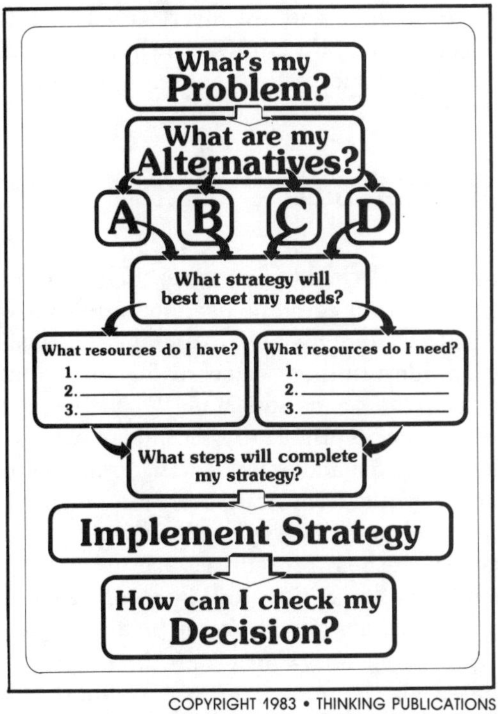

FIGURE 7.1 PROBLEM SOLVING MODEL CHART (Reprinted with permission)

The third part of the class meeting is a time for adolescents to compliment themselves and one another. Professionals should be prepared to model compliments, since the adolescents receiving intervention often have received few compliments. Compliments should focus on actions (e.g., "I like the way you said 'Good morning' to me.") rather than on physical attributes (e.g., "I like your shirt."). Initially, compliments may feel uncomfortable to adolescents. However, even this discomfort has an advantage, because compliments can be used very successfully to eliminate insults among adolescents grouped together. For every insult from one adolescent to another, have the adolescent follow it with a compliment. In our clinical experiences, giving compliments is so aversive, initially, for adolescents that it extinguishes the "put-down" behaviors. Once adolescents have seen professionals model compliments (including self-compliments), have received a number of compliments during intervention, and have been "forced" to give compliments following insults, they gradually begin voluntarily to make positive comments about themselves and fellow peers. Once that begins, group cohesiveness often becomes stronger, adolescents seem more willing to take risks to change communication behaviors, and emotional support of one another may become evident inside and outside of the intervention sessions.

The class meeting will take approximately the first five to ten minutes of the session if there are no issues and the meeting consists only of a review of objectives and compliments. The meeting may last the entire session if the issues or problems are weighty and are intertwined with the adolescents' intervention goals and objectives. Flexibility on the part of the professional will be an absolute necessity for successful implementation of the discussion.

Selected Specific Methods

Many volumes would be needed to delineate the many specific methods (i.e., procedures and materials) that could be used for thinking, listening, speaking, nonverbal communication, and survival language. Methods abound and vary with the theoretical underpinnings selected for intervention. Instead of attempting to present many methods superficially, a few representative methods will be presented with some depth. These methods have been selected because they are ones we advocate for adolescents with language disorders. They are consonant with our theoretical constructs presented in Chapter 2, and with the recommended general program type of learning strategies.

Within each specific method, procedures are described, materials are discussed, areas of emphasis are delineated, general program types that could best incorporate the method are cited, sample bridging questions that could be asked by the adult providing intervention are listed, and potential strategies that could be mediated for the adolescent are summarized. The selected specific methods are these:

1. Referential communication activities
2. Simulation and role playing activities
3. Narrative skill building activities.

Referential Communication Activities During referential communication activities, also known as "barrier activities," the communication functions of giving and getting information are emphasized. To perform these functions, adequate expression and comprehension of messages are required. This ability to express and to comprehend informative messages is a function repeated many times by competent communicators throughout a typical day. However, adolescents with language disorders often have difficulty engaging in precise message formulation and reception. Referential communication activities increase this precision (McKinley and Schwartz, 1985).

Referential communication activities are appropriate for all stages of adolescence. By altering the content and the level of difficulty, the activities become adaptable to any age and ability level.

Procedure Referential communication activities require a minimum of one speaker and one listener. They are seated near one another with a physical barrier (i.e., a screen) between them. The speaker and the listener have identical sets of materials that are concealed from each other by the screen. The speaker explains to the listener how to construct or reconstruct an identical two or three-dimensional model that the listener cannot see.

Barrier activities may involve more than one speaker and one listener simultaneously. One speaker may give directions to many listeners. Numerous speakers could collaborate on sending a clear message to one or many listeners; this is a common communication experience (e.g., a committee deciding how to word a statement; two parents agreeing on what to say after their child has misbehaved). Another option for including more than one speaker and one listener during referential communication activities is to appoint an observer(s). The observer is free to study the model the speaker is describing and to observe the responses of the listener. The observer can often see first-hand when and why any communication breakdowns are occurring. The format of assigning "speaker-listener-observer" roles is based upon the idea that people can more easily focus on the relation between speaker (message) and listener (response) when not enmeshed in one of those roles (Shantz, 1981). It may be that "vicarious" role reversal occurs by the observer, thus making it an effective experience.

Whatever combination of participants is used during barrier activities, the outcome is natural communication. There is a reason for the speaker to formulate a message and a reason for the listener to attempt to understand it. All participants, including any observers, are afforded the opportunity to observe the effects of adequate and inadequate communication.

A number of variations during referential communication activities may be utilized with adolescents. These are summarized in the list below.

1. <u>Questions for clarification versus no questions</u> Questions for clarification should be allowed initially between the listener and the speaker. They should not only be encouraged, but modeled by the adult providing intervention. If the adolescent's message has been too general, Robinson (1981) has found that saying, "I've got n [4, 2, or however many] like that. I'm not sure which one you mean. Can you help me?" is more

effective than either saying, "Which one?" or guessing which referent the speaker intends (e.g., "Is it this one?").

As participants become more proficient in producing and comprehending messages, occasional sessions might be held during which questions for clarification are not allowed. During and after these sessions, adolescents should discuss and bridge their experiences (e.g., How did the rule of "no questions" affect your understanding of the message? Was the activity more or less difficult when questions were not allowed? What question(s) would you have asked if you could have? In what other situations have you been where you were not allowed to ask questions for clarification?).

2. State versus state-restate The usual sequence of events during barrier activities is for the speaker and the listener to compare models after the message has been given and questions for clarification, if allowed, have been asked. Another option is for the listener to restate the entire message to the speaker before the comparison of models is shared. The restatement may also be accomplished sequentially (i.e., as the speaker gives one part of a step-by-step message, the listener restates the information). Restatement may allow for identification of the source of any communication breakdowns and permit repair.

3. Gestures versus no gestures Initially, gestures that help to clarify the spoken message may be allowed, especially for adolescents who need the activity to be as concrete as possible. Gestures might be particularly tempting to use when spatial orientation is an important attribute to describe. Disallowance of gestures which substitute for description (e.g., pointing to a piece of the model rather than describing it) should be enforced most of the time. However, occasional use of gestures will allow the opportunity for discussion concerning how the oral message becomes modified with and without accompanying gestures.

4. Partial message versus complete message When adolescents begin referential communication activities, they are more likely to be successful if partial messages are sent and received in sequential order. Later on, speakers should be required to send the entire message at once, and listeners should be required to receive the whole message prior to beginning the response. This requires memory strategies, thus making the level of the task more difficult.

5. Questions for information versus clarification This variation of referential communication activities requires the listener to ask questions for information rather than questions for clarification. The speaker in turn supplies responses to these questions rather than initiating the content of the message. For example, if "wh" questions are allowed, then the questions might include: What shapes are used? What size is the triangle? and Where is it placed? The activities could also be structured to require the listener to ask Yes-No questions. The speaker remains in control of the

model to be duplicated. However, the listener must employ careful questioning strategies to obtain all the necessary information to complete the activity successfully.

Materials Materials for referential communication activities may be either two or three-dimensional. In both cases, the materials should be sophisticated enough so they do not cause embarrassment to the adolescent. Regardless of the material selected, two or more identical sets will be needed.

The adult providing intervention should mediate for the adolescent that the model constructed or reconstructed with the materials is secondary to the communication process occurring. Referential communication has not been successful until the speaker and the listener share a common meaning for the message. When communication breakdowns occur, they should be analyzed and repaired.

Depending upon the focus of the barrier activity, the materials may be natural or contrived. For example, actual objects may be used (i.e., natural materials), and the speaker must describe to the listener how to orient them to one another. On the other end of the spectrum, materials may be contrived, such as drawing two-dimensional representations of objects.

An additional material that is sometimes desirable during referential communication activities is a tape recorder. With a tape recorder, the speaker's message can be recorded and replayed to prevent discrepancies between what was perceived to have been communicated versus what actually was communicated.

Areas of Emphasis The most common areas of emphasis during referential communication activities are speaking and listening. The role of the adolescent engaged in the activities may alternate between speaker and listener, or one role may be assigned throughout. Regardless of the specific content of an activity, ongoing opportunities are available for producing and comprehending clear messages.

If the content of the referential communication activities is carefully planned, then areas of emphasis may also include thinking behaviors, nonverbal communication, and survival language. For example, thinking may be emphasized more specifically if the materials selected require application of spatial, quantitative, and qualitative concepts. Nonverbal communication may be emphasized if messages that could be more easily communicated with gestures, or a combination of gestures and oral language, are utilized. For example: Give each adolescent a group of pictures illustrating such actions as someone waving a flag, starting a lawn mower with a pull rope, and bouncing a ball. Through gestures, the adolescent can communicate to the receivers what picture is to be matched. Also, using the format of gestures versus no gestures (cited under "Procedure" above), provides a means for focusing upon the area of nonverbal communication.

An emphasis on survival language behaviors during referential communication activities is best accomplished when tasks from the adolescent's natural environment are planned. Activities chosen should relate as closely as possible to situations in which the adolescent would actually be placed. For example, have the adolescent give a message about how to find several items in a storage closet or drawer.

General Program Types Referential communication activities are most commonly used during a learning strategies program. The activities assist adolescents to discover strategies they might use to send or to receive messages more effectively. Referential communication activities may also be used in conjunction with a basic skills program and with a functional curriculum program when survival language content is stressed. Usually, referential communication activities would not be compatible with a tutorial program.

Bridging Questions Speech-language pathologists using referential communication activities might consider asking these bridging questions during or after the activities:

1. In what other situations has it been important to communicate a message clearly?
2. Tell me about a time when you were talking and a breakdown in communication occurred, i.e., you were the cause of the breakdown. What were the consequences?
3. Tell me about a time when you were listening and a breakdown in communication occurred, i.e., you were the cause of the breakdown. What were the consequences?
4. Give an example of when you asked a question for clarification. Did it prevent a communication breakdown?
5. You have just been prevented from using gestures and eye contact when saying your message. When else are you prevented from using nonverbal communication?

Strategies to Mediate A partial list of strategies that the speech-language pathologist could mediate during referential communication activities include these:

1. Visualizing the information being spoken or listened to (i.e., seeing the model "in your mind")
2. Using a plan to organize the information (i.e., what is most important to say first, next, last?)
3. Concentrating attention on the speaker when in the role of a listener (i.e., blocking out distractions)
4. Knowing how and when to ask a question for clarification
5. Using appropriate concepts (e.g., spatial, quantity, quality) to make messages concise

6. Taking the listener's perspective when producing a message.

Simulation and Role Playing Activities Simulation includes activities that "... are designed to teach participants to deal more effectively with life situations" (Fine, 1983, p. 11). Activities represent the real world and allow adolescents nonthreatening, nonembarrassing opportunities to practice communication behaviors before entering actual situations.

During role playing, participants "make believe" that a constructed situation is real and react to it in a spontaneous manner (Buchan, 1972). The constructed situation may simulate a real life or an imaginary situation. The key factor in role playing is spontaneity. In simulation, participants may be spontaneous or use a structured script.

The overlap between simulation and role playing is great. Both share theoretical constructs based upon Inhelder and Piaget's (1958) premise that knowledge is born of action and that anything is understood only to the extent that it is reinvented. Both share common procedures and require participants, a scene, and action.

Simulation and role playing activities can be used during early adolescence, through middle adolescence, and into late adolescence. This presumes that the simulations and role plays will be based upon situations appropriate to a given age level.

Procedure The general sequence of steps for simulation and role playing are these (Chesler and Fox, 1966):

1. Preparation and instruction
2. Dramatic action and discussion
3. Evaluation.

Preparation and instruction include problem selection, warm-up, and instructions given to the participants and audience members. Problem selection may be done before the intervention session by the speech-language pathologist, or it may arise from concerns expressed by adolescents. The problem may be serious or light; past, present, or future-oriented; controversial or noncontroversial. Once the problem has been selected, a warm-up exercise may be advisable. Warm-up is "... the process of getting an individual or group to loosen up and ready to participate actively in the session" (Buchan, 1972, p. 56). The warm-up exercise may be a simple dramatization (e.g., calling on pairs to introduce each other or to describe their favorite food), or the warm-up exercise may involve a pretense of being something (e.g., a machine) or doing something (e.g., painting a wall). Whatever is chosen, the warm-up process should be short. It should also help adolescents to become more receptive to suggestions and to reduce inhibitions (Thompson, 1978). The last aspect of the procedure, instructions, should specify the scene and the exact role that participants are to play, e.g., is the participant to play a nice teacher or a grouchy one; should an angry tone of voice be used, or a calm one, or neither? Instructions should also be given to audience members not acting out dramatic roles. What, specifically, should they be observing while they watch the role play?

The second step of simulation and role playing includes both the enactment of the drama and the interpretation of the action. Dramatic action may be enhanced by the techniques of role reversal, mirroring, and modeling (Buchan, 1972). In role reversal, one person exchanges roles with another to facilitate seeing the other person's perspective. For example, if one adolescent is role playing a student, and another one is role playing a parent, they might subsequently change roles. Role reversal generates alternative solutions in a problem situation and makes it possible for adolescents to demonstrate how they would like to be treated in a given situation.

In mirroring, the adult leading intervention assumes the place of one of the adolescents who had been role playing a character. Then, the adult repeats the scene just played while the adolescent observes, i.e., as if seeing himself or herself in a mirror. Mirroring permits adolescents an opportunity to see what their communication behaviors are, not what they *think* they are.

In modeling, the speech-language pathologist demonstrates appropriate use of a communication behavior after another adolescent has displayed the behavior inappropriately. Modeling shows how a particular behavior should be applied within a specific communicative context. At the conclusion of the action, it is important to have adolescents dissociate with the roles that they assumed. Once this dissociation has occurred, a discussion should ensue that encourages the application of desirable communication behaviors observed during the simulation or the role play.

The final step of the simulation and role playing procedure is evaluation. During evaluation, the speech-language pathologist and the adolescents review the successes and failures of the role playing or simulation experience. Do additional reenactments of the scene have to be played to practice appropriate communication behaviors? The purposes and effects of simulation and role playing should be evaluated by the speech-language pathologist to determine what evidence there is to show that adolescents have learned new communication behaviors.

Materials Before dramatic action of the simulation or role play commences, the scene should be set carefully. The physical setting should be established (e.g., the location of doors, windows, and furniture; the sounds, smells, lighting, and temperature of the setting). Speech-language pathologists may make the setting concrete by using the actual objects being described for the scene, or abstract by using no props and asking adolescents to imagine how the scene would look, sound, feel, and smell. Obviously, a combination of concrete and abstract aspects may be used. Objects or people may also be used in an abstract way during the simulation, e.g., a table may be used to represent a city park; an adolescent may play an auxiliary role such as a mailbox or a tree, if it is important to the action. In addition to establishing firmly the physical setting, the time of day and the date should be determined, when necessary to do so, before the action begins.

Whether materials are concrete or abstract during simulation and role playing, they are more natural than contrived. Adolescents should recognize the physical scenes that are set as ones that closely approximate their daily communication situations.

An additional material that is frequently helpful is videotape and its related equipment. It can be very beneficial to tape the role playing or simulation activities, then to analyze the action by watching the tape during discussion and evaluation. However, videotape should be used cautiously if it is a first experience for adolescents. Many people can remember their own shock the first time they observed themselves on a screen. Adolescents should first become accustomed to seeing themselves engaged in normal activities on videotape before observing themselves in role playing or simulation.

Areas of Emphasis The most common areas of emphasis during simulation and role playing are speaking, listening, and survival language. Speaking opportunities are afforded during participation in a role and in follow-up discussions. Listening opportunities are present when playing a role and when observing others as an audience member. Survival language behaviors are almost always foremost when engaging in simulation activities, e.g., language needed in a restaurant, in a post office, in a bank.

Like referential communication activities, careful planning can result in areas of emphasis also encompassing nonverbal communication and thinking behaviors. For example, during setting of the scene, participants could be instructed to stand too far apart from each other for effective communication (instruct the adolescents specifically where to stand); audience members can be instructed to observe and to discuss primarily the nonverbal communication behaviors of the participants. Thinking behaviors can be emphasized during problem situations that have a multitude of alternative solutions, or during discussion when hypothetical questions are asked.

General Program Types Simulation and role playing would not be used with a tutorial program, and would have limited use with a basic skills program. Role playing and simulation are most common during learning strategies and functional curriculum program types. Role playing and simulation allow adolescents the opportunity to see the consequences of communication when a situation is reenacted from several different perspectives. The adolescent has the opportunity to analyze which communicative interaction was most successful and why (i.e., what strategies were being used at the time?). Within a functional curriculum program, simulation is one of the best methods for preparing adolescents to develop adequate communication for a variety of common situations.

Bridging Questions Speech-language pathologists might consider asking these bridging questions during or after role playing and simulation activities:

1. In the role play you just completed, you had to take the perspective of another person. When else is it important to take the perspective of another person? How is this helpful?
2. Perspective has as its root word "spec" which means to see. What other words do you know that have "spec" as a root? Do all of the words have something to do with seeing?
3. In the role plays you just completed for the selected problem today (describe the problem), there were several different alternatives. Describe other problem situations that have alternative answers. Do any problem situations have only one solution? Defend your answer.
4. In the simulation activity you just completed, you used hypothetical thinking (e.g., if this happened, then this would be appropriate to say; if that happened, then that would be appropriate to say). Where else have you used hypothetical thinking at home? When with your friends?
5. In the last role play, one of the characters was told to be very egocentric. This means to hold only to your point of view and not to take the perspective of someone else. Describe a time when you or someone you know has been egocentric. What were the consequences of being egocentric?

Strategies to Mediate A partial list of strategies that the speech-language pathologist could mediate during role playing and simulation activities include these:

1. Taking the perspective of the listener (i.e., how might saying or doing something affect the feelings of another person involved in the role playing or simulation activity?)
2. Considering alternatives to the same problem situation
3. Memorizing certain standard scripts (e.g., introduction, greeting)
4. Imagining yourself in the situation, saying and doing what you think is best
5. Listening for relevant details of what other characters are saying
6. Thinking about two or more sources of information (if there are three or more participants in the role play).

Narrative Skill Building Activities A wide array of discourse-level skills are needed for successful participation in social and academic pursuits, including instructions, reports, explanations, and story telling during conversation. As children reach adolescence, the ability to comprehend and to produce larger units of language becomes increasingly important for peer acceptance and academic survival. Whereas younger children often receive help from teachers and parents to fill-in narrations, adolescents are often not helped, and their "... discourse disarray [may be viewed] as basically inconsiderate, thoughtless, inattentive, or willfully dense" (Garnett, 1986, p. 45)

Narrative skill building activities can be used during early, middle, and late stages of adolescence. Narration activities should be chosen with the adolescent's social-emotional level and interests in mind.

Procedure Westby (1985) has suggested three levels of activities for enhancing narrative skills. Goals for each level have been summarized as follows (Westby, 1985):

1. "Provide exposure to literate language. Structure interactions to facilitate reporting.
2. Facilitate understanding of relationships among character traits, emotions, and events. Require child to structure the narrative.
3. Facilitate comprehension of more complex embedded narratives. Facilitate metanarrative skills." (p. 208)

Although it is desirable for adolescents to be performing at the highest level of activity, they may need to acquire more concrete behaviors before abstract abilities such as metanarrative skills develop. Obviously, activities recommended at the early, more concrete, level (Westby, 1985) to provide exposure to literate language for young children (e.g., "show and tell" time, dramatization of nursery rhymes) are not appropriate at the adolescent level. However, exposure can be promoted through activities such as listening to "Books on Tape" that are of interest to adolescents; watching movies, home videos, or Public Broadcasting System literary presentations based upon any of the "Books on Tape" (e.g., *The Other Side of the Mountain*, Valens, 1975); and listening to old time radio dramatizations such as Orson Wells' "War of the Worlds."

Adolescents should be assisted to report on stories like those cited above, as well as personal stories, using scaffolding techniques for narrative development. "Scaffolding is the use of leading questions that help the speaker organize [the] story" (Page and Stewart, 1985, p. 25). Garnett (1986) has suggested that a chart listing major elements of a story can be used as a guide for narrators and for discussion after the story. Table 7.9 suggests the content of this chart for adolescents. Younger adolescents, or those less skilled in narration, should be guided to use the concrete scaffolding items first (e.g., setting, events), both when listening to stories and when telling them. As narrative skills emerge, abstract elements of a story (e.g., theme, moral) should receive focus. When these more skilled adolescents hear stories that they retell, they should be able to answer all of the questions listed in Table 7.9. When they tell stories, the beginning is marked by a description of setting and the ending is marked by a conclusion, but the elements listed in between vary in sequence and in whether they need to be included.

TABLE 7.9 A SUGGESTED CHART OF STORY ELEMENTS TO BE USED AS A GUIDE FOR NARRATORS

Elements of a Story

Beginning Setting of story
- Who are the main characters?
- Where does the story take place?
- When does the story take place?

Theme of the story
- What is the main idea (theme) of the story?

Response to the story
- Did you like the story? Why or why not?

Events of the story
- What happens to the characters?

Goal(s) of the characters
- What are the characters trying to do?

Motive(s) of the characters
- Why are the characters trying to reach the goal(s)?

Attempts
- What happens when the characters try to reach the goal?

Reactions of the characters
- What are their feelings?
- What are their plans?

Ending Conclusion
- How does everything turn out?
- What lesson (moral) did you learn from the story?

Similar scaffolding could be developed for narrations which are not stories, such as the structure an adolescent uses for giving an oral report in class. For example, these questions could be asked: What is the main idea? What is the problem? What are some solutions? What can other people do to help? How can I summarize my report? The list of example questions is useful when the organizational scheme for the report is problem/solution. Different questions would need to be asked if another organizational scheme is used (e.g., chronological order, compare and contrast, cause and effect). Verbal scaffolding questions might initially be specific to a single report and later be phrased more generically, like the questions for stories in Table 7.9. As adolescents become familiar with various elements of narration and practice logical sequencing of the elements, they should be encouraged to remind themselves of the questions to be answered during the narration. Reliance on a chart, or on someone to ask the questions of them should be discouraged.

Page and Stewart (1985) and Westby (1985) emphasize the importance of direct instruction in improving cause-and-effect relationships as a general means to developing narration skills. Emphasis should be on relationships that are most essential to stories, including the effects of the environment on people, animals, and events; the effects of various types of people (e.g., the "do-gooder," the "villain") and animals on events; the effects of events on feelings and conversely, the effects of feelings on events; and the knowledge that much behavior is intentionally planned. Through mediation and discussion, adolescents should be presented with questions such as these:

1. How do you identify emotions?
2. What causes feelings?
3. What do people do when they feel a certain way?
4. What would you predict (*character name*) will do in this situation? Why?

At the highest level of narration, adolescents should discuss themes, plots, and/or morals of stories (Westby, 1985). They should talk about the structure of narratives and how to vary structure intentionally for different purposes, i.e., metanarrative skills. Adolescents might tell stories from the perspectives of different characters, or tell a similar story with different endings. For example, *Choose Your Own Adventure* books, *Twist-A-Plot* books, and similar series allow each story to be completed in several dozen ways. A *Choose Your Own Adventure* book could be read to the adolescent, followed by informational and critical listening questions concerning characters and events. At the frequent decision points within the story, the adolescent can be asked which choice to select and why. Following completion of the story once, or in a number of different ways, the adolescent can reformulate it using the assistance of self-imposed scaffolding questions.

Throughout narrative skill building activities, professionals should be particularly aware of oral expression difficulties that interfere with clear formulation or reformulation, e.g., word retrieval problems, verbal mazes, inappropriate use of sentence fragments, nonspecific language including lack of pronoun references. These problems must be addressed before adequate narrative skills can be expected. Many specific remediation procedures for oral expression problems exist in the literature, and professionals should avail themselves of these resources (e.g., Simon, 1980; Wiig, 1982b).

Materials The primary materials needed for narrative skill building activities are books, audio cassette tapes, and playback equipment. The books and tapes selected should provide models for well-structured narrations. Secondary-level English teachers are a good resource for selecting quality literature that is of interest to most adolescents. When the selected books are not available on tape, service groups in high schools are often willing to assume responsibility to tape the necessary books. In addition to professionally recorded "Books on Tape" and amateur productions, there are some nonfictional lectures on audio tape that could be used with adolescents to study narrations that are not stories (e.g., Leo Buscaglia's [1982] tape program entitled *LOVE*).

When books not on tape are used for narrative skill building activities by professionals, they should be read to the adolescent, or paraphrased, so the primary task remains one of listening, not reading. In some cases, it might be desirable for the adolescent to follow along in the book as it is being read, so that both auditory and visual modalities are used. Usually, it is not appropriate that during oral language intervention the primary task of adolescents should be that of reading stories.

Areas of Emphasis Speaking and listening are the most often emphasized areas during narrative skill building activities. Listening is primary when reformulation tasks are presented; speaking is necessary during both formulation and reformulation tasks.

As with the other two specific methods already described, thinking and nonverbal communication can be focused upon if the tasks are structured appropriately. For example, requesting the adolescent's underlying reasoning for why a particular choice was made within a *Twist-a-Plot* story places emphasis on thinking during the activity. Asking the adolescent to predict how the facial expression just described in the story will affect the feelings of another character places emphasis on nonverbal communication.

Survival language skills are often not emphasized if the narrative activities focus on fiction, as they frequently do. However, narrative tasks which involve formulating or reformulating reports or explanations, for example, might focus almost exclusively on survival language (e.g., the weather report announces an impending hurricane that affects the adolescent's geographical area).

General Program Types Narrative skill building activities are most common within a basic skills program. Current intervention activities for narration emphasize a hierarchy of skills which must be acquired. Narrative skill building activities are also compatible with a learning strategies program when the activities emphasize *how* to formulate or reformulate narratives effectively (e.g., using a scaffolding technique).

A functional curriculum program would make use of narrative skill building activities infrequently, only when activities are organized to emphasize an area within survival language. A tutorial program does not utilize narrative skill building activities unless the adolescent's teachers in the classroom happen to be emphasizing them as part of the curriculum.

Bridging Questions Adults providing intervention might consider asking these bridging questions during or after formulation or reformulation tasks:

1. In the story, one of the main characters felt very (*emotion*). When is a time you felt that way? What event led to your feeling that way?
2. What happens when the setting of a story is never explained? Think of a time someone tried to tell you something and you did not know the setting. Think of a time you tried to tell someone else a story and forgot to tell them the setting.
3. In some stories, you can predict how the characters will feel or act next. When (besides in stories) do you predict something that will happen? How can predictions help you?
4. Sometimes reports are organized by describing the problem and then giving solutions. What are some topics you could organize that way? Sometimes it is easier to organize reports by the order of events (i.e., first, next, last). What are some topics you could organize that way? Sometimes reports are organized by comparing how things or ideas are the same and how they are different. What are some topics you could organize that way?
5. The group has been talking about cause and effect. Tell me something funny that happened to you. Together, let us figure out what caused it to be funny.

Strategies to Mediate A partial list of strategies that the professional could mediate during narrative skill building activities include these:

1. Asking key questions of yourself to help organize the narrative (i.e., scaffolding)
2. Listening for the major organizational structure of a narrative
3. Using cohesion devices to connect ideas in the narrative together (i.e., to make the narrative easier for listeners to understand)
4. Predicting outcomes of events as a way to remember "what happens next"
5. Describing the setting of a story first, before much action is begun
6. Pretending you are a character in the story, and everything happens to you as you retell the story from that character's perspective.

Commercial Resources For Adolescents

Many commercial resources, both computer-assisted and traditional, have been developed for adolescents in the last decade. Because of the burgeoning number of computer-assisted instructional programs (CAI) appropriate for adolescents, they will be addressed separately, later in this section. Table 7.10 summarizes some of the traditional resources that professionals might consider when intervening with adolescents. The table is not intended to be a critique of the commercial resources available, but rather a summary of key information. Each commercial resource has this summary information: Resource name, author(s), publisher, copyright, area(s) of modification, stage of adolescence (i.e., at which the resource is appropriate), documentation, natural versus contrived procedures, and natural versus contrived materials. Several of the columns in Table 7.10 are self-explanatory; however, the latter three may not be. A description of these three categories follows.

The term "documentation" refers to whether the commercial resource includes information concerning the philosophical tenets, theoretical premises, or literature support underlying the material. A cursory glance at Table 7.10 will reveal that many commercial resources fail to provide documentation for users. The lack of documentation is alarming because the resource may conflict with theoretical constructs of other approaches and resources utilized during intervention. If a resource does not have documentation, then users should spend considerable time before choosing the resource for a given adolescent, to make certain that it is appropriate to use.

Natural versus contrived materials refer to how similar or dissimilar the materials are to everyday situations. Materials can be aligned on a continuum from natural to contrived. The most natural material for an adolescent would be none, or materials identical to those located in actual communication situations (e.g., real money, real job application forms, real menus from restaurants). Absence of materials is also considered natural, because much of the time when normal adolescents are engaged in conversations no materials are selected by them, i.e., a group of adolescents frequently carries on a conversation removed from the here-and-now. Contrived materials refer to those that are artificial to everyday contexts (e.g., flash cards used to learn new vocabulary). While it might be tempting to think that naturalistic materials are always better than contrived, the materials depend on the objectives and the adolescent. Contrived materials are often good for teaching strategies. They can act as a catalyst for generating more naturalistic discussion among adolescents. In our clinical experiences, we have found it disastrous to attempt a discussion with early adolescents without the assistance of some contrived material that triggers their interest in bridging questions. On the other hand, adolescents should be able to communicate appropriately when naturalistic materials are used, by the time they are dismissed from intervention.

Natural versus contrived procedures refer to how similar or dissimilar the procedures are to everyday situations. Natural procedures for adolescents include those which replicate most closely daily communication situations, e.g., conversing with a friend, asking a teacher a question in the classroom. On the other end of the continuum are contrived procedures which differ the most from daily communication situations. For example, use of a drill-and-practice exercise is one in which people do not typically engage in a daily situation.

TABLE 7.10 TRADITIONAL COMMERCIAL RESOURCES FOR ADOLESCENTS

Program	Areas of Modification	Stage of Adolescence	Documentation	Natural/ Contrived Materials	Natural/ Contrived Procedures
ALP: Active Listening Program. van der Laan, C. Thinking Publications, Eau Claire, WI (1986).	Listening	Early Middle Late	Yes	Contrived	Contrived
COMMUNICATE. Mayo, P., and Waldo, P. Thinking Publications, Eau Claire, WI (1986).	Listening Speaking	Early Middle	Yes	Contrived	Natural/ Contrived
Communication Workshop. Zakim, S. Linguisystems, Inc., Moline, IL (1986).	Listening Speaking Nonverbal Communication	Early Middle Late	No	Contrived	Natural/ Contrived
CoRT Thinking Lessons. deBono, E. Pergamon Press, New York, NY (1981).	Thinking	Early Middle Late	Yes	Contrived	Natural
Communicative Competence: A Functional-Pragmatic Language Program. Simon, C. Communication Skill Builders, Tucson, AZ (1980).	Thinking Listening Speaking	Early Middle Late	Yes	Natural/ Contrived	Natural/ Contrived
Daily Communication: Strategies for the Language Disordered Adolescent. Schwartz, L., and McKinley, N. Thinking Publications, Eau Claire, WI (1984).	Thinking Listening Speaking Nonverbal Communication Survival Language	Early Middle Late	Yes	Natural/ Contrived	Natural/ Contrived

TABLE 7.10 CONTINUED

Program	Areas of Modification	Stage of Adolescence	Documentation	Natural/ Contrived Materials	Natural/ Contrived Procedures
FILE: File of Intermediate Language Exercises. Richard, G. Linguisystems, Inc., Moline, IL (1983).	Speaking	Early Middle Late	No	Contrived	Natural/ Contrived
HELP: Handbook of Exercises for Language Processing (Volumes I and II). Lazzari, A., and Peters, P. Linguisystems, Inc., Moline, IL (1980).	Listening Speaking	Early Middle Late	No	Contrived	Contrived
In Other Words. Agency for Instructional Technology, Bloomington, IN (1983).	Listening	Early Middle	No	Contrived	Contrived
Interview. Cornelius, Jr., E. Longman, Inc., New York, NY (1981).	Listening	Middle Late	No	Natural	Contrived
The Language of Humor. Ertmer, D. Linguisystems, Inc., Moline, IL (1984).	Thinking	Early Middle	Yes	Contrived	Contrived
LAPSS: Listening and Auditory Processing for Secondary Students. Delfosse, A. Linguisystems, Inc., Moline, IL (1985).	Listening Speaking Survival Language	Early Middle Late	No	Natural/ Contrived	Natural/ Contrived
Let's Talk: Developing Prosocial Communication Skills. Wiig, E. Charles E. Merrill Publishing Co., Columbus, OH (1982).	Speaking	Early Middle Late	Yes	Contrived	Contrived

TABLE 7.10 CONTINUED

Program	Areas of Modification	Stage of Adolescence	Documentation	Natural/ Contrived Materials	Natural/ Contrived Procedures
Let's Talk: Intermediate Level. Wiig, E., and Bray, C. Charles E. Merrill Publishing Co., Columbus, OH (1984).	Speaking	Early Middle Late	Yes	Natural/ Contrived	Natural/ Contrived
Listening In and Speaking Out-Intermediate. James, G., Whitley, C., and Bode, S. Longman, Inc., New York, NY (1980).	Listening Speaking	Early Middle	No	Natural	Contrived
Listening In and Speaking Out-Advanced. Bode, S., Whitley, C., and James, G. Longman, Inc., New York, NY (1981).	Listening Speaking	Middle Late	No	Natural	Contrived
Listening Skills Development. Eggleston, P., and Riggs, R. The Oregon Teaching Center, Redmond, OR (1982).	Listening	Early	No	Contrived	Contrived
MEER: Manual of Exercises for Expressive Reasoning. Zachman, L., Jorgensen, C., Barrett, M., Huisingh, R., and Snedden, M. Linguisystems, Inc., Moline, IL (1982).	Thinking Listening Speaking	Early Middle Late	No	Contrived	Contrived
Mind Benders. Harnadek, A. Midwest Publications Co., Pacific Grove, CA (1978).	Thinking	Middle Late	No	Contrived	Contrived
PROBLEM SOLVER. Waldo, P. Thinking Publications, Eau Claire, WI (1986).	Thinking Speaking	Early Middle Late	Yes	Contrived	Natural/ Contrived
Referential Communication: Barrier Activities for Speakers and Listeners (Parts One and Two). McKinley, N., and Schwartz, L. Thinking Publications, Eau Claire, WI (1985).	Thinking Listening Speaking	Early Middle Late	Yes	Contrived	Natural

TABLE 7.10 CONTINUED

Program	Areas of Modification	Stage of Adolescence	Documentation	Natural/ Contrived Materials	Natural/ Contrived Procedures
SCRIPTING: Social Communication for Adolescents. Mayo, P., and Waldo, P. Thinking Publications, Eau Claire, WI (1986).	Speaking	Early Middle	Yes	Contrived	Natural/ Contrived
Semantic Fitness. Keffer, C., and Long, C. Linguisystems, Inc., Moline, IL (1986).	Thinking Speaking	Middle Late	No	Contrived	Contrived
Situational Language: A Pragmatic Approach to Problem Solving. Huisingh, R., Barrett, M., Zachman, L., Jorgensen, C., and Snedden, M. Linguisystems, Inc., Moline, IL (1984).	Thinking Speaking	Early Middle Late	No	Natural/ Contrived	Natural/ Contrived
Skillstreaming the Adolescent: A Structured Learning Approach to Teaching Prosocial Skills. Goldstein, A., Sprafkin, R., Gershaw, N., and Klein, P. Research Press, Champaign, IL (1980).	Thinking Speaking Nonverbal Communication	Early Middle Late	Yes	Contrived	Natural/ Contrived
Teaching Functional Academics: A Curriculum Guide for Adolescents and Adults with Learning Problems. Bender, M., and Valletutti, P. Pro-Ed, Austin, TX (1982).	Survival Language	Middle Late	No	Natural	Natural/ Contrived
Transfer Activities: Thinking Skill Vocabulary Development. Mayo, P., and Gajewski, N. Thinking Publications, Eau Claire, WI (1986).	Thinking	Early Middle	Yes	Contrived	Natural/ Contrived

TABLE 7.10 CONTINUED

Program	Areas of Modification	Stage of Adolescence	Documentation	Natural/ Contrived Materials	Natural/ Contrived Procedures
Warm-up Exercises: Calisthenics for the Brain (Books I and II). Kisner, R., and Knowles, B. Thinking Publications, Eau Claire, WI (1984 and 1985).	Listening Speaking	Early Middle Late	No	Contrived	Contrived
Words, Expressions, Contexts: A Figurative Language Program. Wiig, E. Charles E. Merrill Publishing Co., Columbus, OH (1985).	Listening Speaking	Early Middle Late	Yes	Natural/ Contrived	Contrived

The professional should select the procedure that is most appropriate for the given adolescent and objective. Adolescents who are initially learning a new behavior may be greatly assisted by using a one-on-one drill-and-practice procedure. However, as behaviors are acquired, it is important to move procedures toward normal communication. Failure to do this will lessen the degree to which behaviors are likely to be transferred. Before dismissal from intervention, adolescents should be able to communicate successfully.

It is our contention that some professionals consistently use contrived materials and contrived procedures with adolescents, and thus fail to move them along the continuum toward more natural contexts. Intervention using contrived materials and procedures would use a high amount of one-on-one work with structured intervention programs. To reiterate, this is appropriate for some adolescents some of the time. However, in our clinical experiences, the benefits of intervention for the adolescent in other situations will not be apparent until procedures and materials become more natural.

Many commercial resources which have contrived materials and procedures can be moved along the continuum toward "naturalistic" through the general procedures of mediation, bridging, and discussion explained previously in this chapter. For example, it is not unusual for some commercial materials to list an objective at the beginning of the activity and a brief summary of the procedures to use. With adolescents, this objective needs to be mediated before and during the activity if changes in communication behaviors that generalize are desired. It is also essential that adolescents bridge the content of the objective that is specified in the commercial resource to other situations. Focusing the activity so that adolescents grasp the meaning of the activity and recognize the application in their lives results in the materials and procedures being less contrived and more natural. If professionals using the commercial materials fail to see the relevance of the prescribed objectives, a general rule is not to use that commercial resource. If the adults providing intervention cannot verbalize a strong rationale for adolescents as to *why* they should learn a particular behavior specified in the commercial resource, then it will not be taught successfully.

Computer-Assisted Instruction and Language Intervention for Adolescents The computer is a professional tool which, if used wisely, can assist the speech-language pathologist in working with adolescents with language disorders. Guidelines for using the microcomputer in language intervention have been proposed by Larson and Steiner (1985). Table 7.11 presents a review of some representative software that may be used with adolescents as part of their intervention sessions. This list of software is not exhaustive and does not provide a critique of the software presented. We would strongly urge speech-language pathologists to review carefully the existing software before purchasing it, since some software packages are disappointing. The software review process can be facilitated by using one of the many existing software review systems such as USERS I and USERS II (Greyerbiehl et al., 1986a; 1986b).

TABLE 7.11 COMPUTER-ASSISTED COMMERCIAL RESOURCES FOR ADOLESCENTS

Software Program	Areas of Modification	Stage of Adolescence	CAI Activity
Birth of the Phoenix. Phoenix Software, Inc., Lake Zurich, IL (1981).	Thinking (Listening)	Middle Late	Instructional Game
Botticelli. Krell Software Corp., Stony Brook, NY (1983).	Thinking (Listening)	Early Middle Late	Instructional Game
Cause and Effect. Collins, M. Hartley Courseware Inc., Dimondale, MI (1985)	Thinking (Listening)	Early Middle	Drill and Practice
Challenging Analogies. Micro Power and Light Co., Dallas, TX (1982).	Thinking (Listening)	Late	Drill and Practice
Connections. Krell Software Corp., Stony Brook, NY (1983).	Thinking	Early Middle Late	Instructional Game
Do I Know Enough? *Solutions Unlimited.* Decision Development Corp., Agency for Instructional Technology, Bloomington, IN (1984).	Thinking (Listening)	Early Middle	Problem Solving
Fact or Opinion. Savitsky, D., and Savitsky, S. Learning Well, Roslyn Heights, NY (1985).	Thinking (Listening)	Early Middle Late	Instructional Game
The Factory. Kosel, M., and Fish, M. Sunburst Communications, Inc., Pleasantville, NY (1984).	Thinking	Early Middle Late	Problem Solving

TABLE 7.11 CONTINUED

Software Program	Areas of Modification	Stage of Adolescence	CAI Activity
Galileo. Krell Software Corp., Stony Brook, NY (1983).	Thinking	Late	Instructional Game
Grammar Examiner. DesignWare Inc., San Francisco, CA (1984).	(Listening)	Late	Combinatorial
Hey Wait! Think, See, So? *Solutions Unlimited*. Decision Development Corp., Agency for Instructional Technology, Bloomington, IN (1984).	Thinking (Listening)	Early Middle	Problem Solving
Letters from the Past. *Solutions Unlimited*. Decision Development Corp., Agency for Instructional Technology, Bloomington, IN (1984).	Thinking (Listening)	Early Middle	Problem Solving
Mind Puzzles. Minnesota Educational Computer Consortium, St. Paul, MN (1983).	Thinking (Listening)	Middle Late	Problem Solving
Money! Money! Hartley Courseware, Inc., Dimondale, MI (1982).	Survival Language (Listening)	Early	Drill and Practice
Plan Ahead. *Solutions Unlimited*. Decision Development Corp., Agency for Instructional Technology, Bloomington, IN (1984).	Thinking (Listening)	Early Middle	Problem Solving

TABLE 7.11 CONTINUED

Software Program	Areas of Modification	Stage of Adolescence	CAI Activity
Plato's Cave. Krell Software Corp., Stony Brook, NY (1983).	Thinking (Listening)	Late	Problem Solving
The Puzzler. Sunburst Communications, Inc., Pleasantville, NY (1984).	Thinking (Listening)	Early	Problem Solving
Rocky's Boots. Robinett, W., and Grim, L. The Learning Company, Portola Valley, CA (1982).	Thinking	Middle Late	Problem Solving
Saving Energy. *Solutions Unlimited.* Decision Development Corp., Agency for Instructional Technology, Bloomington, IN (1984).	Thinking (Listening)	Early Middle	Problem Solving
Survival. *Solutions Unlimited.* Decision Development Corp., Agency for Instructional Technology, Bloomington, IN (1984).	Thinking (Listening)	Early Middle	Problem Solving
The Whitewater Canoe Race. *Solutions Unlimited.* Decision Development Corp., Agency for Instructional Technology, Bloomington, IN (1984).	Thinking (Listening)	Early Middle	Problem Solving
Who Says So? *Solutions Unlimited.* Decision Development Corp., Agency for Instructional Technology, Bloomington, IN (1984).	Thinking (Listening)	Early Middle	Problem Solving

Each software package listed on Table 7.11 has been reviewed as to the primary areas of modification it can address, i.e., thinking, listening, speaking, nonverbal communication, and survival language. In the "area of modification" column, a word in parentheses means that by presenting the software program in a different way than what it was originally designed for, it could enhance that area. For example, many programs demand reading by the user; the professional could read or paraphrase the information for the adolescent, thereby enhancing listening. The software programs were reviewed for appropriateness of use with adolescents in early, middle, or late stages of development. The last column on the table presents the computer-assisted instructional activity that the software package is designed to enhance:

1. *Drill and Practice* This approach provides repetition on concepts, tasks, or skills already taught, but in which additional practice is needed. For example, practice using a number of grammatical constructions is a drill-and-practice activity.
2. *Simulation* Simulation activities could be used when real-life situations would be unsafe, expensive, or difficult to arrange. In language intervention, a simulation may serve as an intermediate step before attempting a less controlled real situation (Larson and Steiner, 1985).
3. *Tutorial* This approach assumes no prior knowledge of a topic and, beginning at the most basic level, proceeds step-by-step to teach a given skill or concept.
4. *Instructional Games* This activity teaches instructional/problem solving tasks using a game format. An example of this software would be text or graphic adventure games.
5. *Problem-solving Activities* This type of software allows the adolescent to enter relatively unstructured information into the computer to investigate and to structure a particular concept or task. Some examples of this approach are word processors, informational retrieval systems, or problems to be solved that are presented in a gamelike situation, e.g., *The Factory* (Kosel and Fish, 1984).
6. *Combinatorial* This approach, as the name implies, combines several types of activities into one program. Many software programs do combine a number of these instructional activities.

Although most of the software packages that appear on Table 7.11 have some accompanying documentation, there is a wide range of variability. For example, *Birth of the Phoenix* (1981) has documentation that is excellent for teaching an adolescent how to engage in an adventure game. Other software packages, such as *Mind Puzzles* (1983), have documentation that provides additional off-the-computer activities to teach the same concept. Programs such as *Botticelli* (1983) present minimal information about instructional use. None of the software reviewed presented information on what theoretical foundation it had been based and if it had been field-tested for effectiveness.

SUMMARY

This chapter summarized direct intervention methods to use with adolescents when modifying communication behaviors. What behaviors to modify first, and lists of potential behaviors to teach were provided. Three general procedures that have wide application to all intervention activities were presented: Mediation, bridging, and discussion. Three specific methods, representative of appropriate procedures and materials to use with adolescents, were outlined: Referential communication activities, simulation and role playing activities, and narrative skill building activities. Commercial resources that could be used during intervention with adolescents, including existing computer software programs, were presented in tabular form. Whether general procedures, specific methods, commercial resources, or a combination of these are used, the primary focus of all direct intervention is to help adolescents to acquire appropriate and effective communication for academic, personal-social, and vocational settings.

DISCUSSION QUESTIONS

1. Discuss additional general intervention procedures under which you would operate during the intervention process with adolescents.
2. Describe additional specific intervention methods that would modify the adolescent's thinking, listening, speaking, nonverbal communication, or survival language behaviors.
3. Select several commercial resources, including at least two computer-assisted instructional packages, appropriate for adolescents. Summarize and critique these resources for language intervention.

SUGGESTED READINGS

Feuerstein, R. *Instrumental Enrichment.* Scott, Foresman, Inc., Chicago, IL, 1980.

McKinley, N. and Schwartz, L. *Referential Communication: Barrier Activities for Speakers and Listeners*. Thinking Publications, Eau Claire, WI, 1985.

Page, J. and Stewart, S. Story grammar skills in school-age children. *Topics in Language Disorders*, 5(2): 16–30, 1985.

Westby, C. Learning to talk—talking to learn: Oral-literate language differences. In: C. Simon (ed.), *Communication Skills and Classroom Success*. College-Hill Press, San Diego, CA, 1985.

CHAPTER 8

Indirect Intervention for the Adolescent

GOALS:

To describe beneficial modifications within the adolescent's educational system

To explain how to implement educational system modifications through applying a consultation model

To describe supportive modifications within the adolescent's environmental system

To explain how to initiate and maintain environmental system modifications through the use of counseling

Indirect intervention involves people from the adolescent's educational and environmental systems in activities that assist the youth to communicate more effectively. Two groups of adolescents can benefit from indirect intervention:

1. The adolescents who have communication disorders accompanied by concomitant problems within the educational and/or environmental systems contributing to their disorders (i.e., the primary problem rests within the adolescent).
2. The adolescents who have been determined during assessment not to have a communication disorder, but for whom the interdisciplinary team

recommends certain modifications at school or at home (i.e., the primary problem rests within the educational and/or environmental systems).

The major vehicle for indirect intervention within the educational system is consultation; within the environmental system, the vehicle is counseling. During consultation and counseling, the speech-language pathologist attempts to affect positive modifications for adolescents, without face-to-face contact with those youth who are having problems. While both consultation and counseling have been presented briefly in preceding chapters, in this chapter their implementation is explained.

The first section of this chapter presents how to consult within the educational system for the purpose of influencing modifications. The second section presents supportive modifications that could be made within the adolescent's environmental system, and ways to implement those changes. Table 8.1 illustrates an overview of indirect intervention for adolescents.

TABLE 8.1 INTERVENTION COMPONENT: INDIRECT SERVICES

Who?	What?	How?
Educational system members	Modifications of the system	Consultation A. Curriculum committee participation B. Content area tutoring C. Adaptation of classroom discourse D. Adaptation of materials
Environmental system members	Modifications of the system	Counseling

EDUCATIONAL SYSTEM

Deficits in the educational system may hamper both groups of adolescents cited in the opening paragraph. When these deficits revolve around language, the deficits must either be modified to meet the existing performance of the adolescent, or the adolescent's performance must be changed to cope with the system's deficiencies. Information presented in this section focuses only on modifications that can be made within the educational system, independently of alterations in the adolescent's performance, or in tandem with those alterations.

Modifications of the Educational System

When the educational system is modified to meet the language needs of adolescents, changes may be proposed in these areas:

1. The organization of curriculum materials
2. The oral language of the educator(s) during classroom discourse
3. The written language of the textbook(s) and/or other printed materials.

The oral language used by the educator to lecture, to impart directions, and to question may be too rapid, complex, or disorganized for the adolescent to comprehend. It may be laden with unfamiliar vocabulary terms or lengthy sentences. These problems may have been documented during assessment, through the self-evaluation of teacher language. (See Appendix G.) Likewise, the written language of the textbook and other printed material may be too complex for the adolescent, or may contain an abundance of novel technical terminology. The textbook and other course materials may be sequenced inappropriately, demand cognitive abilities that exceed the adolescent's present capacity, or require written responses that surpass the adolescent's ability level. (See Appendix I for how to analyze the curriculum.) For the adolescent to succeed in a course having one or all of these problems, modifications may need to be made.

How to Modify the Educational System: Consultation

Consultation is the method through which speech-language pathologists bring about modifications in the oral language of educators, the written language of classroom resources, and the organization of curriculum materials. A consultation model may be viewed as inferior if colleagues are accustomed only to direct intervention services for adolescents. Speech-language pathologists may first need to convince administrators of the merit of consultation before progress can be made. Educational systems that were analyzed to be relatively open, flexible, and responsive when subjected to the "Structure of the Educational System Checklist" (see Appendix F) may be quicker to accept a consultation model than closed, rigid systems that have preconceived ideas of what speech-language pathologists do. When an educational system is slow to accept the idea of consultation, speech-language pathologists could attempt to persuade administrators to allow a trial period after which the effectiveness of the model would be evaluated jointly.

Triadic Model of Consultation At least three individuals are involved in what has been called the triadic model of consultation (Tharp, 1975; Tharp and Wetzel, 1969). These people include: (1) the consultant, who has the content and process knowledge related to the problem (i.e., either a communication disorder within the adolescent or a curriculum deficiency related to language within the educational system); (2) the consultee, who maintains some control over the reinforcers and plays a natural role within the locale of the client; (3) the client, who has the problem behavior in need of change. For purposes of this text, we are assuming that the speech-language pathologist is functioning in the consultant's role.

Consultees are usually regular and special educators involved in programming for the adolescent, although they may be other members of the educational system (e.g., administrators, social workers, school psychologists). If the consultation model is just being initiated in a setting, it may be best to involve those educators who agreed to be placed on the list of teachers who welcomed mainstreamed students in their classes. (See Appendix H.) The assumption is that those individuals would be most receptive to consultation.

Occasionally, regular and special educators are not the consultees, but the clients, because they are the ones who have the problem to be resolved (e.g., poor classroom discourse skills, disorganized scope and sequence of objectives). In such situations, the immediate supervisor of the regular or special educator may become the consultee who helps to reinforce for the client (i.e., the teacher) what the interdisciplinary team recommends and the consultant trains. When the assistance of an immediate supervisor is enlisted, it should be done discreetly, or the speech-language pathologist will risk destroying the relationship needed with the regular or special educator to affect changes. Since most speech-language pathologists are at the same status level as regular and special educators, assistance from the administrative level should be recruited in the spirit of implementing the recommendations of the interdisciplinary team for the benefit of a student.

The collaborative approach to consultation used during program planning (see Chapter 6) is continued during intervention, whether the problem rests primarily within the adolescent or the educational system. The consultant provides support for the educator to implement changes in the classroom that are recommended by the interdisciplinary team. This difficulty may stem from the adolescent's communication disorder or from inherent problems with the language or the organization of the curriculum. When consultation involves adolescents with communication disorders, the consultant may train the educators to intervene appropriately with the problem behaviors.

The consultant should be aware that consultees will be in one of seven "stages of concern" during consultation (Hall and Loucks, 1978):

1. *Awareness* Little concern is demonstrated toward the changes needed to benefit the adolescent.
2. *Informational* A general interest is shown in learning about the needed changes.
3. *Personal* Analysis is made by consultees of the effects of the needed changes on their present role and status, and whether the changes present potential conflicts with personal commitments.
4. *Management* Attention is given to how to implement the changes, realizing they may affect scheduling, efficiency, and organization within the classroom.
5. *Consequences* Attention is focused on the relevance of changes to the adolescents and on evaluation of outcomes.
6. *Collaboration* A willingness to coordinate and cooperate with others in the use of the new procedures is expressed.
7. *Refocusing* A consideration of inducing other major changes and proposing alternatives to the existing form of previous changes is apparent.

Identification of a consultee's "stage of concern" is essential for the consultant to formulate appropriate expectations. If a consultee is at an awareness level, it is too early to expect support for modifications in the oral language of instruction, the written language of classroom resources, or the organization of curriculum materials. Beginning consultation sessions would develop awareness in the consultee, and supply information about the proposed modifications. Consultees would need to be given time for personal analysis and only then would they be ready to receive assistance in how to implement and evaluate the changes. Once a consultee has reached the collaboration stage, that person can begin supporting changes within other settings, along with the speech-language pathologist.

Idol, Paolucci-Whitcomb, and Nevin (1986) have proposed six principles of consultation that may heighten a colleague's stages of concern and improve acceptance of the consultant:

1. *Active listening facilitates meaningful interactions from all participants.* Techniques such as "door openers" (i.e., an invitation to talk), passive listening (i.e., keeping quiet), and acknowledgment responses (i.e., evidence of attending to the message) are critical to use (Gordon, 1980).
2. *Oral and written communication must rely on common nonjargon language.* The probability of shared meaning is increased when appropriate

language is used that is familiar to all participants in the triadic model.

3. *Positive nonverbal language is required to implement collaborative consultation.* Consultants should perceive subtleties of nonverbal communication and make adjustments as needed to increase the comfort level of the participants (e.g., Does the consultee prefer to meet with the consultant across a desk or seated next to the consultant in chairs?).

4. *Collaborative consultation relies on people who use appropriate interview skills.* Both the consultant and the consultee should feel free to direct the oral interaction to gain necessary and desired information.

5. *Cooperative goal structures underlie conflict resolution through collaborative consultation.* Frequently, disagreements arise over professional turf issues (e.g., "That's a speech problem [i.e., not my problem]"). Agreeing on cooperative goals helps to resolve conflict. When arguments do occur, they should be viewed as opportunities for eliciting useful information from each other.

6. *Situational leadership guides the implementation of collaborative consultation.* Leadership occurs in a "give-and-take" fashion in collaborative consultation. The style of leadership adjusts, depending on the skill and attitude levels of the consultant and consultee. Four situational leadership styles have been identified (Hersey and Blanchard, 1982). They are described from the consultant's perspective in the next paragraph.

The four leadership styles can be summarized as telling, selling, participating, and delegating (Hersey and Blanchard, 1982). When the consultee is inexperienced or insecure, and does not have a positive attitude about the proposed changes to be made, telling may be the best leadership style for the consultant to use. Telling encompasses giving specific information to the consultee and modeling tasks. When the consultee is inexperienced or insecure, but has a positive attitude toward the changes to be made, selling might be used. The consultant sets goals and provides support, but there is joint control of the task. The third style, participating, is used when the consultee has the necessary experience and abilities, but lacks a positive attitude toward the changes. The consultant facilitates goal accomplishment and demonstrates trust that the consultee can make the needed changes. Special attention should be given to ensure that these consultees receive credit for their ideas and accomplishments. The last leadership style, delegating, is reserved for those consultees who have the necessary expertise and a positive attitude to implement changes. The consultant plays the role of a support person rather than the role of an instructor. Table 8.2 illustrates the leadership style to select based upon the consultee's needs. Readers are also urged to consult Hersey and Blanchard (1982).

The leadership style of the consultant may need to adjust as the ability and attitude of the consultee changes. To initiate or to maintain meaningful and positive changes, ongoing feedback between the consultant and consultee dur-

TABLE 8.2 CONSULTATION LEADERSHIP STYLE TO SELECT BASED UPON THE CONSULTEE'S ABILITIES AND ATTITUDES

CONSULTANT	CONSULTEE	
Leadership Style	Ability	Attitude
Telling	Absent	Negative
Selling	Absent	Positive
Participating	Present	Negative
Delegating	Present	Positive

ing regularly scheduled meetings is crucial. This feedback should focus on the behaviors involved in the changes, not on the people. Both positive and negative comments about behaviors should be shared. Whenever the consultant and the consultee agree to try new behaviors, clarification of the rationale is needed as to why changes are being requested.

Specific feedback from the consultee to the consultant concerning the adolescent's behavior is necessary to a successful consultation model. The consultee should report, either orally or in writing, the effect on the adolescent of suggested changes in the setting. The impact of these changes on adolescents should be evaluated by either the consultee or the consultant, or both. Evaluation of the adolescent might consist of an oral interview (group or individual), a written questionnaire, or documentation of student performance.

When consultees have been trained to intervene with an adolescent's problem communication behaviors, a specific feedback system should be devised for that student by the consultant. Usually such a system consists of daily or weekly behavioral checklists that the consultee maintains. It may also include space after the checklist for anecdotal comments. The feedback system should be purposely simple and require a minimum of time for the consultee to complete. The lengthier the feedback system, the greater the risk of the consultee not following through on documenting the adolescent's performance. (See Appendix N for a sample feedback system called "The Daily Performance or Multiband Chart" reprinted with permission from Idol, Paolucci-Whitcomb, and Nevin, 1986.) At the adolescent level, this feedback system should be shared with the youth whenever it is operative (e.g., daily, weekly). This allows all three participants of the triadic model (consultant, consultee, client) to remain informed of current progress and to redesign the focus of consultation as needed.

Consultants should maintain a written log of all consultation contacts by noting the date, content of the meeting, and both objective and subjective observations about modifications occurring in the classroom. (See Appendix N for a sample consultation log form.) In addition, any feedback forms used by the consultee to document student performance should be kept on file. Readers may consult *Collaborative Consultation* (Idol, Paolucci-Whitcomb, and Nevin, 1986) for additional examples of consultation forms.

In summary, the consultation model may be used whenever modifications within the educational system are desirable. It is as applicable to promoting major modifications within the system, such as those that emerge from curriculum committees, as it is to supporting minor changes, such as adaptation of classroom materials that are under the control of one teacher. Important modifications of the educational system that might be suggested during consultation to benefit adolescents are summarized in the next four sections.

Curriculum Committee Participation Broad modifications in specific content areas can be made when the curriculum is formally reviewed by a committee appointed by administration. This formal review generally occurs every few years, and it is frequently linked with new textbook selection.

Through consultation, the speech-language pathologist should make known to administrators, to department heads of specific academic areas, and to classroom teachers that individuals in the discipline of communication sciences and disorders are uniquely qualified to appraise the language and cognitive demands of curricula as they affect students with language disorders and learning disabilities. We urge speech-language pathologists to volunteer for curriculum committees. In some settings, the voluntary request to serve on a curriculum committee appears so novel that approval is quick; any willing professional *wanting* to be at the meetings is a welcomed addition. In other settings the voluntary request is suspect, and speech-language pathologists may need to lapse into an information dissemination campaign to educate others as to how the discipline may contribute positively to the outcomes of the curriculum committee. Frequently, speech-language pathologists can make inroads on elementary level curriculum committees before they can on those at the secondary level. One phone call from the elementary principal to the secondary principal may remove roadblocks more quickly than other approaches, assuming that the elementary principal speaks positively about the benefit of input from speech-language pathologists. In settings where speech-language pathologists have already proven the discipline's contribution to curriculum committees, they may be asked to participate even before a request is submitted.

Once appointed to serve on a curriculum committee for a specific academic area, or for a specific grade level, the speech-language pathologist should analyze the language and cognitive demands of the curriculum on students by using procedures suggested in Chapter 5. If the curriculum is implemented with both normal and disordered students, a cross-section of performance may be needed from both groups. Through these types of efforts, some settings have begun alternative curriculum options for students. For example, rather than expecting all seventh graders to participate in one structured sequence of activities for English with identical textbooks, an optional seventh grade English course is developed that accommodates students who would have extreme difficulty with the regular curriculum, but who are not so impaired that they require special education. This "school within a school" concept may be a particularly viable option for at-risk adolescents and for "gray area" students, i.e., those with intelligence quotients that are too high for placement in programs for retarded individuals and too low for placement in learning disabilities programs. Many of these students are marginal communicators, but they may not qualify for speech-language programs. Through curriculum committees, changes in the system can be made to benefit the marginal communicators, as well as those already identified as having language disorders. The speech-language pathologist can be a primary advocate for these modifications.

When committees are formed to review and to modify curricula in special education areas, speech-language pathologists should become involved. It is a rare special education curriculum that does not include language or communication as an area to teach. However, the scope and sequence of objectives may not be organized appropriately. Important objectives may be missing. Language goals may be buried in other areas of the curriculum. Thus, teachers could fail to grasp the strong language component contained within those goals (e.g., comprehension of the concepts of "left-right" is a goal tucked in the "Gross Motor" area of the curriculum). Through participation of speech-language pathologists on special education curriculum committees, these curriculum deficits can be repaired.

Content Area Tutoring In Chapter 6, we advocated the use of peer tutors for adolescents with communication disorders and suggested a system for organizing peer tutoring. Speech-language pathologists may advocate that a similar system be devised by classroom teachers for content area tutoring, e.g., in math or biology. The speech-language pathologist would not organize the peer tutoring for content areas, but rather, during consultation might suggest that such a system be implemented for certain adolescents. The trials and errors of establishing the peer tutoring system within the speech-language program might also be shared.

If classroom teachers who are initiating a peer tutoring system are unfamiliar with resources for peer tutoring, references should be shared by the speech-language pathologist, e.g., Klausmeier, Jetter, and Nelson, 1972; Koskinen and Wilson, 1982a; 1982b. Myrick and Erney (1979) offer a plan of action for training peer facilitators in an academic class. Throughout their text, they summarize "Guidelines for Training" that would permit educators to use an organized approach to orienting and training peers with minimal investment of planning time and effort. Another advantage of sharing *Youth Helping Youth: A Handbook for Training Peer Facilitators* (Myrick and Erney, 1979) is that these authors summarize studies that have documented the efficacy of peer tutoring programs.

During consultation time, the speech-language pathologist should determine with other educators which, if any, adolescents with communication disorders might need a peer tutor in a specific content area. Assuming that one or more of these adolescents does need a tutor, the speech-language pathologist should volunteer to train the content area facilitators about specific communication disorders. Even though the content area tutor will not be working on the adolescent's communication directly, the tutor should know what to expect from the adolescent with a disorder and how to respond appropriately.

Adaptation of Classroom Discourse Maintaining appropriate participation in classroom-setting activities demands interactional "work" between the educator and the student. When educators or adolescents have poor interactional skills in the classroom, modifications in discourse may be warranted.

Educator Requests Requests made by educators are often indirect (e.g., "Don't you know you're supposed to begin reading Chapter 6 as soon as the bell rings?" is said to stop a student from finishing a written assignment) (Donahue, 1985). To derive the illocutionary force of indirect requests, a great deal of shared knowledge is required. When this shared knowledge is absent, educators should consider the use of direct requests.

Educators should be helped to control the semantic and syntactic complexity of their requests. Requests should be simplified or reformulated to match the student's conceptual level. In other words, educators using effective instructional techniques match the level of their questions with the level of student comprehension. For example, if they are asking what Blank, Rose, and Berlin (1978) call a Level IV question (i.e., a question involving reasoning about perception, such as "Why do most citizens pay taxes?"), they may need to simplify to a lower level question. Level I questions match perceptions (e.g., "How did our textbook define taxes?"). Level II questions require elective analysis of perception (e.g., "Think of services that are paid for by tax dollars."). Level III questions elicit the reordering of perception (e.g., "How do people find out if they owe taxes?"). Silliman (1984) pointed out that specific differences between Level III and Level IV questions still need clarification.

When indirect requests are used, the educator should ensure that the adolescent derives the meaning. Rather than assuming that requests for action are understood, the teacher might ask the adolescent to explain what is expected. Educators should avoid simply asking, "Do you understand?" since the polite response is "yes," and there is evidence that some youth with learning disabilities are excessively polite (Donahue, 1981). As an alternative, they could ask, "What do you understand you are to do?" or "What are you going to do?" The tone of voice used should convey interest, not intimidation. As the adolescent reexplains the task to the educator, the teacher can provide additional explanatory comments as necessary.

Educator Response to Questions for Clarification How the educator responds to student requests for clarification, even those that seem unnecessary at the time, will set the learning tone in the classroom. Perhaps all of us can remember a teacher in our past who ridiculed and embarrassed students for asking a question or for confessing to a lack of understanding. Students attempting to survive in these classrooms quickly learned that they were safer to say nothing at all and to suffer the consequences (e.g., completing an assignment incorrectly) than to risk the ire of the teacher.

When consulting with educators, speech-language pathologists should encourage them to remain receptive to student questions, to share that receptive attitude with students, and to resist making the assumption that the students' questions are ridiculous and irrelevant. For example, at times, directions are ambiguous to students, but may not appear that way to educators because of their familiarity with the material. Rather than reacting negatively, educators might pursue a student's line of thinking by countering with a question like, "What is confusing you about the instructions?" or "What words in the directions are new to you?"

When student requests for clarification are global (e.g., "I don't get it. Say it again."), educators should help adolescents to isolate the information that was not understood, and then restate the question more precisely. Often, students *do* understand some of the spoken instructions or parts of the lecture; however, they lack the necessary skill to ask a specific question concerning what was *not* understood.

For adolescents with language disorders, question asking behavior may be complicated by the degree of mismatch between discourse rules in the regular classrooms versus those in resource programs. If the resource room is informal, and students are allowed to ask questions whenever they arise, students may have difficulty adjusting to regular educators who expect questions for clarification only at particular times (e.g., before or after class, at the *end* of instructions rather than midway). Thus, the adolescent who blurts out questions informally may be judged by the classroom teacher as bumbling or rude (Donahue, 1985). A plan of action should be established that gives the educator a consistent, constructive method of responding to the adolescent's inappropriate communication (e.g., a signal system might be devised between the consultee and the client so that the client knows the behavior is inappropriate; behaviors might be charted, shared with the consultant, and connected to a consequence).

Consultants should assist consultees to realize that adolescents are not always being intentionally rude when questions for clarification are asked. Adolescents may need to ask questions at the time they occur to them, before the questions are forgotten. Teachers should be encouraged to allow students to ask questions at the time they arise, even if this means a change in classroom protocol.

Consultants should also help consultees appreciate those times when the client is communicating appropriately when asking questions. Incidents of appropriate communication by the client should be praised by the consultee. Likewise, consultants should model praise for consultees when they ask appropriate questions during consultation meetings.

Adjustment of Speaking Styles Good teaching involves adjustment of the form and content of messages to reflect an awareness of the needs and feelings of students. Messages are appropriately simple or complex, and stated with tactfulness. When selecting discourse style for the classroom, "... teachers use a combination of prior knowledge about the expected linguistic and cognitive abilities of their students along with immediate verbal and nonverbal feedback. In this way they adjust their speaking styles to fit the presumed capabilities of the children they teach." (Nelson, 1984, p. 175).

Students who are not within the educator's expected group norm for language facility will have difficulty succeeding in that teacher's classroom. Occasionally, educators will overshoot the majority of the group, as reflected by such student comments as "Nobody understands what's going on. I think Mr. B. talks to himself most of the time." They may also undershoot, as reflected by comments such as "This class is so easy it's boring. She must think we are babies."

Consultants should encourage educators to use several speaking styles for class members. For example, if an explanation of a process or a concept brings perplexed looks from some of the students, the educator should reexplain the information using concrete, simplified language. At times, the rate of delivery may need to be slowed down for students to capture main ideas; key phrases may need to be repeated several times orally and written on the blackboard.

Style is also influenced by the presence of verbal mazes, false starts, and revisions. If spoken language is excessively cluttered with these features, clarity of messages may be impaired. Consultants should explain to consultees how clear messages and clear questions, free from clutter, assist learning. A positive reminder to organize the message or question, then to say it clearly the first time, is usually received better than a criticism of the speaker's style.

Adaptation of Materials To grasp information presented within a course, adolescents may need certain adaptations of the material. Speech-language pathologists may play a major advocacy role for these changes during consultation. Four major adaptations are summarized below.

Variety of Modalities Speech-language pathologists should encourage educators to use a combination of input modalities when giving directions or presenting information. Information should be seen and heard by adolescents; it should also be conveyed kinesthetically, if feasible. For example, if the teacher is attempting to explain the concept of "density," the students might be told what density is, have the word and definition displayed on an overhead projector or blackboard, and have an opportunity to hold objects that are the same weight, but of different densities (e.g., a pound of styrofoam packing chips and a pound of butter). The majority of students will benefit from this variety of modalities. However, an occasional student will find the combination of modalities overwhelming and be too sensorily bombarded to learn. For such a student, selection of the strongest modality is advisable whenever crucial information is imparted.

A primary means for teachers to input information both auditorily and visually is to use printed listening guides while they are lecturing. The listening guide should summarize main ideas, relevant details, and new vocabulary presented in the lecture. This information should be arranged to correspond chronologically with the lecture, and items should be spaced liberally to allow for additional data to be added by the students. The advantage of listening guides is that they remove the pressure from those students who struggle to record notes. The guides prove to be particularly helpful when adolescents identify essential ideas and study for tests. Contrary to the belief that adolescents will not listen if the information is spread before them on guides, listening appears to become better and more efficient; students are able to concentrate on the ideas being presented rather than on the mechanics of note taking.

Note Taking Options In addition to, or instead of, using listening guides to ease the difficulty of note taking for some adolescents, a "buddy system" could be initiated by the classroom teacher. Students who take concise, well-organized notes could share them with the adolescents struggling to grasp the information presented during lectures. This sharing may be accomplished through machine or hand copying of notes, or through use of carbon paper in the "buddy's" notebook.

Another option is to allow adolescents to audio tape classroom lectures, then to take notes while relistening to the information. The advantage of this option is that the student can start and stop the tape as needed to capture main ideas in writing. Tape recorders that have variable speeds, but do not distort the spoken message, are useful for those adolescents who need to slow the rate of the teacher's speech, or for those who could speed up the rate without destroying comprehension.

The disadvantage of tape recording is the time that it takes to relisten to the lectures. Frequently, the adolescents who need to tape record are the same students who fall behind in their school work. Time may not be available during the school day to relisten to lectures. Unless there is flexibility to take the tapes home after school, this option may be undesirable.

Another potential disadvantage of tape recording might be a perceived infringement of academic freedom by classroom teachers. After all, the tapes will possibly be heard by school colleagues and family members. Some teachers may refuse to allow taping in their classes, despite the best possible advocacy on the part of the speech-language pathologist. Speech-language pathologists should be aware that Section 504 states that reasonable accommodations must be made for students with disabilities. Perhaps if teachers are made aware of Section 504 requirements, they would be less likely to resist the taping of their lectures (D. Vetter, Personal Communication, 1986).

Books on Tape Another useful application of audio cassette tape is to record the adolescent's textbooks. This will permit the student to listen and relisten to the printed information required within specific content areas. Since many educators are too busy to tape their textbooks, several other options should be explored. A number of states, as well as the Library of Congress, have books on tape already recorded for visually handicapped students, and these tapes might be available to students with learning problems. A phone call to your state department of education can verify whether textbooks on tape are available.

If textbooks on tape must be created, then youth groups interested in service projects should be contacted. These groups might be housed within a school setting (e.g., the Honor Society, Future Nurses of America, the Drama Club) or they may be community-based (e.g., 4-H, Boy Scouts, Girl Scouts). Whatever group, or groups, might become involved in taping books, they should be adequately trained by the speech-language pathologist and/or other knowledgeable educators. Training should consist of explaining the mechanics of the process (e.g., how close to speak from the microphone, how to adjust the sound level of the recording) as well as consist of practicing the use of appropriate rate, volume, inflection, and pronunciation. If an actual recording studio can be secured for taping, that would result in the highest quality of production. However, if a studio is not available, arrangements should be made to have the taping done in a quiet room, free from excessive echoing.

In addition to modifying printed textbooks by recording them on audio tape, speech-language pathologists should advocate for other printed information to be delivered orally to adolescents who need it. For example, if written tests are an unfair assessment of the student's knowledge because poor writing skills interfere with test responses, then an alternative might be to have tests administered orally. Student responses can be dictated, or recorded verbatim. Who will be responsible for this adaptation (e.g., the speech-language pathologist, another professional in special education, a classroom teacher) should be determined during consultation sessions.

Color Coding Textbooks Adolescents who possess some reading skills, or who are willing to read along with an audio cassette tape, can be aided further by color coding their textbooks. Several colors should be used for the coding, e.g., yellow highlight is used for main ideas; blue highlight is used for relevant details; green highlight is used for new vocabulary words. The meaning of each color should be determined before coding begins and should be adhered to by all participants. If multiple books from different subject areas are being coded, there should be agreement among all of the professionals regarding the system of coding.

Initially, classroom teachers should do the color coding, since they are most familiar with their expectations for student performance. However, during consultation meetings, a plan should be devised whereby the adolescents are gradually taught to color code the textbook themselves. The plan should include designation of who will be responsible for teaching adolescents this skill.

Sometimes the greatest resistance to color coding comes from those administrators who rigidly enforce a "no marks in books" policy. This seems most apparent when new textbooks have just arrived. Consultation with these administrators should emphasize the ongoing need of certain adolescents within a setting for color coding. When those adolescents depart from the setting, others with similar needs will replace them. Beginning the color coding plan with older, more worn, textbooks is generally more acceptable than using new books, yet the plan will usually be successful enough to prove its effectiveness to administrators.

The four adaptations of materials just described (Variety of Materials, Note Taking Options, Books on Tape, and Color Coding Textbooks) represent only some of the many adaptations that can be recommended during consultation. Several excellent resources provide additional ideas for secondary level classroom modifications (DeMier, Wise, and Marcum, 1982; Oklahoma Project, 1982; Project STILE, 1979).

ENVIRONMENTAL SYSTEM

Like the educational system, certain modifications within the adolescent's environmental system may be warranted. The last half of this chapter will describe what modifications might need to be made and how to implement those changes.

Modifications of the Environmental System

When the environmental system is modified to meet the language needs of adolescents, changes may be proposed in these aspects:

1. The oral language of persons within the environmental system
2. The structure of learning environments away from the adolescent's school program (if enrolled in one)
3. Parental attitudes and feelings toward their child
4. Siblings' or peers' attitudes and feelings toward the adolescent.

The oral language of parents, siblings, peers, and others within the environmental system may be too rapid and too complex for the adolescent to comprehend. Frequent repetition of information may be necessary before the adolescent appears to comprehend. Even so, communication breakdowns may be common. The need for repeating information and for repairing breakdowns often tries the patience of those interacting with the adolescent, thus potentially influencing their feelings and attitudes negatively toward the adolescent. Intervention to change the oral language of persons within the environmental system may greatly reduce their frustration and the adolescent's.

The learning environment at home and, if applicable, at the adolescent's place of employment should match the documented learning style for how the adolescent learns best. (See Appendix C.) The flexibility to modify the learning environment is often present, and changes may be made quickly once information about the adolescent's needs has been shared.

Positive parental attitudes and feelings toward the adolescent should be acknowledged and reinforced. Emotional support to modify negative attitudes and feelings should be offered. Negative attitudes and feelings may stem from parental concerns about their adolescent with a disability. Among their concerns are issues such as "Will my child ever gain employment that allows self-sufficiency?" and "Will my child be taken advantage of sexually because of being easily persuaded?" They now realize the permanency of certain disabilities and know that their child may or may not ultimately be an independently functioning adult.

Similarly, siblings of the adolescent should be praised for their positive attitudes and feelings, and should be offered emotional support to modify their negative attitudes and feelings. Resentment is often the most consistently overriding reaction toward a sibling with a disability, because the normal child feels that the parents are doing more for that child (Wentworth, 1974). Jealousy, hostility, and embarrassment are also common feelings. Grief may be exhibited by some siblings' knowing that people with disabilities may experience discrimination and inappropriate treatment, and others may express grief over being denied a normal sibling. Both siblings and peers may need to be taught ways to interact constructively with the adolescent who has a communication disorder.

How to Modify the Environmental System: Counseling

Counseling is to the environmental system what consultation is to the educational system. As noted by Mowrer (1982), counseling has long been recognized as part of the speech-language pathologist's job. Professionals such as Johnson (1946), Van Riper (1947), Luper and Mulder (1964), Anderson and Newby (1973), Moncur and Brackett (1974), Webster (1977; 1976), Simpson

(1982), and McFarlane, Fujiki, and Brinton (1984) have advocated the use of counseling as a means of working with family members and peers. Most counseling takes one of three formats: (1) informational programs or meetings to provide family members and peers with facts about the adolescent's handicapping condition; (2) programs or conferences to assist parents to deal with and understand their own problems and those of their child; (3) training programs to help family members and peers to develop effective teaching skills (Vander Zanden and Pace, 1984). Within any of these formats, counseling may include providing information about communication disorders, obtaining information from environmental system members about the adolescent, or providing release and support for feelings. This description is identical to that of counseling directly with the adolescent.

Theories of Counseling You may be saying, "Not more theories!" We would like to reiterate that nothing is as practical as a "good" theory. There are at least five major theoretical camps in counseling. The first is psychoanalytical theory which, according to Downing (1975), was influenced by S. Freud, Jung, and Adler. This theoretical camp emphasizes unconscious or conscious forces behind behaviors, early childhood experiences, the labeling of past experiences, and a directive approach during the therapy process. Because of the need for extensive training to implement this approach, it is usually used in psychotherapy rather than counseling.

The second camp is the phenomenological approach, which has been most widely applied by Rogers (1961) in his client-centered therapy, and by Perls (Perls, Hefferline, and Goodman, 1965) in Gestalt theory. The phenomenological approach, developed somewhat as a reaction to the rigidity of the psychoanalytical approach, focuses on the person's perception in the present environment rather than in the past or future. In client-centered therapy the assumption is that the person is rational, good, and capable of logically reasoning through situations. The therapy process is nondirective. Gestalt therapy emphasizes the whole person: The mind and body are the same, not separate, in relating to the environment. The therapy approach in Gestalt therapy is more directive than non-directive, and is implemented by applying a series of verbal and nonverbal procedures in a group therapy process.

The third theoretical camp, behavioral theory (Bandura and Walters, 1963) arose because of the inability of the psychoanalytical and phenomenological approaches to measure and evaluate therapeutic outcomes. According to behavioral theory, speech-language pathologists would work only with specific, observable, objective, and measurable variables. This theory's underlying assumption is that human behavior is determined by its immediate consequences in the environment; behavior is learned therefore it can be unlearned. In this approach, values, feelings, and thoughts are ignored by the speech-language pathologist who analyzes goals, directs strategies, evaluates outcomes, provides positive reinforcement, and arranges environmental contingencies.

The cognitive-behavioral approach is the fourth theoretical camp, and it emphasizes rational thinking and problem solving. The two major proponents are Ellis (Ellis and Harper, 1972), in rational-emotive therapy, and Glasser (1965) in reality therapy. Rational-emotive therapy maintains that people are born rational into an irrational world. They teach themselves to become more irrational as they incorporate the world's values into their belief system. The underlying assumption is that if you change the way you think, you can change your belief system, which changes behavior. In reality therapy, the approach is rational, logical, and learning-oriented with an emphasis on the present. The therapeutic approach is very judgmental and confrontive because the therapist judges the value of a behavior based on the therapist's perceptions of reality.

The last camp is the transactional analysis approach, which falls midway between the phenomenological and the cognitive-behavioral camps. It is like the cognitive-behavioral camp because it focuses on reality, logic, and learning, but it uses many of the Gestalt therapy techniques of emphasizing the client's perspective. Transactional analysis uses a group therapy process in which verbal and nonverbal techniques are used.

Variables Affecting Counseling The theories utilized when working with family members or peers would be contingent upon the speech-language pathologist's training and competency. Obviously, the speech-language pathologist needs to take into account a number of variables before counseling begins. A partial list of variables that affect counseling include the following:

1. The coping strategies available to family members and peers (e.g., If family members have good coping strategies and need to be encouraged to continue to use them, then the speech-language pathologist might use a client-centered approach to counseling. If the family members have poor coping strategies, then a more directive confrontive approach like reality therapy might be used to introduce the need to develop better coping strategies.)

2. The type and degree of the reaction of parents, siblings, and peers to the target adolescent (e.g., If siblings and peers react negatively to the adolescent, then they might benefit from a transactional analysis approach, especially considering the variety of transactional analysis materials available for children and youth [Freed, 1977; 1976; 1974]. If siblings and peers already react positively to the adolescent, then they might benefit from client-centered therapy.)

3. The past history of the parent-educator relationship (e.g., If the relationship is amenable, then reality therapy might be used. If the relationship is already full of conflict, then the confrontation in reality therapy may destroy the last hope for a constructive parent-educator relationship; instead, a client-centered approach might be used.)

4. The specific characteristics of the family, such as racial group, income level, marital status of parents (e.g., If lower socio-economic family members prefer not to discuss their feelings and expect to have professionals present them with a structured approach to solving a problem, then a viable approach might be behavioral therapy. If family members prefer to discuss their feelings, then a client-centered approach might be beneficial.).

The last item on the list above deserves special consideration. Sue (1981) labels counseling as ". . . a white, middle-class activity that holds many values and characteristics different from those of Third World groups" (p. 28). During counseling, there is typically an emphasis on verbal communication using standard English, an imposition of class-bound values (e.g., strict adherence to time schedules; an ambiguous or unstructured approach to problems; the seeking of long-range solutions and goals), and an assumption of culture-bound values by the counselor (e.g., using an analytic cause-effect approach; distinguishing between mental and physical well-being; encouraging verbal/emotional/behavioral expressions). These characteristics of counseling may be sources of conflict and misinterpretation by family members and peers who are not white middle-class, unless adjustments are made by the counselor to accommodate other language systems (i.e., in addition to standard English), different class-bound values, and alternative culture-bound values. Even when appropriate adjustments are made, ". . . cross-cultural helping cannot be approached through any one theory of counseling" (Sue, 1981, p. 52).

Counseling Parents Speech-language pathologists should be aware that parents of adolescents may appear to be or are uninvolved or uninterested in their older child's needs because the parent-educator relationships may have been characterized by conflict in the past. Also, parents may remain uninvolved because of the lack of continuity in parent education programs; a paucity of resources available commensurate with parent and family needs; and parent burnout.

Some parents may be angry about insensitive handling of them or their child, inadequate professional services, or incompetent management of the adolescent's program (McFarlane, Fujiki, and Brinton, 1984). Speech-language pathologists should first consider whether the parents' anger is justifiable. If it is, understanding the parental perspective should be an impetus to offering more appropriate services. If it is not, that realization may be an important source of support while interacting with the angered parents. Whether the parents are justifiably angry or not, speech-language pathologists should not become defensive, but should continue treating parents as they would like to be treated when expressing anger.

There are four basic principles to adhere to when working with parents of adolescents (Christensen and DeBlassie, 1980): (1) all those parenting the adolescent should be involved in the counseling process because it avoids the distortion that can occur when one parent reports the session to another; it helps to clarify their reactions toward each other and their child; and it can aid mutual understanding; (2) parents usually need support during the first meeting; (3) parents need to be shown effective ways of expressing feelings and giving feedback in the first sessions; and (4) parents should be informed of community agencies. When parents are feeling "in trouble" coping with their adolescent child's communication, more intensive, one-on-one counseling conferences may be needed. Otherwise, group informational and support meetings (see Chapter 3) and training programs may be adequate to meet parental needs.

Training Programs In recent years, a number of parent training programs have become increasingly popular across the nation. These programs have been taught by a variety of professionals, either singly or in teams. Among these professionals are speech-language pathologists.

Gordon's *Parent Effectiveness Training (PET)* (1970) is an example of one such training program in which parents are taught to use the language of acceptance, to be active listeners, to use "I messages," to establish problem ownership, and to implement a "no lose" method of resolving parent-child conflict. These and related skills are developed through the use of discussions, role model demonstrations, and role playing. Another example is Dinkmeyer and McKay's *Systematic Training for Effective Parenting for Teens (STEP Teen)* (1983), in which parents are brought together in a structured framework of discussions, readings, and activities to change negative family behavior.

According to Barret (1982), one major shortcoming of these types of parent training programs is that the major emphasis is on the parent; the adolescents are left at home and become the unwilling recipients of their parent's new behaviors. Barret (1982) designed a training program to assist parents that included adolescents, with the purpose being for all participants to communicate more effectively. The training program is called *Improving Familytalk: Educating Families to Work Better*, and is designed for four two-hour sessions. Each session has three components: Lecture, experiential, and personal learning. In session one, the lecture emphasizes viewing ". . . the family as a system in which faulty communications are a reflection of the system as a whole rather than the result of a rebellious adolescent or an antiquated parent" (Barret, 1982, p. 179). Following the lecture, the members of the group are asked to complete a paper-pencil task in which they identify three strengths and three weaknesses in their family communication, and to finish the sentence, "I would like to change the communication in my family by . . ." (Barret, 1982, p. 180). Last, the members form small mixed groups (adults and adolescents) in which they listen to answers generated in the paper-pencil task and make comments. The last fifteen minutes are spent summarizing insights gained in the session.

In session two, the lecture phase attempts to increase the participants' awareness of styles and concepts of effective communication. Participants are put into groups of six, separating parents and children, and they each role play being a helpee or helper. The lecture then continues, followed by an experiential component wherein family members use their new communication skills to discuss minor problems. In session three, the lecture and small group discussion consist of reflecting on family expectations. Then, using Gordon's (1970) problem-solving model, solutions to family conflicts are presented. In session four, the main emphasis is on building self-esteem in the family. This type of workshop enhances family education, which allows parents and adolescents to practice effective communication.

A study by Robin et al. (1977), using a similar family education format, revealed positive results. In this study, parents and normal adolescents were taught to resolve conflicts using problem solving and communication skills. Problem solving was defined as: Defining the problem, listing alternative solutions, evaluating the solutions, and planning implementation. Communication skills were defined as: Clear expression and reception of meaning, appropriate emotive attentive style, and reflective listening. Twenty-four mother-adolescent dyads were assigned to a treatment or control group. The twelve dyads assigned to the treatment group received five sessions of therapy, during which modeling, guided practice, role playing, feedback, and social reinforcement were utilized to teach problem solving and communication skills. The results revealed improved problem solving and communication skills in families where there had been parent-adolescent conflict.

In addition to training parents about communicating with their adolescent children, some attention should be given to expressed learning styles as revealed by completion of the questionnaire in Appendix C. The results of the questionnaire should be explained to parents, and implications for changes that could be made in the adolescent's study habits at home might be discussed. For example, if the adolescent has an expressed preference for a certain location at home for studying, or a requested temperature, light level, or sound level, then parents should help to structure the environment at home to accommodate how their child learns best.

Parents should be careful to modify the home environment for studying only in ways that it helps the adolescent to study best, not in ways that the adolescent *prefers*. It is conceivable that how the adolescent prefers to study (e.g., with the TV and dim lights while eating popcorn) is not how the adolescent learns best. However, when modifications truly benefit the adolescent's studying, parents should be encouraged to make and maintain those alterations in the home learning environment.

Counseling Siblings Parents are not alone in their need for counseling; siblings may have similar needs. Helping professionals should organize and conduct sibling groups for brothers and sisters of adolescents with communication disorders. Speech-language pathologists may or may not provide the leadership for the group. If a related professional (e.g., guidance counselor, psychologist) functions as the group's coordinator, then speech-language pathologists should remain in contact with that person and be readily available as a resource person. If no such sibling group exists within an agency, speech-language pathologists might function as strong advocates for the initiation of the service.

Wasserman (1983) has identified four specific concerns expressed by sibling groups:

1. *The need for information* Siblings should be informed about communication disorders, their characteristics and consequences.
2. *The need to understand and to resolve emotional reactions* The emotional reactions of siblings are inconsistent, but when negative reactions predominate, counseling may be particularly imperative.
3. *The need for sibling self-identity and role definition* These are important if normal siblings are to develop a separate identity from their brother or sister with a disability. Also, the role the normal sibling is to assume for the care of the sibling with a disability should be defined carefully (e.g., Is the sibling to be a tutor at home? If so, how should tutoring be conducted?).
4. *The need for effective coping strategies* Normal siblings may need assistance to develop appropriate strategies to cope with their brother or sister with a disability. For example, the sibling group may share ways that the question, "What am I going to say to my new boyfriend/girlfriend about my brother's (or sister's) problem?" could be answered.

Sessions that emphasize and incorporate both informational and therapeutic components allow each of these four concerns to be addressed.

Chinitz (1981) suggests that a starting point for sibling group discussion is exploring individual differences of their own and that of the sister or brother with a disability. Next, factual information about specific disorders could be introduced such as etiology, associated characteristics, and special resources needed for the adolescent with a communication disorder. Within the sibling group, ample opportunity should be provided to identify and resolve both positive and negative aspects of living with a sibling with a disability.

Visits to the classroom and intervention sessions of the adolescent with a communication disorder are encouraged, and are conducted unobtrusively so that normal siblings learn about special needs and activities. According to Chinitz (1981), one of the major advantages to having sibling groups was that ". . . the children offered each other suggestions for solving problems they had been unable to resolve on their own" (p. 22). In addition, sibling group members become attuned to individual differences, receptive to information on the etiology and nature of handicapping conditions, and aware of intervention strategies for the adolescent with a disability.

Counseling Peer Groups Similar to sibling groups, peer groups should be established that will emphasize disseminating information to peers who may not be knowledgeable about disabilities and human differences. With a competent discussion leader conducting the group sessions, peers can analyze their own differences and those of others. They should discuss the impact of a disability upon the adolescent's life style, and the way they can be supportive and encouraging of adolescents who have a disability.

Dinkmeyer and Muro (1971) found that peer group counseling was more beneficial than individual counseling, because adolescents are more comfortable talking about feelings, attitudes, and beliefs in peer groups than with an adult. Peer tutoring and counseling have been found to be advantageous for secondary students. Using this approach, the adolescent with a communication disorder benefits and learns from the interaction with a normal adolescent. Likewise, the normal adolescent learns about human differences and the impact the communication disorder has on the adolescent.

SUMMARY

Indirect intervention by the speech-language pathologist entails working with those educational and environmental system members who frequently interact with the adolescent. The adolescent may have a communication disorder, or the primary problem may have been identified to be within the educational and/or environmental systems (i.e., the interdisciplinary team recommended certain modifications at school or home).

During indirect intervention, the speech-language pathologist consults with educators and counsels family members and peers concerning the changes suggested by the interdisciplinary team. Modifications within the educational system might include reorganization of curriculum, organization of content tutoring, changes in classroom oral discourse, and adaptations of written materials. These modifications are initiated and maintained through the use of a collaborative consultation model.

Modifications within the environmental system might include adapting oral language, restructuring the adolescent's learning environment, altering negative feelings and attitudes toward the adolescent, and reinforcing positive feelings. Environmental system modifications are made through counseling parents, siblings, and peers.

Through the indirect intervention efforts of the speech-language pathologist, important changes in the adolescent's educational and environmental systems can be made. Although the involvement of the adolescent is indirect, the benefits are direct, and may be powerful.

DISCUSSION QUESTIONS

1. Discuss how you would implement a collaborative consultation model within various employment settings.
2. Analyze a junior high school textbook from a content course (e.g., science, English). Discuss language and cognitive demands of the textbook that might be inappropriate developmentally for early adolescents. How should the content of the textbook be modified to make it more appropriate for early adolescents?
3. You are counseling the parents of an adolescent about their vocational concerns for their son with a language disorder. Their son recently lost his job as a grocery store carry-out boy because of inappropriate communication with customers. Discuss the various directions that the counseling session may take and your corresponding responses. Determine the theory(s) of counseling on which your responses are based.

SUGGESTED READINGS

Donahue, M. Communicative style in learning disabled children: Some implications for classroom discourse. In: D. Ripich and F. Spinelli (eds.), *School Discourse Problems.* Little Brown/College-Hill Press, San Diego, CA, 1985.

Idol, L., Paolucci-Whitcomb, P., and Nevin, A. *Collaborative Consultation.* Aspen Publishers, Inc., Rockville, MD, 1986.

McFarlane, S., Fujiki, M., and Brinton, B. *Coping with Communicative Handicaps: Resources for the Practicing Clinician.* Little Brown/College-Hill Press, San Diego, CA, 1984.

CHAPTER 9

The Follow-up Component

GOALS:

To provide a rationale for engaging in follow-up activities

To present a critique of the literature on existing follow-up studies

To explain direct and indirect follow-up activities

The final component in the prototype delivery model is follow-up. Follow-up was defined in Chapter 3 as any activity designed to measure the real and perceived benefits of speech-language programs. Follow-up is being used in this chapter in the broadest sense, since it entails gathering information on benefits during the intervention process and after the adolescent has received services. The major reason for accumulating follow-up data on adolescents is to determine the efficacy of services. In addition, follow-up data are needed to demonstrate accountability, especially cost effectiveness and time efficiency. Once gathered, the data should be shared with professionals so that they may learn about the effectiveness of various treatment plans (Vetter, 1985).

During direct follow-up, the adolescents themselves are involved. During indirect follow-up, the adults who come in contact with the adolescents would be the informants. These adults (e.g., educators, parents) would inform the speech-language pathologist of their perceptions of the benefits that the adolescents received from direct speech-language services. The educators would also inform the speech-language pathologist about the value of the consultation model, when it was used. In addition, family members who participated in counseling activities would be asked to evaluate the effectiveness of these services.

Table 9.1 illustrates a comprehensive direct and indirect follow-up proce-

TABLE 9.1 FOLLOW-UP COMPONENT

	Who?	What?	How?
DIRECT	Adolescents Early Middle Late	Baseline data Benefits of program	Study design Survey methodology A. Interviews B. Questionnaires
INDIRECT	Adults and peers familiar with adolescent	Benefits of services for adolescents Benefits of consultation model Benefits of counseling	Survey methodology A. Interviews B. Questionnaires

dure. Data regarding the efficacy of services should be collected periodically during the time that speech-language services are being provided and after the services have been terminated.

The discipline of communication sciences and disorders recognizes the need for follow-up information, but few studies have been published. A review of the literature revealed that of those published, only a few studies have been conducted on adolescents (Aram, Ekelman, and Nation, 1984; DeAjuriaguerra et al., 1976; Garvey and Gordon, 1973; Griffiths, 1969; King, Jones, and Lasky, 1982; Strominger and Bashir, 1977; Weiss, Hansen, and Heubelein, 1979). Of those studies cited, Weiner (1985) states that retrospective studies, particularly, contain problems in experimental design. Some of the problems in design have been the size of the sample, the kinds of subjects in the sample, the type and consistency of the information available from the initial evaluation, and the events that occurred between the initial evaluation and the follow-up evaluation. Even when the investigators had control over some aspects of the study design, certain factors remained problematic, such as the availability and willingness of the potential subjects to participate and the time and money available for the study.

GUIDELINES TO CONSIDER WHEN DESIGNING A FOLLOW-UP STUDY

Assuming that the investigator has willing subjects, time, and money to conduct a follow-up study, then what criteria should be followed in the designing of such a study? According to Weiner (1985), the study should be designed to be prospective and longitudinal rather than retrospective and cross-sectional. A prospective study would allow for direct interactions with the clients in conjunction with talking to their family members or teachers (i.e., direct and indirect follow-up). The baseline data could be standardized for all participants in group follow-up studies. The study should use a multivariate approach, that is, an assessment of various factors on outcome (e.g., type of language disorder; intelligence; a comparison of the types of intervention programs, if several are used). A longitudinal study would allow for data to be collected from the same subjects at specified intervals.

An alternate, more limited, and less costly approach might be to have a coordinator who would be responsible for planning and executing a follow-up study by collaborating with persons at a large number of facilities (Weiner, 1985). Currently, people are already employed in regional special education centers, or in state departments of education, who have as part of their job description the tracking of students. Usually this tracking consists of following students while they are in the educational system (e.g., how many children who were enrolled in early childhood special education programs continue to receive special education through the elementary years). A reasonable extension of this person's position responsibilities would be to coordinate the tracking of students during and beyond the secondary level. Another potential coordinator is the individual within the state department of education who is responsible for educational demographics. Educational demographers are concerned with the movement of people through the educational system, preschool through graduate school. They tend to view education as a continuum, not as discrete units (Hodgkinson, 1985). Demographers have models already intact for collecting data on what happens to various groups of children (e.g., how many minority students drop-out from high school). These models have applicability to collecting data on students enrolled in special education, including those students who received speech-language intervention through the secondary years.

Another approach would be to have the speech-language pathologist coordinate a series of well-designed, single-subject studies (McReynolds and Kearns, 1983; Weiner, 1985). A discussion of single-subject design studies will be presented later in this chapter. The approach of implementing single-subject studies or using a coordinator would take less time, effort, and money than a prospective, longitudinal, large sample study.

If during the assessment and intervention process (explained in Chapters 4, 5, 7, and 8) the clinician has systematically and rigorously selected and implemented clinical methods with the adolescent, then follow-up is a relatively straightforward task. "Unfortunately, a belief has persisted for many years that clinical practice and rigorous experimental research are discrete endeavors" (Vetter, 1985, p. 55). We concur that sound clinical practice should parallel well-designed experimental research.

DIRECT FOLLOW-UP

What to Investigate During Direct Follow-up

The procedures for conducting a follow-up study should be directed toward the recipient of language intervention. It is important to consider carefully the types of data needed, to make an accurate evaluation of the success or failure of intervention for the adolescent. Some of the areas in which baseline assessment data might be gathered are presented in Chapter 4: Case history information (i.e., type and extent of speech-language services that have been received to this time, as well as medical, environmental, and educational history); cognitive functions; production and comprehension of linguistic features; discourse abilities (i.e., conversations and narrations); general intelligence.

The adolescent's communication performance should be evaluated periodically during intervention. During each intervention session, data are collected on how well the adolescent is attaining the criterion stated in each objective. At periodic intervals (e.g., once a year), selected formal tests and informal assessment procedures, identical to those used for the baseline, should be readministered.

It is also critical to collect information on the adolescent's perceptions of the benefits of having received intervention. Perceived benefits of language intervention as related to academic, personal-social, and vocational success should be documented on a periodic basis. How to accomplish this is explained in the next section.

How to Conduct Direct Follow-up

Before collecting data on the results of the various intervention activities provided to adolescents, professionals must protect the student's rights and welfare in accordance with the U.S. Department of Health and Human Services Regulations (45 CRF 46, Protection of Human Subjects) and the guidelines of various professional codes of ethics. When conducting interviews or sending questionnaires, investigators should follow the policies that have been established for conducting survey research projects:

1. Adolescents or adult respondents must be advised at the beginning of the procedure that all information shall be kept confidential and shall not be identified with the respondent.

2. At the outset of the procedure, the adolescent and/or adult respondent shall be advised about the purpose of the research as well as who is

sponsoring it (informed consent).

3. At the beginning of the project, the speech-language pathologist shall include the importance of the knowledge to be gained and why the value of the information to be gained outweighs any risk to the informant.
4. Adolescents shall be informed that participation in the follow-up study may not provide any direct benefits to them.

Study Design How to conduct direct follow-up activities should include the selection of a study design, i.e., single-subject or group design.

Single-Subject Design The scientific practitioner approaches the clinical process as if it were a well-designed single-subject experiment. Comprehensive data on how to establish single-subject experimental designs have been presented (Connell and Thompson, 1986; Kearns, 1986; McReynolds and Kearns, 1983; McReynolds and Thompson, 1986; Vetter, 1985); therefore, those data are not reiterated here.

Vetter (1985) discussed the process for establishing the systematic evaluation of a treatment program. This approach would determine the efficacy of speech-language intervention with adolescents. One of the first steps for establishing the systematic evaluation of a treatment program is to isolate the adolescent's problems. This is accomplished by using several sources of information: (1) obtaining client report data from cumulative records and interviewing the adolescent and the close observers of the adolescent; (2) administering only formal assessment instruments that provide data needed to plan intervention procedures; and (3) administering informal procedures carefully, to ensure that the same attention to detail and the same concern for reliability and validity have been followed as when using a formal test. Note that these data may be obtained by using the procedures in Chapter 4.

According to Vetter (1985), a second step in the systematic approach to evaluating a treatment program is to determine the relevant behaviors or attitudes that need to be changed in the client. This is accomplished by observing the client and determining the relevant measurable behaviors of interest. In Chapter 7, Tables 7.2 through 7.6 listed a number of relevant behaviors that speech-language pathologists might consider when facilitating oral communication in adolescents.

A third step is to assess the baseline behaviors of the client, that is, to determine the presence (frequency of occurrence) or absence of the behaviors of concern. Vetter (1985) noted two major functions for gathering baseline data: ". . . as the reference point against which change may be evaluated and as a source of information that contributes to the overall assessment of the client's communication behaviors" (p. 59). The client should be observed several times (at least three and probably more) to determine the frequency of occurrence of the behavior or behaviors to be modified. The clinician may observe several behaviors at the same time, thus obtaining multiple baseline data. Once a single baseline or multiple baselines have been obtained, the clinician must then implement the intervention program that the adolescent will receive.

A number of different designs are available for studying treatment effectiveness. One of the most popular is the pretest/post-test format, or the AB experimental design. Using this design, the clinician establishes a baseline of behavior (pretest, or A), administers the treatment, and then evaluates if any change from the baseline has occurred (post-test, or B). Using this or other similar procedures, the clinician can estimate the change in communication behaviors associated with treatment of the adolescent. By replicating treatments across adolescents who receive intervention, the clinician can begin to draw some conclusions about the effectiveness and efficiency of a particular intervention program for adolescents with similar communication disorders.

Group Design When analyzing the effectiveness of treatment in a group of adolescents, remember that it is also important to isolate the adolescents' problems and to determine relevant behaviors to be modified. Baseline data can best be obtained by administering a selected battery of formal and informal assessment procedures to all the adolescents. (See Chapter 4.) Additional tests can be administered to individual adolescents at the speech-language pathologist's discretion. The battery should contain a standard case history form and, at a minimum, one formal test on language production and comprehension. Several spontaneous language samples should be obtained under different communication conditions. The spontaneous language samples should be analyzed for syntactic, semantic, and pragmatic features. An intelligence test, such as the *Wechsler Intelligence Scale for Children (Revised) (WISC-R)* (Wechsler, 1974) or *Wechsler Adult Intelligence Scale (WAIS)* (Wechsler, 1955), should be administered by a qualified professional.

All students entering secondary-level speech-language programs would complete the battery to provide baseline entrance data. These data are used as reference points when selected tests and informal procedures are readministered upon exit from the secondary intervention program.

Survey Methodology Whether the speech-language pathologist is establishing a single-subject or a group design, survey methods may be desirable. Survey methodology seeks to collect data from any population or sample of individuals and includes, but is not limited to, interviews and questionnaires.

Interviews Using an interview procedure, professionals can collect data on the adolescent's perceptions of benefits derived from current or past language intervention. Major factors to consider when interviewing are summarized below:

1. *Obtaining Consent* The speech-language pathologist must ask permission of the adolescent (and the adolescent's parent[s], if a minor) to con-

duct the interview. The speech-language pathologist must provide a written description of the statement that will be made to the adolescent in securing informed consent and a copy of the questionnaire from which the oral questions will be asked. (A sample form for informed consent is in Appendix O.)

If one wishes to audio or video tape the interview, then additional written permission to record must be obtained before the interview begins, and the adolescent (and the adolescent's parent[s], if a minor) must be informed about how the recording will be used. If the interview is not to be taped, then the interviewer should know how to record answers accurately and rapidly so that the personal interaction is not destroyed. A date should be established well in advance of the interview, and then the date should be confirmed a few days before the interview is to take place. The interviewer should be prompt and have a copy of the questions available for the adolescent to read if the adolescent so desires.

2. *Engaging in Professional Conduct* In Chapter 5, a series of interviewing procedures for use with family members was presented and may be consulted for suggestions when interviewing adolescents. The interview with an adolescent should always be considered a professional situation that demands professional planning and conduct on the part of the interviewer. Speech-language pathologists should state the purpose of the interview, specify how the adolescent was chosen to be interviewed, and assure anonymity and confidentially.

3. *Conducting Interviews* During personal or face-to-face interviewing, the interviewer gathers information in the physical presence of the respondent. This method of conducting interviews has the greatest credibility among respondents, because it is the most trusted of the various forms of interviewing. In the personal interview, the interviewer has greater control over the respondent's behavior than when sending a questionnaire. Personal interviewing allows the interviewer to clarify a statement or to probe for additional information. Spontaneous probes are necessary when the response is irrelevant to the question asked, is unclear, seems incomplete, or is suspected of being untrue (Adams, 1958). A personal interview also allows for observations of body language, e.g., facial expressions.

   The major disadvantages to personal interviewing are the high costs in time and money. Another disadvantage is that the respondent may not be available when the interviewer is available. Finally, the interviewer may project bias into the interviewing process. Some of the sources of interviewer bias are: Writing responses incompletely or inaccurately, suggesting responses to the adolescent, conveying a demeanor that is unsuited to the situation, and dressing unsuitably (e.g., looking like a teen-ager).

Another type of interview, the telephone interview, has been used extensively since 1970 because ninety-eight percent of American households have telephones. Telephoning is far less costly and time consuming than the face-to-face interview. Also, it is geographically flexible and may be free of many perceptual biases (e.g., biases stemming from observation of personal appearance, living conditions). However, a telephone interview usually does not have the credibility that the face-to-face interview appears to have. It can be disruptive to the adolescent and give a feeling of invasion of privacy.

A telephone interview would not be used when adolescents are currently enrolled in speech-language programs. However, when the follow-up study involves interviewing adolescents who have been terminated from speech-language intervention, and who have relocated geographically, the telephone interview may be the best procedure. Whether the speech-language pathologist attempts to interview the adolescent in a personal, face-to-face interview or in a telephone interview, careful consideration must be given to how the instructions are stated: They should be clear and concise. Also, the questions should be asked in an orderly fashion and in a conversational manner. They should be topically arranged, jargon free, and open-ended. The adolescent should not be led to conclusions by the interviewer. It is too easy for adolescents to tell the professional what they think that professional wants to hear, rather than what they are feeling or thinking. Questions that may be highly emotional or personal should be left to the end of the interview. The interviewer should arrange for sufficient time for discussion of any issues pertinent to the adolescent.

Questionnaires Another method for surveying the adolescent's perceived benefits of speech-language services is to send a questionnaire. The questionnaire is far less costly than either form of oral interview and is the most free of perceptual bias. However, the speech-language pathologist has no control, or at best minimal control, over whether the adolescent will respond to the questionnaire. If the adolescent does elect to respond, the reply may come very slowly. Also, in an interview the speech-language clinician can rephrase questions for clarity or probe for additional information if it is warranted. Neither of these is possible when sending a questionnaire to an adolescent. However, when large samples are needed, the questionnaire may prove to be the most effective and efficient method. The speech-language pathologist should consider the following guidelines when designing, writing, and sending the questionnaire:

1. The language used in the questionnaire should not be above a third-grade reading level; it should not be condescending or disorganized.
2. All of the questions should be pretested in a pilot study. This procedure would eliminate as many problems as possible before questionnaires are

sent to a larger group of informants.

3. The questionnaire should be as short as possible so that it is not too time-consuming. It should also be as interesting as possible so that the adolescent responds.
4. A brief letter of transmittal and explanation, requesting the adolescent's participation in the project and outlining the purpose and scope of the project, should accompany the questionnaire. Adolescents should be informed of their rights as human subjects and of the confidentiality of all data. An adolescent's act of responding to the questionnaire may be considered evidence of informed consent to participate in the study. A sample cover letter is included in Appendix P.
5. The respondent should be able to answer the questions in a few words, or with a numerical scale, not in a long narrative.
6. The questionnaire should be accompanied by a self-addressed, stamped return envelope.

A sample questionnaire is provided after the cover letter in Appendix P. The questionnaire should be modified to meet the unique needs of the agency using it. Additional questions may be added, or irrelevant questions deleted.

Even if adolescents are still attending school when the follow-up questionnaire is being used, investigators should send the questionnaire to their homes rather than to give it to them at school. It is less likely to become lost if sent home. Usually, there is more privacy in responding to a questionnaire at home than in school.

After the questionnaire has been sent, the returns will need to be monitored. It may be necessary to send a follow-up questionnaire. According to Babbie (1981), an acceptable response rate for a questionnaire is as follows: Fifty percent response rate is adequate for analysis; sixty percent response rate is good; seventy percent response rate or more is very good. These criteria should be taken into account when analyzing the results and generalizing from them to a larger population.

Most adolescents who have received speech-language services will not be tracked for any longer then five to ten years after graduating from the speech-language program. Remember that during this time they have become adults and should not be referred to as adolescents in any correspondence.

INDIRECT FOLLOW-UP

What To Investigate During Indirect Follow-up

Those individuals who have direct contact and are familiar with the adolescent who received or is receiving speech-language services may serve as informants. These individuals may be educators, family members, or employers. Whatever their role, they are being asked to provide information about their perceptions of the benefits derived by the adolescent from having received speech-language services. In addition to presenting data on their perceptions of adolescents who received direct intervention, members of the educational system might also be asked to provide data on how well the consultation model worked, if it was implemented. Also, family members would be contacted to provide data on how valuable counseling was for them.

How to Conduct Indirect Follow-up

Some of the best procedures for obtaining information about the informants' perceptions of the benefits of speech-language services to the adolescent are the same as those used in the direct follow-up. These procedures would consist of face-to-face and telephone interviews and mailed questionnaires. The general guidelines for conducting interviews and designing questionnaires are the same for the indirect informants as for the adolescent. Differences would exist only in the specific content of the questions and the language level of the questions. The family would be informed, during a staff meeting on their child, about the possibility of collecting follow-up data. They would be informed as to when and how the data would be collected. Informed consent forms would need to be signed by both the adult and the adolescent, if specific data are gathered about that adolescent.

Although the speech-language pathologist may be the primary person involved in collecting follow-up data on the adolescent, it is advantageous to involve the school district administrators in collecting data, too. The administrators should become involved in collecting and analyzing data from teachers and parents, since they may bring another perspective to the over-all process. Even more importantly, administrators may be made more aware of the type and extent of services provided by speech-language pathologists. Thus, follow-up activities would further promulgate information dissemination, the first component of the prototype delivery model.

IMPACT OF FOLLOW-UP DATA

Once the data have been collected, they must be analyzed carefully. Using an integrated software package such as *Appleworks* (Lissner, 1985), speech-language pathologists could keep data on the adolescents in the database component; or they could analyze the data in terms of differences between pretest and post-test results by using the spreadsheet component.

The data could be analyzed for effectiveness, efficiency, and affectivity (Idol, Paolucci-Whitcomb, and Nevin, 1986). The program's effectiveness could be measured by determining how many of the students' individualized objectives were achieved. Efficiency would be ascertained by determining whether the objectives were achieved within a designated amount of time. Affectivity would be measured by finding out whether the adolescent actually enjoyed participating in the program.

A critical use of the follow-up data is to determine the efficacy of services. This determination will allow for enlightened decisions concerning changes that are needed in the prototype service delivery model for adolescents. Goals or objectives established by the speech-language pathologist for the service delivery model that were unrealistic or inadequate should be altered or terminated. Given these data, professionals should identify new goals and objectives. In essence, the analyzed data, once disseminated, can be used to make short- and long-range improvements in the prototype delivery model, across a variety of settings.

SUMMARY

The follow-up component is perhaps one of the least implemented of the six prototype delivery model components. Few follow-up studies have been conducted on adolescents, and problems abound in those that have been done. To modify this situation, speech-language pathologists should implement both direct and indirect follow-up procedures. A direct follow-up procedure involves the adolescent, to determine the benefits derived from speech-language services. Data may be collected using single-subject and group design and survey methodology. Indirect follow-up procedures would involve obtaining information from an adult or a peer who is familiar with the adolescent. Information would be gathered through an interview or a questionnaire to ascertain perceptions of the benefits of speech-language services. Analyzed data would be used to make modifications in the delivery of speech-language services to adolescents and to share with colleagues so that they, too, could make appropriate alterations in their programs.

DISCUSSION QUESTIONS

1. Discuss how you might use computer technology to assist you in tracking students from: (1) the elementary to secondary level, and (2) the secondary to post-secondary level.
2. Design a single-subject study that would document accountability of your clinical intervention program with an adolescent.
3. You have completed follow-up procedures and demonstrated the efficacy of secondary-level speech-language programming. Discuss with whom you would share these data, what to report, and how to disseminate the information.

SUGGESTED READINGS

McReynolds, L., and Kearns, K. *Single-subject Experimental Designs in Communicative Disorders.* University Park Press, Baltimore, MD, 1983.

Vetter, D. Evaluation of clinical intervention: Accountability. *Seminars in Speech and Language*, 6(1): 55–65, 1985.

Weiner, P. The value of follow-up studies. *Topics in Language Disorders*, 5(3): 78–92, 1985.

APPENDIX A

Secondary-Level Referral Form:

Communication Disorders

SECONDARY-LEVEL REFERRAL FORM: COMMUNICATION DISORDERS

Course or Specialty: ____________ Educator: ____________________

Date Completed: ______________ Total of All Ratings: ____________

Using the following scale, mark the following statements regarding the communication behavior of ________ (student) in your classroom.

5 - Almost Always
4 - Frequently
3 - Sometimes ("50 - 50")
2 - Infrequently
1 - Almost Never
NA - Not Applicable / No Chance to Observe

Thinking

____ 1. The student organizes and categorizes information.

____ 2. The student sequences data in a logical order.

____ 3. The student identifies and solves problems independently.

____ 4. The student finds, selects, and utilizes information for assignments.

____ 5. The student thinks about ideas and events that are not just in the "here and now."

____ TOTAL

Listening

____ 1. The student understands complex sentences and multiple meaning words.

____ 2. The student indicates comprehension of main ideas presented.

____ 3. The student follows a sequence of directions even if asked only once.

____ 4. The student identifies relevant supporting details and records them in a notebook and/or systematically retrieves them on request.

____ 5. The student uses critical listening skills such as detecting fact from opinion, evaluating a speaker's argument, and recognizing propaganda.

____ 6. The student effectively listens by asking questions and making comments during conversations.

____ TOTAL

Speaking

____ 1. The student plans what to say, sequences it in a logical way, and produces the resultant sentence(s) with few verbal mazes.

____ 2. The student uses grammatically intact sentences; sentence fragments are appropriate to the context (e.g., the student answers with a single word in response to a question such as, "Where is he going?").

____ 3. The student easily finds words to communicate as precisely and accurately as possible and avoids use of low informational words (e.g., "stuff," "things," "whatchamacallit").

____ 4. The student gives directions, makes reports, tells or retells stories, and explains processes in detail with clarity and accuracy.

____ 5. The student provides relevant and complete answers to questions.

____ 6. The student interacts orally with educators and other students, being considerate of their feelings, taking turns speaking and listening, and initiating and maintaining conversations.

____ 7. The student displays normal voice characteristics with regard to pitch, volume, and quality (e.g., lack of chronic hoarseness, breathiness).

____ 8. The student displays normal fluency characteristics (i.e., lack of word or syllable repetitions, prolongations of sounds, silent gaps within words).

____ TOTAL

Nonverbal Communication

____ 1. The student interprets and uses correct body movements and facial expressions.

____ 2. The student follows rules for social distance when talking.

____ TOTAL

Survival Language

____ 1. The student demonstrates comprehension of basic spatial and temporal concepts.

____ 2. The student demonstrates the ability to obtain and to keep a job with his/her present level of communication skills (i.e., Would you hire this student given the way the individual talks and listens?).

____ 3. The student demonstrates sufficient language to cope with daily living situations such as job applications, shopping, using the telephone, and interpreting signs and labels.

____ 4. The student understands and uses figurative language acceptable to the peer group.

____ TOTAL

Thinking Total: ________

Listening Total: ________

Speaking Total: ________

Nonverbal Communication Total: ________

Survival Language Total: ________

TOTAL OF ALL RATINGS (A): ________

TOTAL NUMBER OF POINTS POSSIBLE (B): ________

PERCENTAGE ([A ÷ B] x 100): ________

- -

I feel confident in this student's ability to function independently once his/her school experience is over. ____

If you rate this item "1" or "2," please comment on how the student's oral communication is contributing to the problem: ____________________

____

____

APPENDIX B

Case History Forms

CASE HISTORY FORM FOR ADOLESCENTS

Interviewer:____________________ Date:____________________

I. Personal Information of Interviewee

A. Name:______________________________________

B. Birthdate:________________ Age:________ Sex: ____M ____F

C. Address:______________________________________

D. Home Phone:________________ Work Phone of Parent/Guardian:________________

E. Education: Highest grade completed____________________

II. Environmental History

A. List and describe below all members of your family. Indicate in the far right column any speech, hearing, or language problems present among other members of the household.

Name	Relationship	Sex	Communication Problem

B. List two friends with whom you enjoy talking.____________________

III. Educational and Vocational History

A. Please list the school subjects you are the best in.

____

B. Please list the school subjects you enjoy the most.

____

C. Please list the school subjects you have the most difficulty in.

____

D. Why do you feel you are having difficulty with these subjects?

____

____

____

E. Are you involved in activities outside of school? ____No ____Yes

If yes, describe:______________________________

F. Do you have any future vocational goals? ____No ____Yes

If yes, describe:______________________________

G. Do you hold a full or part-time job? ____No ____Yes

If yes, describe:______________________________

IV. Health History

A. List below: (1) major illnesses, diseases, or operations; (2) age at the time of each; and (3) resulting health complications or handicaps.

Illnesses/diseases/accidents	Age	Resulting handicaps

B. Were you hospitalized for any of the above conditions?
____No ____Yes

If yes, where?______________________________

For how long?______________________________

C. Have you received, or are you now receiving rehabilitation treatment such as radiation therapy, physical therapy, occupational therapy? Describe the reason for, type, duration, and result of treatments:

____

____

D. Are you currently under a doctor's care? ____No ____Yes

If yes, for what? ______________________________

E. Are you currently taking any medication? ____No ____Yes

If yes, what kind? ______________________________

For what? ______________________________

How much? ______________________________

How often? ______________________________

F. Do you have any known allergies? ____No ____Yes

If yes, describe: ______________________________

G. Do you have any known drug sensitivities? ____No ____Yes

If yes, describe: ______________________________

H. Have you had seizures? ____No ____Yes

If yes, how often? ______________________________

When was the most recent seizure? ______________________________

I. Do you have any known hearing problems? ____No ____Yes

If yes, describe: ______________________________

J. Have you had a past history of ear infections? ____No ____Yes

If yes, describe: ______________________________

K. Do you have any known visual problems? ____No ____Yes

If yes, describe: ______________________________

Glasses worn? ____No ____Yes

V. Speech, Language, and Hearing History

A. Describe the present problem: ______________________________

____

B. How long has there been a problem? ______________________________

____

C. What do you think caused the problem? ______________________________

____

D. What types of speech and language services have you received?

____

How long have you received them? ______________________________

How do you feel about the services you received? ______________

____

E. Were you ever dismissed from speech and language therapy?

____No ____Yes

If yes, why? ______________________________

____

F. How do you feel about your present speech and language problem?

____

G. Are you understood when you speak? ____No ____Yes

If no, describe: ______________________________

H. Do you understand when others talk to you? ____No ____Yes

If no, describe: ______________________________

____

I. Do you avoid speaking situations? ____No ____Yes

If yes, describe: ______________________________

J. Are there times or situations when your problem is better or worse?

____No ____Yes

If yes, describe: ______________________________

____

VI. Please provide in the space below any additional information that may be useful in evaluating your communication skills and in planning an intervention program.

THINKING, LISTENING, AND SPEAKING SUPPLEMENTAL CASE HISTORY

Student: ______________________________ Age: ____________

Examiner: ______________________________ Date: ____________

I. Feelings and Attitudes

A. Thinking

1. What is thinking? ______________________________

2. How important on a scale from 1 to 5 is thinking in your life?

1	2	3	4	5
Not at all Important		Sometimes Important		Extremely Important

3. Whom do you know that you consider to be a good thinker?

____

What makes you feel __(name)__ is a good thinker? ____________

____

____

4. Have you ever felt you would like to think better? ____No ____Yes

If yes, in what situations? ______________________________

____

____

5. What interferes with your ability to think clearly? ____________

____

____

B. Listening

1. What is listening? ______________________________

2. How important on a scale from 1 to 5 is listening in your life?

1	2	3	4	5
Not at all Important		Sometimes Important		Extremely Important

3. Whom do you know that you consider to be a good listener?

____

What makes you feel ____(name)____ is a good listener? __________

____

____

4. Have you ever felt you would like to listen better? ____No ____Yes

If yes, in what situations? ______________________________

____

____

5. What interferes with your ability to listen? ______________

____

____

C. Speaking

1. What is speaking? ______________________________

2. How important on a scale from 1 to 5 is speaking in your life?

1	2	3	4	5
Not at all Important		Sometimes Important		Extremely Important

3. Whom do you know that you consider to be a good speaker?

____

What makes you feel __(name)__ is a good speaker? __________

____

____

4. Have you ever felt you would like to speak better? ____No ____Yes

If yes, in what situations? ___________________________

____

____

5. What interferes with your ability to speak? _______________

____

____

II. Current Need for Thinking, Listening, and Speaking

A. Academic Environment

How often are you required to think, listen, and speak in classroom situations? Use this scale:

1 = Frequently
2 = Occasionally
3 = Seldom
4 = Never

Courses/Subjects	Think	Listen	Speak
________________	____	____	____
________________	____	____	____
________________	____	____	____
________________	____	____	____

Comments: ___________________________________

____

B. Social Environment

How often are you required to think, listen, and speak in daily living situations (e.g., with friends, with family members)? Use this scale:

1 = Frequently
2 = Occasionally
3 = Seldom
4 = Never

Situations	Think	Listen	Speak
______________	_____	_____	_____
______________	_____	_____	_____
______________	_____	_____	_____
______________	_____	_____	_____

Comments: ____

____

C. Vocational Environment

How often are you required to think, listen, and speak in a job situation (e.g., with co-workers, with customers)? Use this scale:

1 = Frequently
2 = Occasionally
3 = Seldom
4 = Never

Situations	Think	Listen	Speak
______________	_____	_____	_____
______________	_____	_____	_____
______________	_____	_____	_____
______________	_____	_____	_____

Comments: ____

____

III. Intervention: Past and Future

A. What intervention have you received in the past for thinking? ___

____

____

For listening? ____

____

For speaking? ____

____

B. Do you feel you need to improve your thinking? ____No ____Yes

Comments: ____

____

Do you feel you need to improve your listening? ____No ____Yes

Comments: ____

____

Do you feel you need to improve your speaking? ____No ____Yes

Comments: ____

____

(Reprinted with permission of THINKING PUBLICATIONS from *Daily Communication: Strategies for the Language Disordered Adolescent* [Schwartz and McKinley, 1984].)

2. LISTENING SURVEY FOR ADOLESCENTS:

Purpose: To recognize individual beliefs and attitudes toward listening

An adaptation of the **Personal Analysis Questionnaire** proposed by Wolff et al. (1983) can assist adolescents in recognizing their individual misconceptions about listening. The questionnaire is reprinted in the appendix and can also be administered orally, requiring the student to listen rather than read.

LISTENING QUESTIONNAIRE

Mark each statement as true or false.

____ 1. Teachers or friends who don't listen to me are too stupid to appreciate my ideas.

____ 2. Teaching students to listen is as foolish as trying to teach them to breathe.

____ 3. I already have developed good listening skills because I have to listen all the time in school.

____ 4. It is more important to be good speakers than good listeners because we learn by talking.

____ 5. It is more important to be good readers than good listeners because we can go back to check material we read.

____ 6. I think I have been adequately trained to listen at school and home.

____ 7. Students should not have to work at listening to class lectures.

____ 8. I can't stand to listen to people who talk about ideas that sound crazy.

____ 9. It doesn't matter if I stop listening because I don't miss much.

____ 10. I'm a good listener when I want to be.

Each true answer reveals a misconception about listening. Have students count their number of **true** responses and compare it to the scale below.

0, 1 = Free of false information about listening
2, 3, 4 = Positive attitude toward listening training
5, 6, 7 = Aware of listening training; misconceptions are warping your thinking
8, 9, 10 = BRICK WALL. Misconceptions have kept listening information from being useful to you

Compare and discuss results within the group.

APPENDIX C

Learning Style Questionnaire

LEARNING STYLE QUESTIONNAIRE

DIRECTIONS TO THE PERSON ADMINISTERING THE QUESTIONNAIRE:

This learning style questionnaire attempts to determine how an adolescent learns best a difficult or new subject, not necessarily how they prefer or like to learn a difficult or new subject. This is NOT a learning style preference inventory where students are assessed as to how they like to learn.

Please inform the student(s) that this is NOT a test but rather a survey to find out how they learn a new or difficult subject best. You should emphasize to them that there are no right or wrong answers. You should read the directions and survey questions to the students. Questionnaires should be given to the students so that they can read along and mark their own copies.

It is preferable to complete the questionnaire on a one-to-one basis but small groups of 3 to 7 may be administered the questionnaire. It is appropriate to rephrase questions and to answer students' questions as you proceed through the survey in order to clarify for better understanding.

It is important to emphasize to students that they are to check and/or rank order items as stated. When rankings are requested, be certain that items are rank ordered and not simply checked. You should have the students fill in the identification information (e.g., name, date of birth) before beginning to answer the questions. You should stress to the students that they should answer the questions as honestly as possible and that they should give their immediate or first reaction to each question.

You should read the directions aloud to the students and answer any of their questions before beginning the questionnaire.

LEARNING STYLE QUESTIONNAIRE

IDENTIFICATION INFORMATION

Student: ______________________________ Current Date: _______________

Sex: _____ Grade:_____ Birthdate: _____ School District: __________

Parent or Guardian: ____

Address: ____________________________________ City: ____________

Home Phone: ____________________ Work Phone: _________________

Adult assisting you to complete this questionnaire: _______________

DIRECTIONS TO THE STUDENT: This is NOT a test. There are no right or wrong answers. The following items are simply a way to find out how you learn best. If an item is unclear, feel free to ask questions of the person administering this questionnaire.

The purpose of this questionnaire is to determine how you *learn best;* not how you *like* to learn a subject. For example, you might like to have the TV on while you are studying, but you study best when it is quiet. Also, you might like to study at night, but you are more productive if you study in the morning. "Learn best" means how you remember information the longest, attend to a task the best, or recall details and main ideas most easily. Knowing how you learn best will help us to help you to be more successful in school.

Before you begin to answer the questions, please write your name, current date, address, and other identification information requested in the space provided above.

I. Answer the following statements honestly about when, where, why, and with whom you learn best.

My most difficult subject is: ________________________________

I learn my most difficult subject best:

A. WHEN

1. Time (Check only one.)
   _____ Morning
   _____ Afternoon
   _____ Night
   _____ Other (Explain): ______________________________

2. Timing (Check only one.)
   ____ Before meals
   ____ After meals

3. Conditions
   a. Sound (Check only one.)
      ____ Quiet
      ____ Radio
      ____ Conversation
      ____ TV
      ____ Music
      ____ Noisy
      ____ Other: (explain): ____________________
   b. Light (Check only one.)
      ____ Dim
      ____ Moderate
      ____ Bright
      ____ Other (explain): ____________________
   c. Temperature (Check only one.)
      ____ Cold
      ____ Cool
      ____ Warm
      ____ Very Warm
      ____ Other (explain): ____________________
   d. Intake (Check only one.)
      ____ Eat food
      ____ Drink liquids
      ____ Chew on something
      ____ Not eat, drink, or chew anything while learning
      ____ Other (explain): ____________________

I learn my most difficult subject best:

B. WHERE?
   1. Place (Indicate your first and second choices.)
      ____ Home ____________________
      Which room/place within your home? (e.g., bedroom, kitchen, living room, etc.)
      ____ School ____________________
      Which room within the school? (e.g., library, study hall, classroom)
   2. Location (Within each place, rank order the locations.
      1 = location where you learn best.)
      a. Home
         ____ Desk/Table
         ____ Bed
         ____ Floor
         ____ Straight Chair
         ____ Soft Chair
         ____ Couch
         ____ Other (explain): ____________________

b. School
- ____ Desk/Table
- ____ Floor
- ____ Soft Chair
- ____ Straight Chair
- ____ Other (explain): ______________________________

I learn my most difficult subject best:

C. WHY? (Rank order 1-4 as to why you learn best. 1 = the strongest reason for learning is because.........)
- ____ I want to
- ____ The teacher expects me to/demands it
- ____ My parent(s) expects me to/demands it
- ____ I'll get a reward such as:
  - ____ money
  - ____ better grades
  - ____ privileges
- ____ Other (explain): ______________________________

I learn my most difficult subject best:

D. WITH WHOM? (Rank order the top four. 1 = the best way to study the subject.)
- ____ Alone
- ____ A partner
- ____ Small Group (3-7)
- ____ Large Group (8 and above)
- ____ Teacher(s)
- ____ Parent(s)
- ____ Sibling(s)
- ____ Other (explain): ______________________________

II. Given the following situations check how you learn best.

A. Inside the classroom

1. Participating in the class (Rank order how you learn best in the classroom. 1 = the way you learn difficult material the best.)
   - ____ Listening
   - ____ Reading
   - ____ Writing
   - ____ Speaking
   - ____ Doing
   - ____ Combination of the above
     Please specify ______________________________

2. Participating in assignments within the classroom (Rank order the top four assignments that help you to learn the information best. 1 = best way to learn via an assignment.)
   - ____ Worksheet Questions
   - ____ Experiments
   - ____ Demonstrations
   - ____ Group Projects
   - ____ Individual Projects
   - ____ Written Reports
   - ____ Oral Reports
   - ____ Other (explain): ______________________________

3. Remembering main points from what the teacher says (Rank order the top four. 1 = the best way to remember main points from what the teacher says.)
   - ____ Repeat the material to yourself
   - ____ Think of a picture in your mind
   - ____ Make up words to remember main points in order
   - ____ Break ideas into smaller chunks
   - ____ Outline what the teacher says in writing
   - ____ Follow an outline that the teacher has provided
   - ____ Use rhyming words to recall main points
   - ____ Put main points into categories
   - ____ Audio tape what the teacher is saying and replay it later
   - ____ Other (explain): ______________________________

4. Taking notes (Check only one.)

   While listening to a lecture I take notes when learning my most difficult subject as follows:
   - ____ Notes are key words
   - ____ Notes are attempts at complete sentences
   - ____ Notes are "doodles"
   - ____ Other (explain): ______________________________

5. Asking questions of the teacher (Check only one.)

   I learn my most difficult subject best if I ask questions:
   - ____ During Class
   - ____ After Class
   - ____ Before Class
   - ____ Other (explain): ______________________________

6. Remembering main points from a textbook (Rank order the top four ways that you learn best from a textbook. 1 = the best way to remember main points from a textbook.)
    - ____ Look at headings and subheadings within the chapters
    - ____ Outline important ideas from the textbook
    - ____ Underline/highlight main points
    - ____ Write down questions to anticipate what a teacher will ask on a test
    - ____ Answer questions at the end of each chapter (if available)
    - ____ Follow along in the textbook as I am listening to an audio tape of the textbook
    - ____ Other (explain): ______________________________

B. Outside of the Classroom

1. Participating in outside classroom assignments (Rank order the top four assignments that help you to learn a difficult subject best. 1 = the best way to learn via an assignment.)
    - ____ Preparing a written report
    - ____ Preparing for an oral report
    - ____ Answering questions from the textbook or worksheet
    - ____ Reading assigned information
    - ____ Other (explain): ______________________________
2. Studying for a test. (Rank order the top four. 1 = the way I study best to take a test.)

    I learn best studying for a test in my most difficult subject when I:
    - ____ Read or reread the textbook the day before
    - ____ Read or reread the textbook 2-3 days before
    - ____ Listen or re-listen to audio tapes of what the teacher said
    - ____ Review the outline of my notes
    - ____ Review the outline provided by the teacher
    - ____ Predict questions to be on the test and answer them
    - ____ Rework problems assigned by the teacher
    - ____ Other (explain): ______________________________
3. I learn my most difficult subject best when I study for ________ minutes each hour before taking a break.

APPENDIX D

Adolescent Conversational Analysis

PROFILE: ADOLESCENT CONVERSATIONAL ANALYSIS

	Appropriate	Inappropriate	Not observed
I. ROLE OF LISTENER			
A. Vocabulary/Syntax			
*B. Main Ideas			
C. Nonjudgmental Manner			
D. Feedback			
II. ROLE OF SPEAKER			
A. Language Features			
1. Syntax			
2. Questions			
3. Figurative language			
4. Nonspecific language			
5. Precise vocabulary			
*a. Word retrieval skills			
b. Verbal mazes			
c. False starts			
B. Paralanguage Features			
1. Suprasegmental features			
*2. Fluency			
*3. Intelligibility			
C. Communication Functions			
1. To give			
2. To get			
3. To describe			
4. To persuade			
5. To express			
6. To indicate			
7. To problem-solve			
8. To entertain			
D. Conversational Rules			
1. Verbal (Topics/Turns)			
a. Initiation			
b. Topic choice			
c. Maintenance			
d. Topic switch			
*e. Turn-taking			
f. Repair/revision			
g. Interruptions			
2. Verbal (Politeness)			
a. Quantity			
b. Sincerity			
c. Relevance			
d. Clarity			
e. Tactfulness			
3. Nonverbal			
a. Gestures			
b. Facial expressions			
c. Eye contact			
d. Proxemics			

38 TOTAL NUMBER OF ITEMS

____ TOTAL NUMBER OF ITEMS MARKED "NOT OBSERVED"

____ TOTAL NUMBER OF ITEMS RATED

____ Number rated as inappropriate ÷ ____ Number of items rated x 100 = ____%

*If consistent problems are evident in this area, conduct additional assessment.

ADOLESCENT CONVERSATIONAL ANALYSIS

Name: ______________________________ Date: ______________

Age: ________ Conversational Partner: ______________________

Setting of Conversation: ________________________________

Materials Present to Elicit Sample: __________________________

(Obtain a minimum of 10 minutes of conversational speech with each partner in each setting. Transcribe exactly the conversational units of each participant. Analyze for the behaviors listed below. Mark "A" for appropriate and "I" for inappropriate behaviors. Determine appropriateness and inappropriateness of a behavior by judging whether or not it is penalizing to the adolescent; a behavior perceived by the clinician as penalizing is marked as inappropriate [Prutting and Kirchner, 1983]. Mark "NO" if a behavior is "not observed" during the sample. Probe any behaviors marked "NO" during directed tasks.)

I. Role of listener in the conversation

A I NO A. Appears to understand the vocabulary and syntactical structures of the conversational partner

Comments:

A I NO B. Appears to follow main idea of conversational topics

Comments:

A I NO C. Appears to listen in a nonjudgmental manner

Comments:

A I NO D. Indicates understanding or lack of understanding of conversational partner by use of verbal and/or nonverbal feedback

Comments:

II. Role of speaker in the conversation

A. Language Features

A I NO 1. Production of a variety of syntactic forms

Comments:

A I NO *2. Production of a variety of questions (Question forms)

Comments:

A I NO 3. Production of figurative language

Comments:

A I NO 4. Production of nonspecific language

Comments:

5. Production of precise vocabulary

A I NO a. Word retrieval skills

Comments:

A I NO b. Verbal mazes

Comments:

A I NO c. False starts

Comments:

*Note: Although questions fall into "II.A.1. Production of a variety of syntactic forms," it is desirable to have more specific information on interrogatives produced by adolescents.

B. Paralanguage Features

A I NO 1. Suprasegmental features (use of vocal inflection, juncture, and rate)

Comments:

A I NO 2. Fluency

Comments:

A I NO 3. Intelligibility

Comments:

C. Communication Functions

A I NO 1. To give information

Comments:

A I NO 2. To get information

Comments:

A I NO 3. To describe an ongoing event

Comments:

A I NO 4. To persuade one's listener to do, believe, or feel something

Comments:

A I NO 5. To express one's own intentions, beliefs, and feelings

Comments:

A I NO 6. To indicate a readiness for further communication

Comments:

A I NO 7. To solve problems

Comments:

A I NO 8. To entertain

Comments:

D. Verbal and Nonverbal Communicational Rules

1. Verbal rules governing topics and turns

A I NO a. Initiation of conversations

Comments:

A I NO b. Topic choice

Comments:

A I NO c. Maintenance of conversational topics

Comments:

A I NO d. Switch of topics using direct or indirect cues

Comments:

A I NO e. Turn-taking

Comments:

A I NO f. Repair/revision when necessary

Comments:

A I NO g. Interruptions

Comments:

2. Verbal rules of politeness

A I NO a. Appears not to talk too much or too little in the situation (quantity)

Comments:

A I NO b. Appears to be honest and sincere

Comments:

A I NO c. Appears to make relevant contributions

Comments:

A I NO d. Appears to express ideas clearly and concisely

Comments:

A I NO e. Appears to be tactful

Comments:

3. Nonverbal rules

A I NO a. Gestures

Comments:

A I NO b. Facial expressions

Comments:

A I NO c. Eye contact/gazing

Comments:

A I NO d. Physical distance from partner (proxemics)

Comments:

APPENDIX E

Narration Analysis

NARRATION ANALYSIS

Name: ______________________________ Date: ______________

Age: __________ Examiner: ______________________________

DIRECTIONS: Place check marks to reflect the highest mode of organization observed for formulated and reformulated tasks.

Cognitive Period	Approximate "Normal" Age of Emergence	Mode of Organization	Tasks: Formulated	Tasks: Reformulated
Pre-operational	2 years	Heaps		
	2 to 3 years	Sequences		
	2 to 3 years	Primitive narrative		
	3 to 4 years	Unfocused chain		
	4 to 5 years	Focused chain		
	5 to 6 years	Narratives		
Concrete	7 to 11 years	Summarization		
Formal	13 to 15 years	Analysis		
	16 years to Adulthood	Generalization		

Description of formulated task: ______________________________

Description of reformulated task: ______________________________

Comments: ______________________________

____

____

APPENDIX F

Structure of the Educational System Checklist

STRUCTURE OF THE EDUCATIONAL SYSTEM CHECKLIST

Name of person completing form: ______________________________

Name of school(s) assessed: ______________________________

Date: ________ Phase of speech-language program: ____ Initiation
____ Maintenance

Interview key personnel as necessary, to obtain information on the questions below. Your answers will summarize the current structure of the educational system and will be useful data for program planning.

I. Response to Educational Reports

A. What have been the primary reponses to national, state, and/or local reports calling for educational reform? (Rank order the top three responses)

_____ General apathy
_____ Some interest in reform
_____ General interest, but lack of concensus on action that should be initiated
_____ Formation of a task force or study committee
_____ Curriculum committees formed to initiate changes
_____ Upgrading of school standards completed, or in the planning stage
_____ Other (Please specify: ______________________________)

B. Who has been leading local educational reform? (If applicable)

____

____

II. Drop-out Rate

A. Summarize the drop-out rate for adolescents in the school setting being assessed for the past three years.

Year	Number of drop-outs	Total percent of drop-outs	Number of drop-outs currently enrolled in speech-language
____	________	________	________________
____	________	________	________________
____	________	________	________________

$$\frac{\text{Number of drop-outs}}{\text{Total number of students eligible to drop-out}} \times 100 = \underline{\quad\quad}\%$$

B. What preventative measures are currently operative in your educational setting to prevent dropping out of school?

____

____

C. Do you perceive a general commitment to modify the educational system to retain potential drop-outs?

____ yes ____ no Explain: ____________________

____

III. Minimum Competency Testing

A. Does the educational setting being assessed have minimum competency testing for graduation? ____ yes ____ no

B. If "no," are there plans to initiate competency testing?

____ Yes, at the state level
____ Yes, at the local level
____ No
____ Don't know

C. If "yes," please summarize the current plan for competency testing.

1. What curricula areas are tested? ____________________

____

2. When are tests given? ____________________

____

3. What happens to students who fail competency testing the first time? ____________________

____

More than one time? ____________________

____

4. What percent of students are failing to pass competency testing after repeated tries? ________

5. How are competency requirements applied to students enrolled in special education programs, including learning disabilities?

____

____

IV. Organizational Framework

A. Is the educational system horizontally structured by age groupings (e.g., freshmen, sophomores, etc.)? ____ yes ____ no

1. If "no," how is the educational system structured for grouping students? ____

____

2. If "yes," how strong do you perceive the peer ties to be within each grade level?

____ Extremely strong (i.e., students in one grade level avoid interacting with those in another)

____ Moderately strong (i.e., students in one grade level prefer to interact only with others at the same level, but do not avoid other levels)

____ Moderately weak (i.e., students in one grade level sometimes choose to interact with those at another level)

____ Extremely weak (i.e., students are not necessarily aware who is at what grade level within the educational setting)

B. Is the educational system vertically structured by program track (e.g., college-bound, vocational-technical education, special education)? ____ yes ____ no

1. If "no," how is the educational system structured with regard to program offerings? ____

____

2. If "yes," how do you think your colleagues view your role in the school?

____ They view me as working only in the special education track and with adolescents who have speech disorders.

____ They view me as someone who works primarily in the special education track, occasionally in the vocational-technical education track, and never in the college-bound track except with adolescents who have speech disorders.

____ They view me as someone who can make significant contributions to students in any track, including those with learning disabilities and language disorders who are in the college-bound track.

V. Interdisciplinary Team Process

A. Who is (are) the key person(s) who makes decisions regarding assignments of professionals to assess adolescents referred for diagnostic testing? ____________________

____

B. How aware is (are) the key person(s) listed above of speech-language services at the secondary level?

____ Very aware; past information dissemination has been successful
____ Moderately aware; some information dissemination has been completed, but more is needed
____ Vaguely aware; information dissemination has been sketchy and/or unsuccessful
____ Other (Please specify: ____________________

____

C. Summarize the number of referrals of adolescents in the past three years and determine how many have included a speech-language evaluation.

Year	Number of Referrals (a)	Number that Included Speech-Language Evaluation (b)	Percent that Included Speech-Language Evaluation (b/a x 100 = ____%)

VI. Criteria

A. Do criteria for entrance and exit into the speech-language program currently exist? ____ yes ____ no

B. If "yes," are you in philosophical agreement with the criteria?

____ Yes, with most of the criteria
____ Yes, with some of the criteria, but not others (Please specify:
____)
____ No, not with many of the criteria, but administrators and/or other speech-language pathologists appear amenable to changes.
____ No, not with many of the criteria and administrators and/or other speech-language pathologists seem unamenable to changes.

C. If "no," are there plans to create criteria?
____ yes ____ no ____ maybe

1. If "yes," who will create the criteria? ____________________

____

By what date? ____

2. If "no" or "maybe," how necessary does your administration perceive criteria to be?

____ Not necessary; they'd prefer to have me use my professional judgement when deciding who is eligible for speech-language services.
____ Somewhat necessary; they like the security and predictability of referring to pre-established criteria for my program, but it's not a priority task to accomplish.
____ Very necessary; they believe criteria are essential for speech-language programs, but have not gotten around to developing them.

ANALYSIS

Based upon your responses, analyze whether the educational system appears open, flexible, and responsive to adolescents who have special needs, and amenable to reform. Also analyze the level of awareness of how speech-language pathologists can contribute to programming for adolescents. Summarize your analysis:

___

___

What change would you make within the system if you could?

(List top priorities)___

___

___

INTERPRETATION

An educational system that is analyzed to be relatively open, flexible, and responsive will generally be more receptive to direct and indirect program planning and intervention that involve modifications within that system. Desired changes you would like to see in the educational system are starting points for the modifications.

APPENDIX G

Teacher Language: Self-evaluation Technique

Student Response Forms

Name: ______________________ Date: ______________________

Teacher: ______________________ Class: ______________________

THIS IS NOT A TEST! ANSWERS WILL NOT AFFECT YOUR GRADE!
PLEASE ANSWER HONESTLY.

Use this scale to rate the lecture or instructions your teacher just gave:

5—Very easy
4—Somewhat easy
3—Neither easy nor hard
2—Somewhat hard
1—Very hard

Rate these characteristics of your teacher's language during the lecture or instructions just finished:

_____ Length of instructions or lecture
_____ Complexity of instructions or lecture
_____ Level of vocabulary
_____ Organization of ideas
_____ Ease of listening
_____ Rate of speech
_____ Tone of voice

Do you have other comments about the teacher's language? What would help you to understand class material better? Write your comments on the back side of this form. Thank you.

APPENDIX H

Adolescents with Communication Disorders—

Attitudinal Scale (ACDA Scale)

Date:

To: Professional Colleagues

From: (Speech-Language Pathologist's Name)

Re: Attached Survey

Attached to this memo is a survey called the ACDA Scale. I would appreciate it if you complete this survey by __(date)__ and return it to my mailbox. The survey should take you five to ten minutes to complete.

The purpose of the survey is to provide information that can help me to improve the speech-language program for secondary-level students. Data will be treated confidentially. If you wish to receive a copy of the summarized data, please let me know and I'll share the results with you.

Please read the directions carefully before completing the ACDA Scale. Contact me if you have questions or concerns at (address/phone number).

ACDA Scale

DIRECTIONS

Read each statement below. You will be using a number between 1 and 5 to indicate how much you agree or disagree with a set of 20 statements.

All answers will be treated confidentially. No individual data will be reported, only group data from a number of teachers and administrators.

NOTE: THERE ARE NO CORRECT OR INCORRECT ANSWERS.

SCALE

(Respond to each of the statements below by choosing the answer that comes closest to how you usually feel or act.)

5—I agree strongly
4—I agree
3—I neither agree or disagree
2—I disagree
1—I disagree strongly

____ 1. Adolescents with communication disorders should be allowed to substitute speech-language intervention for a content area course (e.g., English).

____ 2. It makes sense to give grades and credit to adolescents receiving speech-language services.

____ 3. Adolescents with communication disorders should be allowed to take tests orally if written language is severely impaired.

____ 4. Adolescents with communication disorders should be allowed to tape record classroom lectures and directions given by teachers.

____ 5. Teachers should provide both oral and written instructions for students.

____ 6. Teachers should supply written listening guides for students to follow during lectures.

____ 7. Speech-language programs are a necessary service for adolescents with communication disorders.

_____ 8. Adolescents with communication disorders should be spending full classroom time modules in the speech-language program, not short fifteen to twenty minute blocks of time.

_____ 9. Speech-language services are as important for adolescents with mild disorders as for those with severe disorders.

_____ 10. The speech-language program is an important resource for adolescents with communication disorders.

_____ 11. Adolescents with communication disorders should be kept in the educational mainstream as much as possible.

_____ 12. Adolescents who feel they have a problem with communication should be able to refer themselves to the speech-language program for testing.

_____ 13. Adolescents with communication disorders are just as intelligent as adolescents without communication disorders.

_____ 14. Adolescents with communication disorders should be expected to meet the same graduation standards as adolescents without communication disorders.

_____ 15. It is possible for an adolescent with a communication disorder to lead a normal life.

_____ 16. Adolescents with communication disorders should be treated the same as anyone.

_____ 17. Adolescents with communication disorders usually make a contribution to society.

_____ 18. The curriculum should be modified to meet the individual needs of adolescents with communication disorders.

_____ 19. Adolescents with severe disorders deserve more curriculum modifications than adolescents with mild disorders.

_____ 20. Adolescents with communication disorders should be expected to modify their behaviors to meet the demands of the curriculum.

THANK YOU FOR YOUR TIME. PLEASE RETURN THIS SCALE TO (person or location).

MAINSTREAMING LIST

The speech-language program is maintaining a list of teachers who are receptive to mainstreaming students with language disorders and to making modifications in curriculum, when necessary, to meet the student's needs. If this is an interest of yours, and you are willing to have your name added to this list, please share your name below. Detach this information from the rest of the attitudinal scale and return it to the speech-language pathologist.

Name: ______________________________

Content area: ______________________________

Grade level(s): ______________________________

APPENDIX I

Curriculum Analysis Form

CURRICULUM ANALYSIS FORM

Date(s) of Analysis: ____________ Examiner Completing Analysis: ____________

Student: ____________ Course: ____________

Grade Level: ____________ Instructor: ____________

I. Textbook Analysis (Use the primary text from the course.)

A. Identifying Information

1. Title: ____________
2. Author(s): ____________
3. Copyright: ____________
4. Year Adopted by School: ____________
5. Readability Level: ____________

a. Is this readability level appropriate for the student?

____ yes ____ no

b. Is this readability level similar to the student's other textbooks?

____ yes ____ no

B. Student Familiarity with Textbook

Check which of the following features are included in the textbook. For any that are present, check whether the student can locate these features upon request and state when they are used.

Check if present	Features	Can the student locate the feature?	When is the feature used?
____	1. Table of contents	____ yes ____ no	____
____	2. Index	____ yes ____ no	____
____	3. Glossary	____ yes ____ no	____
____	4. Appendix	____ yes ____ no	____
____	5. Bibliography	____ yes ____ no	____
____	6. Unit or chapter objectives	____ yes ____ no	____
____	7. Review questions and/or practice exercises	____ yes ____ no	____
____	8. Italicization of words (varying print styles)	____ yes ____ no	____
____	9. Graphic aids (charts, tables, graphs, maps)	____ yes ____ no	____

Is this textbook significantly different from others that the student is reading? ____ yes ____ no

If "yes," how is it different? ________________________________

____

II. Classroom Analysis

A. Organization of the Course

1. Which topical arrangement typifies this course? (Check one.)

   ____ Sequential (independence among topics)

   ____ Spiral (dependence among topics)

2. If "sequential" arrangement is primary, have all units been problematic for the student, or only some? (Check one.)

   ____ All

   ____ Some

3. Does the course have significantly different requirements in comparison with the student's other courses?

   ____ yes ____ no

   If "yes," explain: ________________________________

   ____

B. Student's Comprehension of Lecture/Instructions

Enlist the assistance of a "good student" in the classroom. Indicate to that student that you would like him/her to take notes during the first ten minutes of a lecture or set of instructions given in the class within the next week. These notes should be copied by the examiner, then compared with the notes taken by the student undergoing assessment. Use the "good student's" notes to answer questions 1 and 2 below; for question 3, use the notes from the adolescent being assessed.

1. What was the main idea presented (or sequence of instructions)?

   ____

2. What were the relevant supporting ideas? ______________________

____

3. Answer the following questions:
   a. Did the student's main idea(s) match the one(s) the "good student" identified?

      ____ yes ____ no

   b. Did the student's relevant supporting details match the ones the "good student" identified?

      ____ yes ____ no

   c. Did the student indicate verbally or nonverbally any words that were not understood?

      ____ yes ____ no

      If "yes," list them: ______________________________________

      ____

   d. Does the student report having difficulty comprehending the lectures/instructions only in this class or also in others? (Check one.)

      ____ Only this course

      ____ This course and others

C. Student's Comprehension of Tests/Evaluations

Obtain a recent test or other evaluation tool administered to the student. With the student present, ask the following questions:

1. What questions were most difficult to answer? ______________

   ____

   Why were they more difficult? _____________________________

   ____

2. What vocabulary items were unfamiliar? ____________________

   ____

   ____

3. How well did you prepare for this test? (Check one.)

____	____	____	____	____
Not at all	Some	Enough	More than usual	A great amount

4. Using the taxonomy from Benjamin Bloom*, what level(s) of thinking was required most often during this test?

____ Memory
____ Translation
____ Interpretation
____ Application
____ Analysis
____ Synthesis
____ Evaluation

5. Are the course tests significantly different from those in other courses that you are taking?

____ yes ____ no

If "yes," how are they different? ______________________________

____

III. Student Attitude Toward the Course

Ask the student the following questions. The examiner should record responses.

A. Do you think the ideas presented in this course are important to learn?

____ yes ____ no ____ sometimes

B. Do you think this course is interesting?

____ yes ____ no ____ sometimes

C. Do you think the teacher makes this course meaningful?

____ yes ____ no ____ sometimes

D. Do you think this course is made simple enough so that you can learn the information?

____ yes ____ no ____ sometimes

E. Do you think the information you learn in this course is useful?

____ yes ____ no ____ sometimes

F. Do you think the information in this course is presented clearly by the teacher?

____ yes ____ no ____ sometimes

G. Do you think the information in this course is presented clearly by the textbook?

____ yes ____ no ____ sometimes

H. Do you feel motivated to do well in this course?

____ yes ____ no ____ sometimes

*Bloom, B. (ed.), Taxonomy of Educational Objectives, The Classification of Education Goals: Handbook I—Cognitive Domain. Longman, Inc., New York (1956).

ANALYSIS

Results should be analyzed to determine the following:

1. Does the textbook for the course appear to be interfering significantly with the student's comprehension?

2. Does the student appear to be having difficulty understanding the teacher's lectures/instructions in the classroom compared with other students at the same level?

3. Do the tests in the class seem to be interfering with class performance because the student does not understand the language in them?

4. Does the student show any positive attitude toward the course to attempt to perform as well as possible?

Results should also be compared with the student's performance on informal assessment tasks which require the student to use informational listening for short, simulated lectures by the speech-language pathologist. If the teacher has made use of the Teacher Language: Self-evaluation Technique (See Appendix G) in the classroom, results should be compared with those findings, i.e., is the student undergoing assessment the only student experiencing difficulty understanding the teacher?

INTERPRETATION

If the "Results" questions 1, 2, or 3 above are answered affirmatively, and the data match those obtained during direct assessment of the adolescent, then the problem rests primarily within the student. However, if data mismatch (e.g., the student demonstrated good informational listening skills when the speech-language pathologist delivered the lecture, but poor informational listening skills in the classroom), the problem may lie within the educational system. Students should demonstrate a positive attitude before examiners conclude that the problem rests primarily within the educational system (see "Results" question 4).

APPENDIX J

Model Contract for Adolescents

COMMUNICATION CONTRACT

UNIT: Following and generating instructions

	GRADES				
	A	B	C	D	F
1. ___(Name)___ will collect ___(Number)___ instructions that are difficult to follow and discuss why they are difficult.	____	____	____	____	____
2. ___(Name)___ will concisely and clearly state ___(Number)___ specific instructions for activities such as how to open a combination locker, how to get from school to home.	____	____	____	____	____
3. ___(Name)___ will describe ___(Number)___ situations where precision in giving instructions if of utmost importance.	____	____	____	____	____
4. ___(Name)___ will describe ___(Number)___ situations where a lack of precision in giving instructions will cause a problem.	____	____	____	____	____

I, _______(name)_______, agree to complete this contract starting on _____(beginning date)_____ and ending on _____(ending date)_____. I understand that my overall contract grade will be determined by averaging the letter grades for each of the four parts of the contract. Evaluation of each objective will be made by the adult who signs this contract.

If I fail to complete this contract by the date listed above, I will undergo the following consequences:

____

____

____ Student's Signature

____ Date

____ Professional's Signature

____ Date

(NOTE TO PROFESSIONALS: Assist students to select an appropriate number of instructions or situations to earn specific letter grades [e.g., ten instructions earn an "A," eight earn a "B," six earn a "C," four earn a "D," and two earn an "F"). Insert these numbers on the lines provided. Have students project the grade they will attempt to earn for each objective and insert the number corresponding to this grade in the stated objective.)

APPENDIX K

Progress Grading Report

PROGRESS REPORT

Name ______________________ Gr. ________ School Yr. ________

Resident School ______________________________________

Host School ______________________________________

Dear Parent,

This is a progress report for students involved in individualized programming. This progress record includes performance in academics as well as work habits. It addresses individualized classes as well as mainstream classes. This report is intended to reflect the student's progress throughout his/her total day so areas of strength can be recognized and assistance provided for areas of weakness. There are two different scales used in this reporting system. One is for academics and one for work habits. Please see the inside pages of this cover sheet for a detailed explanation of these progress scales.

Sincerely,

____

Reprinted with permission of Cooperative Educational Services Agency #4 (Northern Cluster), LaCrosse, WI.

REPORTING SYSTEMS

ACADEMIC

Academic work is evaluated by the following criteria:

1. Attempts but cannot perform with assistance

2. Performs with assistance or supervision

3. Performs without assistance

4. Performs without assistance with more than acceptable quality, speed and accuracy

5. Performs with more than acceptable quality, speed and accuracy with high initiative and adaptability to a variety of situations

6. Can lead or teach others

WORK HABITS

Work habits are evaluated by the following criteria:

Never—Unacceptable

Seldom—Needs Improvement

Usually—Good

Always—Excellent

PROGRESS REPORT

Student ______________________ School Yr. __________

Teacher ______________________ Prog. Period____ Gr.____

Resident Dist. ______________________ Credit Area __________

ACADEMIC WORK

Subject Area(s) ______________________

We are working on:	Performance 1	2	3	4	5	6

Qtr. Gr. __________ Sem. Gr. __________ Credit Earned __________

(Grades are based on daily work)

Subject Area(s) ______________________ Credit Area __________

We are working on:	Performance 1	2	3	4	5	6

Qtr. Gr. __________ Sem. Gr. __________ Credit Earned __________

(Grades are based on daily work)

COMMENTS:

____

____

____

white—district yellow—parent pink—teacher

PROGRESS REPORT

Student ______________________ School Yr. __________

Teacher ______________________ Prog. Period____ Gr.____

Resident Dist. ______________________ Credit Area __________

ACADEMIC WORK

Subject Area(s) ______________________

We are working on:	Performance 1	2	3	4	5	6

Qtr. Gr. __________ Sem. Gr. __________ Credit Earned __________

(Grades are based on daily work)

WORK HABITS	Never—Unacceptable	Seldom—Needs Improv.	Usually—Good	Always—Excellent	Not Eval.
1. Seeks help when appropriate					
2. Works independently					
3. Accepts criticism					
4. Assumes responsibility					
5. Acknowledges and accepts rights of others					
6. Observes rules and regulations					
7. Exhibits self control					
8. Completes assignments on time					
9. Follows oral directions					
10. Follows written directions					

COMMENTS:

____

____

white—district yellow—parent pink—teacher

EXPLANATION OF WORK HABITS EVALUATED

1. **Seeks Help When Appropriate**
   a. seeks help when clarification of an academic assignment is needed
   b. seeks help in solving personal and interpersonal problems when needed
2. **Works Independently**
   a. completes assignments on his/her own
   b. does not seek unneeded assistance
3. **Accepts Criticism Directed Toward Behavior on Academic Work in a Positive Manner**
   a. listens without overreaction
   b. initiates corrections willingly
4. **Assumes Responsibility**
   a. brings required materials to class
   b. maintains locker, notebooks and work area in orderly manner
   c. accepts rightful blame and consequences for actions
   d. attends class regularly
   e. comes to class on time
5. **Acknowledges and Accepts Rights of Others**
   a. works without distracting others
   b. gains permission before using property of others
   c. uses materials of others and returns without damage
   d. refrains from touching others inappropriately
6. **Observes Rules and Regulations**
   a. observes rules of classroom, playground, and lunchroom
   b. observes rules of IMC and all other school property
   c. complies with directives given by any school staff
7. **Exhibits Self Control**
   a. avoids inappropriate behaviors, even when upset
   b. refrains from engaging in excessive physical or verbal activity
   c. remains on task, even when others are misbehaving
   d. doesn't complain
8. **Completes Assignments On Time**
9. **Follows Oral Directions**
   a. attends to verbal instructions both visually and auditorily
   b. applies group directions to self
   c. follows directions the first time they are given
10. **Follows Written Directions**
    a. reads written directions before proceeding
    b. completes tasks according to directions

Success in life or on a job will not be achieved without the proper work habits.

Attendance:

Quarter	1	2	3	4	Total
Days Present					
Days Absent					
Times Tardy					

Parent's Signature Date

____ __________

____ __________

____ __________

Dear Parent:

Please sign above so we know you have had a chance to review your child's progress report.

Please return only the cover sheet; keep the enclosed progress report sheets.

Return the cover sheet to:

____

Thank you!

APPENDIX L

Graduation Policy from One Educational Agency

EEN* GRADUATION POLICY (Hansen, 1985)

A diploma indicating graduation status will be awarded to EEN students when they have satisfactorily completed an individually designed Prescribed Course of Study (PCS). The diploma would be identical to those received by Non-EEN students.

The PCS will follow the school board policy governing the total number of credits required for graduation. When a student attends a secondary level consortium program the option is available for the student to follow the host district graduation requirements rather than the resident district requirements. If this choice was made the student would receive a diploma from the host district and not the resident district.

The unit of time used to determine what constitutes a credit for EEN students will be the same standard applied to credits earned by Non-EEN students.

The requirement for a specific number of credits per individual subject areas shall be satisfied through one or any combination of courses taught in the EEN programs, substitute courses and required regular education courses.

Courses taught in the EEN Programs when part of the student's IEP, shall receive credit and meet subject area requirements. The grades received from courses taught in the EEN Program will not be considered in honor roll calculations or in grade point averages for class rank.

A prior approval process will designate the acceptable regular education substitute courses for required courses.

An alternative diploma option will be available for specific circumstances. An Occupational Preparation diploma will be awarded EEN students whose total number of credits meets the district's graduation requirements but due to specific educational needs is not able to meet the requirement for number of credits required per subject area. This student will satisfactorily achieve a set of competencies in an occupational preparation area.

A Certificate of Achievement will be awarded to those students who satisfactorily complete their Individual Educational Plans (IEP's) without adhering to the district credit requirements.

The PCS will designate a diploma option and will develop a long range Course Selection Plan. It will include an accounting of credits earned and credits needed to complete the diploma option selected. When applicable the PCS will also make a determination regarding a student's participation in the district's Competency Based Testing Program.

The EEN student's transcripts will list all courses taught in the same manner as they are listed on the transcripts for regular education students. Courses taught in the EEN Program will not be designated as EEN courses or indicate a student's handicapping condition or special education status. The courses receiving credit from an Exceptional Education program will, however, be designated by an asterisk. An explanation will be provided which will indicate that all courses marked with an asterisk were taught as an individualized course of study.

The EEN transfer student's credit standing upon enrollment will follow the school district's transfer student policy for Non-EEN. All subsequent credit requirements will follow the district's EEN Graduation Policy.

---

*EEN = Exceptional Educational Need, a generic term for children with special educational needs, including speech-language, in Wisconsin state statute 115.

Reprinted with permission of Dawna Hansen, Director of Special Education, Cooperative Educational Services Agency #4 (Northern Cluster) LaCrosse, WI.

APPENDIX M

Tutor Application Form

TUTOR APPLICATION FORM

I. Identification Information

Name: ____________________

Address: ____________________
Street City State Zip Code

Telephone: ____________ Age: ______

Homeroom: ____________ Grade: ____

II. Schedule

Please attach your class schedule to this form.

How often can you tutor per week? ____________

What days and time periods are you available?

Days	Time Periods
Monday	____________
Tuesday	____________
Wednesday	____________
Thursday	____________
Friday	____________

When will your available time periods change? ____________

III. Experience

Have you ever worked with other teen-agers who have disabilities?

Yes ____ No ____

If yes, describe those experiences: ____________

____

Why do you desire to participate in the tutoring program? ______

____

____

What interests, skills, talents, or strengths do you have that you could share with the classmate you tutor? ____________________

____

IV. Parental Permission

Please obtain a parent's signature to indicate approval of your participation in the peer tutoring program.

My child, ____________________ (name of child), has my permission to participate in the peer tutoring program coordinated by the speech-language pathologist ____________________ (name of professional) for ______ hours per week.

____________________ Parent's Signature ____________ Date

V. References

Please list the names of two teachers who could provide a recommendation on your ability to tutor a peer successfully.

APPENDIX N

Consultation Feedback Forms

(Reprinted with permission of Aspen Publishers, Inc., from *Collaborative Consultation* (Appendix 8-A and Exhibit 8-6) by Idol, N., Paolucci-Whitcomb, P., and Nevin, A., 1986.)

Appendix 8–A

The Daily Performance or Multiband Chart

Multiple Bands

Each band is labeled to represent one of five behaviors. For example, five behaviors might be:

- oral reading accuracy
- oral reading rate
- oral reading comprehension
- acquisition of isolated sounds
- written reading comprehension

This multiband chart was designed to monitor multiple behaviors. Its advantage is that teachers can evaluate performance for up to five behaviors on a single sheet of paper. The multiband chart is used in conjunction with the instructional format sheet to record daily behaviors.

The Abscissa

This reflects the time spent in school. Each heavy line labeled *M* represents the Monday of each school week, with the intermittent lines representing Tuesday, Wednesday, Thursday, and Friday. The tick marks are used to record the date (month and day) of each Monday. For example, Monday the first of September would be marked 9/1.

The Ordinate

This is divided into ten spaces that may be arbitrarily labeled to represent the expected range of data that will be recorded for each individual behavior. *For example*, oral reading accuracy might range from 80 to 100 percent. Reading rate might range from 40 to 100 cwpm. The criterion for each behavior is represented as a red line drawn the length of each band at the corresponding number. (In lieu of a red line, a yellow marking pen can be used to color in the top portion of the band that represents the area falling at criterion or above.)

Baseline Data

This is the first set of data recorded that describes the basic instructional plan without added interventions. It is labeled condition A, (A) , with the arrow pointing to the first day of data collection. It is entered on the top band of the chart (i.e., the space without lines).

Interventions

Each additional intervention that is decided upon is, of course, described on the Instructional Format Sheet and labeled with successive alphabet letters. The same letters are recorded in the multi-band chart. The arrows point to the exact data points that designate the first day of instruction under the new condition. The circled letter is recorded in the band that represents the behavior for which the intervention was selected. For example, soundsheet drill may be selected in an attempt to improve reading accuracy. If it is the first intervention to be tried for any of the behaviors on the chart, it is labeled (B) and drawn in the band representing reading accuracy. Then, an intervention line is drawn vertically to cross over all bands. This line is drawn between the day line of the previous condition and the day line of the new condition.

Books

The title of the book that is being used is written in the blank space above the first band. When a second book is started, the new title is recorded. A red line is drawn the width of the chart, crossing all five bands.

Figure 8A–1 The Daily Performance (Multiband) Chart

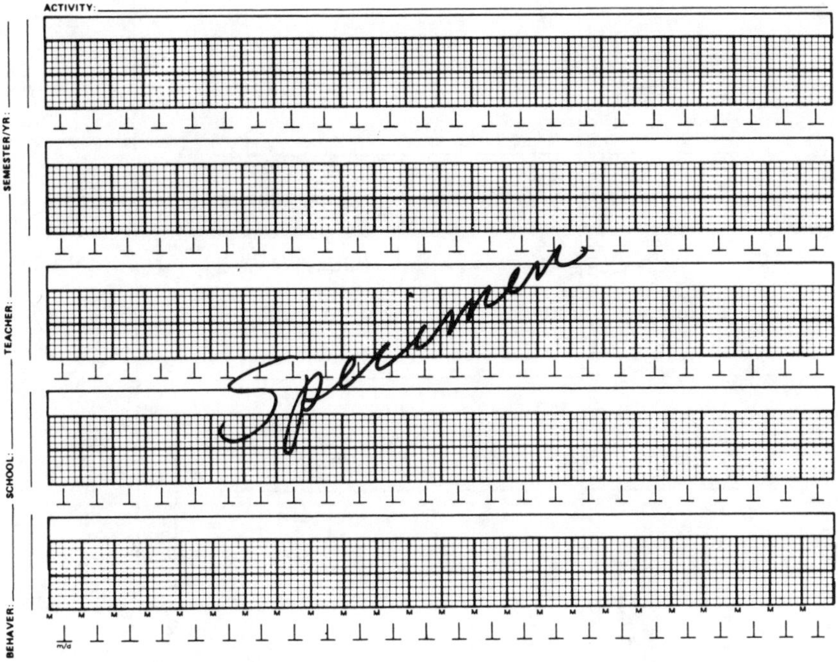

Exhibit 8–6 Consultation Log for Consultant Recording of Self-Perceptions of the Consultation Process

CONSULTATION LOG

Consultant ____________

Who did you meet?	Date: ______		Purpose of Conference		How did you feel about the conference?			Additional comments
	Start time	Finish time	Expected outcome (consultation step, etc.)	Actual outcome (What was actually accomplished?)	Positive	Neutral	Negative	

Note: This form was originally developed by Phyllis Paolucci-Whitcomb, University of Vermont.

APPENDIX O

Sample Consent Form

SAMPLE CONSENT FORM

1. I have freely consented to take part in a study being conducted by ______(name)______ who is a speech-language pathologist at (agency name) ________________________.

2. The study has been explained to me and I understand the explanation that has been given and what my participation will involve.

3. I understand that I am free to discontinue my participation in the study at any time without penalty.

4. I understand that the results of the study will be treated in strict confidence and that I will remain anonymous. Within these restrictions, results of the study will be made available to me at my request.

5. I understand that my participation in the study does not necessarily ensure any beneficial results to me.

6. I understand that, at my request, I can receive additional explanation or information about the study from the person identified above.

7. I understand that I am entitled to receive a copy of this statement.

8. I understand that if I have any complaints about my treatment in this study, I may call or write to: ______(name, address, and phone number of the agency administrator)______. Although this person will ask my name, I understand that all complaints will be kept in confidence.

Signed: ________________________________ Date: ________________

NOTES: A copy of the signed consent form should be given to each subject. For questionnaires, the return of the questionnaire constitutes informed consent; this form does not need to be used.

Informed consent of children:

Up to sixth grade—parental consent, child's assent

Junior high—parental consent, child's assent or consent as appropriate

High school—parental consent and student's consent

Informed consent for anyone for whom there is a guardian:

Guardian's consent and participant's assent

APPENDIX P

Sample Cover Letter and Questionnaire

SAMPLE COVER LETTER FOR A QUESTIONNAIRE TO BE SENT TO AN ADOLESCENT (OR ADULT) WHO CAN READ AT A THIRD-GRADE LEVEL

Dear ______________________________:

We are collecting information from people who were in the speech-language program in high school. We have very little information about people like you. We would like you to help with a project. The project will study the benefits of the speech-language program while you were in high school. It will take you about ____ minutes to complete the questionnaire I have sent.

This questionnaire has been approved by the Review Board for the Protection of Human Subjects. If you have any complaints about your participation in this study, please contact ________________ at ________________.

Your participation in the project is completely voluntary. You may refuse to participate. It will not be held against you. If you decide not to participate, then throw the questionnaire away.

It is all right to ask for help to read the questionnaire. You may also ask someone to explain unfamiliar words. However, you should decide the answers to the questions by yourself. Send your questionnaire back to me in the self-addressed envelope.

The questionnaire is anonymous. Please do not write your name or address anywhere on the questionnaire or the return envelope. Your information will be combined with that of others. Your cooperation is very important for the success of this study. I hope you will participate in the study. If you have any questions about this study, contact me at ________________. Thank you for your cooperation.

Sincerely,

____
Speech-Language Pathologist

SAMPLE SPEECH-LANGUAGE FOLLOW-UP QUESTIONNAIRE

I. Personal Data

Date of Follow-up: ______________________

Middle/Junior High School Attended: ____________________________

High School Attended: ____

Number of Years in Secondary-Level Speech-Language Programs: ____ years, from 19____ to 19____.

Are you the sole head of the household for tax purposes?

____ yes ____ no

Are you living independently from your parents? ____ yes ____ no

Number of Dependents: _________

Age at Time of this Follow-up:

____ less than 20 years of age

____ 20 to 25 years of age

____ 25 to 30 years of age

____ more than 30 years of age

II. Educational/Employment Data

Educational Status: (Check one.)

____ Credits toward high school diploma, but diploma is not yet earned

____ High school diploma

____ 1 to 2 years of vocational-technical education after high school

____ 1 to 3 years of college education

____ Earned B.S. or B.A. degree from college

____ Other (Specify: ____)

Work Experience: (Check one.)

____ Less than 3 years of part-time employment

____ More than 3 years of part-time employment

____ Less than 3 years of full-time employment

____ More than 3 years of full-time employment

____ Other (Specify: ____)

Employment Skill Level: (Check one.)

____ Primarily unskilled (little or no training required for job)

____ Semi-skilled (trained on the job)

____ Vocationally/technically skilled (trained in school 1 to 3 years after high school)

____ Professional (trained at the bachelor's degree level or more)

____ Other (Specify: ____________________________________)

Number of Paid Jobs (held at the same time, or at different times): (Check one.)

____ 3 or less jobs

____ 4 to 6 jobs

____ 7 to 10 jobs

____ More than 10 jobs

Average Income Earned:

A. Per Hour: (Check one.)

____ Minimum wage

____ Between minimum wage and $1 beyond minimum wage

____ $1 to $2 beyond minimum wage

____ $2 to $3 beyond minimum wage

____ $3 to $4 beyond minimum wage

____ More than $4 beyond minimum wage

B. Per Year (Individual): (Check one.)

____ Less than $5,000

____ $5,000 to $10,000

____ $10,001 to $15,000

____ $15,001 to $20,000

____ $20,001 to $25,000

____ Over $25,001

C. Per Year (Joint Income): (Check one, if applicable.)

____ Less than $5,000

____ $5,000 to $10,000

____ $10,001 to $15,000

____ $15,001 to $20,000

____ $20,001 to $25,000

____ Over $25,001

III. Benefits Received from the Speech-Language Program

Use this scale for the questions below.

1	2	3	4	5
Not at all	A little bit	Some	Quite a bit	A great amount

A. On a scale from 1 to 5, how much do you think your participation in the speech-language program helped you in school? ____

B. On a scale from 1 to 5, how much do you think your participation in the speech-language program helped you to relate better to people? ____

C. On a scale from 1 to 5, how much do you think your participation in the speech-language program helped you to perform better at work? ____

IV. Additional Comments

____

____

____

____

____

REFERENCES

Adams, J. *Interviewing Procedures: A Manual for Survey Interviewers.* Univ. of N. Carolina Press, Chapel Hill, NC, 1958.

Adams, W. Adolescence. In: S. Gabel and M. Erickson (eds.), *Child Development and Developmental Disabilities.* Little Brown and Company, Boston, MA, 1980.

AERA, APA, and NCME (American Educational Research Association, American Psychological Association, and National Council on Measurement in Education). *Standards for Educational and Psychological Testing.* American Psychological Association, Washington, DC, 1985.

Agency for Instructional Technology. *Solutions Unlimited [Computer program].* AIT, Bloomington, IN, 1984.

Algozzine, B., Christenson, S., and Ysseldyke, J. *Probabilities Associated with the Referral to Placement Process.* Institute for Research on Learning Disabilities, Univ. of Minn., Minneapolis, MN, 1981.

Alley, G., and Deshler, D. *Teaching the Learning Disabled Adolescent: Strategies and Methods.* Love Publishing, Denver, CO, 1979.

Allington, R., and Fleming, J. The misreading of high-frequency words. *J. Spec. Ed.* 12(4):417-421, 1978.

Anderson, V., and Newby, H. *Improving the Child's Speech. 2nd Ed.* Oxford University Press, New York, 1973.

Andrews, M., and Shank, K. Some observations concerning the cheering behavior of schoolgirl cheerleaders. *Lang. Speech & Hearing Serv. Sch.* 14(3):150-156, 1983.

Anglin, J. *Word, Object, and Conceptual Development.* Norton, New York, 1977.

Applebee, A. *The Child's Concept of Story.* University of Chicago Press, Chicago, IL, 1978.

Aram, D., Ekelman, B., and Nation, J. Preschoolers with language disorders: 10 years later. *J. Speech & Hear. Res.* 27(2):232-244, 1984.

Aram, D., and Nation, J. Preschool language disorders and subsequent language and academic difficulties. *J. Comm. Dis.* 13:159-170, 1980.

Arlin, P. Cognitive development in adulthood: "A fifth stage?" *Develop. Psychol.* 11(5):602-606, 1975.

Arwood, E. *Pragmaticism: Theory and Application.* Aspen Systems, Rockville, MD, 1983.

ASHA Ad Hoc Committee on Instrument Evaluation. *Report of the committee submitted to the Executive Board.* Aug., 1986.

ASHA. Speech-language-hearing services in the public schools—A class act. *ASHA.* 28(5): 18-21, 1986.

ASHA. Prisoners: A neglected population? *ASHA.* 26(6):19-22, 1984.

Ashear, V., and Snortum, J. Eye contact in children as a function of age, sex, social and intellectual variables. *Develop. Psychol.* 4(3):479, 1971.

Atkins, C., and Cartwright, L. Preferred language elicitation procedures used in five age categories. *ASHA.* 24(5):321-323, 1982.

Austin, J. *How to Do Things with Words.* Oxford University Press, London, 1962.

Babbie, E. *Survey Research Methods.* Wadsworth Publishing Co., Belmont, CA, 1981.

Backland, P., Booth, J., Moore, M., Parks, A., and Van Rheenen, D. *State Practices in Speaking and Listening Skill Assessment.* Speech Communication Association, Annandale, VA, 1982a.

Backland, P., Brown, K., Gurry, J., and Jandt, F. Recommendations for assessing speaking and listening skills. *Commun. Educ.* 31:9-17, 1982b.

Baggett, L. *Behavior that communicates understanding as evaluated by teen-agers.* Paper presented at the American Personnel and Guidance Association Convention. Las Vegas, NV, March 30-April 3, 1969.

Bakan, D. Adolescence in America: From ideal to social fact. *Daedalus* 100(4):981, 1971.

Balsam, D. *The Print Shop [Computer program].* Broderbund Software, San Rafael, CA, 1984.

Bandura, A., and Walters, R. *Social Learning and Personality Development.* Holt, Rinehart and Winston, New York, 1963.

Barker, L. *Listening Behavior.* Prentice-Hall, Englewood Cliffs, NJ, 1971.

Barret, R. Improving family talk: Educating families to work better. *The Humanist Educator* 20(4):178-186, 1982.

Bart, W. The factor structure of formal operations. *Br. J. Educ. Psychol.* 41:40-77, 1971.

Bart, W., Baxter, J., and Frey, S. The relationships of spatial ability and sex to formal reasoning capabilities. *J. Psychol.* 104:191-198, 1980.

Benedict, R. Continuities and discontinuities in cultural conditioning. In: W. Martin and C. Stendler (eds.), *Readings in Child Development.* Harcourt, Brace, New York, 1954.

Berzonsky, M. Formal reasoning in adolescence: An alternate view. *Adoles.* 13(50):279-290, 1978.

Biklen, D., and Bogdan, R. Handicapism in America. *WIN,* October 28, 1976.

Birdwhistell, R. *Kinesics and Context.* Univ. of Pennsylvania Press, Philadelphia, PA, 1970.

Birth of the Phoenix [Computer program]. Phoenix Software, Inc., Lake Zurich, IL. 1981.

Blackwell, P., Engen, E., Fischgrund, J., and Zarcadoolas, C. *Sentences and Other Systems: A Language and Learning Curriculum for Hearing-impaired Children.* The Alexander Graham Bell Association for the Deaf, Washington, DC, 1978.

Blalock, J. Persistent auditory language deficits in adults with learning disabilities. *J. Learn. Dis.* 15(10):604-609, 1982.

Blalock, J. Persistent problems and concerns of young adults with learning disabilities. In: W. Cruickshank and A. Silver (eds.), *Bridges to Tomorrow. Vol. 2.* Syracuse University Press, Syracuse, NY, 1981.

Blanck, P., and Rosenthal, R. Developing strategies for decoding "leaky" messages: On learning how and when to decode discrepant and consistent social communications. In: R. Feldman (ed.), *Development of Nonverbal Behavior in Children.* Springer-Verlag, New York, 1982.

Blank, M., Rose, S., and Berlin, L. *The Language of Learning: The Preschool Years.* Grune and Stratton, New York, 1978.

Bloom, B. (ed.). Taxonomy of educational objectives: The classification of educational goals. In: *Handbook I: Cognitive Domain.* Longman, Inc., New York, 1956.

Bloom, L., and Lahey, M. *Language Development and Language Disorders.* John Wiley & Sons, New York, 1978.

Blue, C. The marginal communicator. *Lang. Speech & Hearing Serv. Sch.* 6(1):32-37, 1975.

Botticelli [Computer program]. Krell Software Corp., Stony Brook, NY, 1983.

Bowerman, M. Semantic factors in the acquisition of rules for word use and sentence construction. In: D. Morehead and A. Morehead (eds.), *Normal and Deficient Child Language.* University Park Press, Baltimore, MD, 1976.

Boyce, N., Godwin, E., and Larson, V. Lord. *Communicative disorders services: Grades 7-12.* Unpublished survey. University of Wisconsin-Eau Claire, Dept. of Communication Disorders, Eau Claire, WI, 1979.

Boyce, N., and Larson, V. Lord. *Adolescents' Communication: Development and Disorders.* Thinking Publications, Eau Claire, WI, 1983.

Boyce, N., and Larson, V. Lord. *Language assessment of the adolescent.* Paper presented at the American Speech-Language-Hearing Association Convention, Los Angeles, CA, Nov. 20-23, 1981.

Brenza, B., Kricos, P., and Lasky, E. Comprehension and production of basic semantic concepts by older hearing-impaired children. *J. Speech & Hear. Res.* 24:414-419, 1981.

Broughton, J. Beyond formal operations: Theoretical thoughts in adolescence. *Teach. Coll. Rec.* 79:87-97, 1977.

Brown, A., and Smiley, S. Rating the importance of structural units of prose passages: A problem of metacognitive development. *Child Devel.* 48:1-8, 1977.

Brown, R. *A First Language: The Early Stages.* Harvard University Press, Cambridge, MA, 1973.

Brown, V. Curriculum development resources. In: L. Mann, L. Goodman, and J. Wiederholt (eds.), *Teaching the Learning Disabled Adolescent.* Houghton Mifflin, Boston, MA, 1978.

Bryan, T. Children's comprehension of nonverbal communication. *J. Learn. Dis.* 10:501-506, 1977.

Bryan, T., Donahue, M., and Pearl, R. Studies of learning disabled children's pragmatic competence. *Topics in Learning and Learning Disab.* 1(2):29-39, 1981.

Buchan, L. *Roleplaying and the Educable Mentally Retarded.* Fearon Publishers, Belmont, CA, 1972.

Buscaglia, L. *Love: A Fresh Dynamic Approach to Developing your Fullest Potential.* Nightingale-Conant Corp., Chicago, IL, 1982.

Buscaglia, L. *The Disabled and Their Parents: A Counseling Challenge.* Charles B. Slack, Thorofare, NJ, 1975.

Carey, S., Diamond, R., and Woods, B. Development of face recognition—A muturation component? *Develop. Psychol.* 16:257-269, 1980.

Carnegie Foundation for the Advancement of Teaching. *High School: A Report on Secondary Education in America.* Harper and Row, NY, 1983.

Carrow, E. *Carrow Elicited Language Inventory.* Teaching Resources, Hingham, MA, 1974.

Chapman, R. Exploring children's communicative intents. In: J. Miller (ed.), *Assessing Language Production in Children.* University Park Press, Baltimore, MD, 1981.

Chapman, R. Some simple ways of talking about normal language and communication. In: J. McLean, D. Yoder, and R. Schiefelbusch (eds.), *Language Intervention with the Retarded: Developing Strategies.* University Park Press, Baltimore, MD, 1972.

Chappell, G. Oral language performance of upper elementary school students obtained via story reformulation. *Lang. Speech & Hearing Serv. Sch.* 11(4):236-250, 1980.

Chesler, M., and Fox, R. *Role-playing Methods in the Classroom.* Science Research Associates, Inc., Chicago, IL, 1966.

Chinitz, S. A sibling group for brothers and sisters of handicapped children. *Child. Today* 10(6):21-23, 1981.

Chomsky, C. *The Acquisition of Syntax in Children from 5 to 10.* MIT Press, Cambridge, MA, 1969.

Christensen, B., and DeBlassie, R. Counseling with parents of handicapped adolescents. *Adoles.* 25:397-407, 1980.

Cole, L. Implications of the position on social dialects. *ASHA.* 25(9):25-27, 1983.

Cole, L., and Campbell-Calloway, M. Resource guide to multicultural tests and materials—supplement I. *ASHA.* 25(9):37-42, 1983.

Cole, L., and Snope, T. Resource guide to multicultural tests and materials. *ASHA.* 23(9):639-649, 1981.

Coles, R. The age of insolence: Those terrible teens. *Family Weekly,* Sept. 4, 1983, pp. 4-5.

Colt, G. The enigma of suicide. *Harv. Mag.* 86(1):47-66, 1983.

Commission on the English Curriculum of the National Council of Teachers of English. *The English Language Arts.* Appleton-Century-Crofts, New York, 1952.

Committee on Language Learning Disorders. Position statement on language learning disorders. *ASHA.* 24(11):937-944, 1982.

Committee on Language, Speech, and Hearing Services in the Schools. Recommended service delivery models and caseload sizes for speech-language pathology services in the schools. *ASHA.* 25(2):65-70, 1983.

Committee on Prevention of Speech-Language and Hearing Problems. Prevention: A challenge for the profession. *ASHA.* 26(8):35-37, 1984.

Committee on the Status of Racial Minorities. Social dialects: Position paper. *ASHA.* 25(9):23-24, 1983.

Comprehensive Tests of Basic Skills. CTB/McGraw-Hill, Monterey, CA, 1968.

Conger, J. *Adolescence and Youth Psychological Development in a Changing World.* Harper and Row, New York, 1973.

Connell, P., and Thompson, C. Flexibility of single-subject experimental designs. Part III: Using flexibility to design or modify experiments. *J. Speech & Hear. Dis.* 51(3),214-225, 1986.

Crager, R., and Spriggs, A., Development of concept utilization. *Develop. Psychol.* 1:415-424, 1969.

Craig, H. Applications of pragmatic language models for intervention. In: T. Gallagher and C. Prutting (eds.), *Pragmatic Assessment and Intervention Issues in Language.* College-Hill Press, San Diego, CA, 1983.

Cromer, R. Child and adult learning of surface structure cues to deep structure using a picture card technique. *J. Psycholing. Res.* 3(6):1-14, 1974.

Cromer, R. Children are nice to understand: Surface structure clues for the recovery of a deep structure. *Br. J. Psychol.* 61(3):397-408, 1970.

Crystal, D., Fletcher, P., and Garman, M. *The Grammatical Analysis of Language Disability: A Procedure for Assessment and Remediation.* Edward Arnold, London, 1976.

Culatta, B., Page, J., and Ellis, J. Story retelling as a communicative performance screening tool. *Lang. Speech & Hear. Serv. Sch.* 14(2):66-78, 1983.

Dagenais, D., and Beadle, K. Written language: When and where to begin. *Topics in Lang. Dis.* 4(2):59-85, 1984.

Damico, J. Clinical discourse analysis: A functional approach to language assessment. In: C. Simon (ed.), *Communication Skills and Classroom Success: Assessment of Language-Learning Disabled Students.* Little Brown/College-Hill Press, San Diego, CA, 1985.

daSilva, W. The formation of historical concepts through contextual cues. In: A. Floyd (ed.), *Cognitive Development in the School Years.* John Wiley and Sons, New York, 1979.

Davelaar, E. Formal operational reasoning and its relationship to complex speech patterns and tentative statement use. *Lang. & Speech* 20(1):73-79, 1977.

Davis, A. Socialization and adolescent personality. In: N. Henry (ed.), *Adolescence, Yearbook of the National Society for the Study of Education. 43:Part 1.* Dept. of Ed., Univ. of Chicago, Chicago, IL, 1944.

DeAjuriaguerra, J., Jaeggi, A., Guignard, F., Kocher, F., Maguard, M., Roch, S., and Schmid, E. The development and prognosis of dysphasia in children. In: D. Morehead and A. Morehead (eds.), *Normal and Deficient Child Language.* University Park Press, Baltimore, MD, 1976.

DeBlassie, R. Counseling with culturally disadvantaged adolescents. *Adoles.* 13(50):221-229, 1978.

DeMier, D., Wise, B., and Marcum, K. *Project ACCESS: Adapting Current Curriculum with Essential Study Skills.* Central Kitsap School District #401, Silverdale, WA, 1982.

DePaulo, B., and Jordan, A. Changes in deceiving and detecting deceit. In: R. Feldman (ed.), *Development of Nonverbal Behavior in Children.* Springer-Verlag, New York, 1982.

Deshler, D., and Schumaker, J. Social skills of learning disabled adolescents: Characteristics and intervention. *Topics in Learning and Learning Disab.* 3(2):15-23, 1983.

Diamond, R., Carey, S., and Back, K. Genetic influences on the development of spatial skills during early adolescence. *Cog.* 13(2):167-185, 1983.

Diedrich, W. Cluttering: Its diagnosis. In: H. Winitz (ed.), *Treating Articulation Disorders for Clinicians by Clinicians.* University Park Press, Baltimore, MD, 1984.

Dimitrovsky, L. The ability to identify the emotional meaning of vocal expressions at successive age levels. In: J. Davitz (ed.), *The Communication of Emotional Meaning.* McGraw-Hill, New York, 1964.

Dinkmeyer, D., and McKay, G. *Systematic Training for Effective Parenting for Teens.* American Guidance Service, Circle Pines, MN, 1983.

Dinkmeyer, D., and Muro, J. *Group Counseling: Theory and Practice.* F. E. Peacock, Itasca, IL, 1971.

Dittman, A. Developmental factors in conversational behavior. *J. Communication* 22:404-423, 1972.

Donahue, M. Communicative style in learning disabled children: Some implications for classroom discourse. In: P. Ripich and F. Spinelli (eds.), *School Discourse Problems.* Little Brown/College-Hill Press, San Diego, CA, 1985.

Donahue, M. Requesting strategies of learning disabled children. *Applied Psycholinguistics* 2:213-234, 1981.

Donahue, M., and Bryan, T. Communicative skills and peer relations of learning disabled adolescents. *Topics in Lang. Dis.* 4(2):10-21, 1984.

Donahue, M., Pearl, R., and Bryan, T. Learning disabled children's syntactic proficiency on a communicative task. *J. Speech & Hear. Dis.* 47(4):397-403, 1982.

Donahue, M., Pearl, R., and Bryan, T. Learning disabled children's conversational competence: Responses to inadequate messages. *Applied Psycholinguistics* 1:387-403, 1980.

Dore, J. Holophrases, speech acts, and language universals. *J. Child Lang.* 2:21-40, 1975.

Dore, J. A pragmatic description of early language development. *J. Psycholin.* 3:343-350, 1974.

Dorval, B. *The development of conversation.* Paper presented at the Biennial Southeastern Conference on Human Development, Alexandria, VA, April 17-19, 1980.

Douvan, E., and Adelson, J. *The Adolescent Experience.* John Wiley and Sons, New York, 1966.

Downing, L. *Counseling Theories and Techniques: Summarized and Critiqued.* Nelson-Hall, Chicago, IL, 1975.

Duker, S. *Listening Readings: Vol. 2.* Scarecrow Press, Metuchen, NJ, 1971.

Duncan, Jr., S., and Fiske, D. *Face to Face Interaction: Research, Methods, and Therapy.* John Wiley and Sons, New York, 1977.

Dunn, L., and Markwardt, Jr., F. *Peabody Individual Achievement Test.* American Guidance Service, Circle Pines, MN, 1970.

Durost, W., Bixler, H., Wrightstone, J., Prescott, G., and Balow, I. *Metropolitan Achievement Tests.* Harcourt, Brace, Jovanovich, New York, 1970.

Durrell, D. *Durrell Analysis of Reading Difficulty.* Harcourt, Brace, Jovanovich, New York, 1955.

Edmondson, W. *Spoken Discourse: A Model for Analysis.* Longman, New York, 1981.

Eisenberg, L. A developmental approach to adolescence. *Children* 12:131-135, 1965.

Eisner, E. Critical thinking: Some cognitive components. *Teach. Coll. Rec.* 66(7):624-634, 1965.

Elder, G. Adolescence in the life cycle: An introduction. In: S. Dragastin and G. Elder, Jr. (eds.), *Adolescence in the Life Cycle: Psychological Change and Social Context,* pp. 1-22. Hemisphere Publishing Corporation, Washington, DC, 1975.

Elkind, D. Understand the young adolescent. *Adoles.* 13(49):127-134, 1978.

Elkind, D. Recent research on cognitive development in adolescents. In: E. Sigmund, S. Dragastine, and G. Elder, Jr. (eds.), *Adolescence in the Life Cycle: Psychological Change and Social Context.* John Wiley and Sons, New York, 1975.

Elkind, D. *Children and Adolescents: Interpretive Essays on Jean Piaget.* Oxford University Press, New York, 1974.

Elkind, D., Barocas, R., and Johnsen, P. Concept production in children and adolescents. *Hum. Dev.* 12:10-21, 1969.

Ellis, A., and Harper, R. *A Guide to Rational Living.* Wilshire Book Co., Hollywood, CA, 1972.

Emerick, L. *The Parent Interview.* Interstate Printers and Publishers, Danville, IL, 1969.

Engler, L., Hannah, E., and Longhurst, T. Linguistic analysis of speech samples: A practical guide for clinicians. *J. Speech & Hear. Dis.* 38(2):192-204, 1973.

Epstein, H. Growth spurts during brain development: Implications for educational policy and practice. In: J. Chall and A. Mirsky (eds.), *Education and the Brain: The Seventy-seventh Yearbook of Education.* University of Chicago Press, Chicago, IL, 1978.

Epstein, H. Phrenoblysis: Special brain and mind growth periods: I. Human brain and skill development. *Developmental Psychobiology* 7: 207-216, 1974.

Epstein, H., and Toepfer, C. A neuroscience basis for reorganizing middle grades education. *Educ. Lead.* 35(8):656-660, 1978.

Eriksen, K. *Communication Skills for the Human Services.* Reston Publishing Co., Inc., Reston, VA, 1979.

Erikson, E. *Identity: Youth and Crisis.* W. W. Norton, New York, 1968.

Fafard, M. *The quality of inservice education in special education.* Paper presented at the Arizona Council for Exceptional Children State Conference. March, 1980.

Fein, D. The prevalence of speech and language impairments. *ASHA.* 25(2):37, 1983.

Ferguson, L. *Personality Development.* Brooks/Cole Publishing, Belmont, CA, 1970.

Feuerstein, R. *Instrumental Enrichment Training Workshop.* Toronto, Ontario, Nov. 22, 1983.

Feuerstein, R. *Instrumental Enrichment.* Scott, Foresman, Chicago, IL, 1980.

Feuerstein, R. *The Dynamic Assessment of Retarded Performers: The Learning Assessment Potential Device, Theory, Instruments, and Techniques.* Scott, Foresman, Chicago, IL, 1979.

Fine, G. *Shared Fantasy: Role-playing Games as Social Worlds.* The University of Chicago Press, Chicago, IL, 1983.

Flin, R. Age effects in children's memory for unfamiliar faces. *Develop. Psychol.* 16:373-374, 1980.

Folb, E. *Runnin' Down Some Lines: The Language and Culture of Black Teenagers.* Harvard University Press, Cambridge, MA, 1980.

Fonosch, G., and Schwab, L. Attitudes of selected university faculty members toward disabled students. *J. Coll. Stud. Personnel* 22:229-235, 1981.

Frassinelli, L., Superior, K., and Meyers, J. A consultation model for speech and language intervention. *ASHA.* 25(11):25-30, 1983.

Freed, A. *The New TA for Kids: Powerful Techniques for Developing Self-esteem.* Jalmar Press, Inc., Sacramento, CA, 1977.

Freed, A. *TA for Teens (and other important people).* Jalmar Press, Inc., Sacramento, CA, 1976.

Freed, A. *TA for Kids (...and grown-ups too...).* Jalmar Press, Inc., Sacramento, CA, 1974.

Freeman, D. *Margaret Mead and Samoa: The Making and Unmaking of an Anthropological Myth.* Harvard University Press, Cambridge, MA, 1983.

French, R. Nonverbal patterns in youth culture. *Educ. Lead.* 35(7):541-546, 1978.

Freud, A. *The Ego and the Mechanism of Defense.* International Universities Press, New York, 1948.

Freud, S. *A General Introduction to Psychoanalysis.* Permabooks, New York, 1953.

Furth, H. *Thinking Without Language: Psychological Implications of Deafness.* Free Press, New York, 1966.

Furth, H., and Youniss, J. Formal operations and language: A comparison of deaf and hearing adolescents. *Int. J. Psycho.* 6:49-64, 1971.

Galda, S. *The development of the comprehension of metaphor.* Paper presented at the Annual Meeting of the American Educational Research Association. Los Angeles, CA, April 13-17, 1981.

Gall, M. *Handbook for Evaluating and Selecting Curricula Materials.* Allyn and Bacon, Boston, MA, 1981.

Gallagher, T. Pre-assessment: A procedure for accommodating language use variability. In: T. Gallagher and C. Prutting (eds.), *Pragmatic Assessment and Intervention Issues in Language.* College-Hill Press, San Diego, CA, 1983.

Gardner, J. *The Turbulent Teens.* Oak Tree Publications, San Diego, 1982.

Garnett, K. Telling tales: Narratives and learning-disabled children. *Topics in Language Disorders* 6(2):44-56, 1986.

Garvey, J., and Gordon, N. A follow-up study of children with disorders of speech and development. *Br. J. Dis. Co.* 8:17-28, 1973.

Gates, A. *Gates Reading Survey.* Bureau of Publications, Columbia University, New York, 1958.

Gates, G. An experimental study of the growth of social perception. *J. Educ. Psychol.* 14:449-461, 1923.

Geers, A., and Moog, J. Syntactic maturity of spontaneous speech and elicited imitations of hearing-impaired children. *J. Speech & Hear. Dis.* 43:380-391, 1978.

Gesell, A., Ilg, F., and Ames, L. *Youth: The Years from Ten to Sixteen.* Harper, New York, 1956.

Gillespie, S., and Cooper, E. Prevalence of speech problems in junior and senior high schools. *J. Speech & Hear. Res.* 16(4):739-743, 1973.

Gilligan, C. New map of development: New vision of maturity. *Am. J. Orthopsych.* 52(2):199-212, 1982.

Glasser, W. *Reality Therapy.* Harper and Row, New York, 1965.

Goldstein, H., Arkell, C., Ashcroft, S., Hurley, O., and Lilly, M. In: N. Hobbs (ed.), *Issues in the Classification of Children, pp. 4-61, Vol. 2.* Jossey-Bass, San Francisco, CA, 1975.

Goodlad, J. A study of schooling: Some findings and hypotheses. *Phi Del. Kap.* 64(7):465-470, 1983.

Goodlad, J., Sirotnik, K., and Overman, B. An overview of "A Study of Schooling." *Phi Del. Kap.* 61(3):174-178, 1979.

Goodman, Y., and Burke, C. *Reading Miscue Inventory: Manual Procedure for Diagnosis and Remediation.* Macmillan, New York, 1972.

Gordon, T. *Leadership Effectiveness Training (LET).* Wyden Books, New York, 1980.

Gordon, T. *Parent Effectiveness Training (PET).* Wyden Books, New York, 1970.

Gray, W., and Robinson, H. (eds.). *Gray Oral Reading Test.* Bobbs-Merrill, Indianapolis, IN, 1967.

Greenfield, P., and Smith, J. *The Structure of Communication in Early Language Development.* Academic Press, New York, 1976.

Greer, J., and Wethered, C. Learned helplessness: A piece of the burnout puzzle. *Excep. Child.* 50(6):524-531, 1984.

Greyerbiehl, D., Schwartz, A., Clymer, E., Owens, A., and Blackstone, S. *User System for Evaluating and Reviewing Software (USERS-I): Screening and Evaluation.* American Speech-Language-Hearing Association, Rockville, MD, 1986a.

Greyerbiehl, D., Chial, M., Schwartz, A., Owens, A., and Blackstone, S. *User System for Evaluating and Reviewing Software (USERS-II): Indepth Review.* American Speech-Language-Hearing Association, Rockville, MD, 1986b.

Grice, H. Logic and conversation. In: P. Cole and J. Morgan (eds.), *Syntax and Semantics: Vol. 3, Speech Acts.* Academic Press, New York, 1975.

Griffiths, C. A follow-up study of children with disorders in speech. *Br. J. Dis. Co.* 4:46-56, 1969.

Gruenewald, L., and Pollak, S. *Language Interaction in Teaching and Learning.* University Park Press, Baltimore, MD, 1984.

Hager, P. *Concept attainment strategies of adolescents in two verbal mediums.* Unpublished master's thesis, Univ. of Wisconsin-Eau Claire, Eau Claire, WI, 1982.

Hains, A., and Miller, D. Moral and cognitive development in delinquent and nondelinquent children and adolescents. *J. Gen. Ps.* 137:21-35, 1980.

Hall, E. *The Silent Language.* Premier Book, Greenwich, CT, 1959.

Hall, G. *Adolescence: Its Psychology and Its Relations to Physiology, Anthropology, Sociology, Sex, Crime, Religion, and Education.* D. Appleton and Company, New York, 1904.

Hall, G., and Loucks, S. Teacher concerns as a basis for facilitating and personalizing staff development. *Teach. Coll. Rec.* 80(1):36-53, 1978.

Hallahan, D. (ed.). Teaching exceptional children to use cognitive strategies. *Excep. Educ. Quarterly* 1(1), 1980.

Halliday, M. *Learning How to Mean: Explorations in the Development of Language.* Elsevior-North Holland, New York, 1975.

Hammill, D., and Larsen, S. *Test of Written Language.* Pro-ed, Austin, TX, 1978.

Hansen, D., *EEN Graduation Policy.* Cooperative Educational Services Agency #4, La Crosse, WI, 1985.

Hartzell, H. The challenge of adolescence. *Topics in Language Disorders* 4(2):1-9, 1984.

Havertape, J., and Kass, C. Examination of problem solving in learning disabled adolescents through verbalized self-instructions. *Learning Disab. Quarterly* 1(4):94-100, 1978.

Havighurst, R. *Human Development and Education.* Longmans, Green and Co., New York, 1953.

Hayes, J. *The Complete Problem Solver.* Franklin Institute Press, Philadelphia, PA, 1981.

Healey, W., Ackerman, B., Chappell, C., Perrin, K., and Stormer, J. The prevalence of communication disorders: A review of the literature. *Final Report.* ASHA, Rockville, MD, 1981.

Hemingway, B., Montague, J., and Bradley, R. Preliminary data on revision of a sentence repetition test for language screening with black first grade children. *Lang. Speech & Hearing Serv. Sch.* 12:153-159, 1981.

Hersey, P., and Blanchard, K. *Management of Organizational Behavior: Utilizing Human Resources.* Prentice-Hall, Englewood Cliffs, NJ, 1982.

Hill, J. *Models for screening.* Paper presented at the American Educational Research Association Annual Meeting, Minneapolis, MN, 1970.

Hilton, J., and Knoblauch, M. *On Television! A Survival Guide for Media Interviews.* AMACON, New York, 1980.

Hiskey, M. *Manual for the Hiskey-Nebraska Test of Learning Aptitude.* Union College Press, Lincoln, NE, 1966.

Hodgkinson, H. *All One System: Demographics of Education—Kindergarten through Graduate School.* Institute for Educational Leadership, Inc., Washington, DC, 1985.

Holinger, P. Violent deaths as a leading cause of mortality: An epidemiological study of suicide, homicide, and accidents. *Am. J. Psychol.* 137:472-476, 1980.

Holinger, P., and Offer, D. Perspectives on suicide in adolescence. In: R. Simmons (ed.), *Research in Community and Mental Health, Vol. II.* JAI Press, Greenwich, CT, 1981.

Hunt, T., and Clawson, E. Dropouts: Then and now. *High Sch. J.* 58:237-251, 1975.

Hymes, D. Introduction. In: C. Cazden, V. John, and D. Hymes (eds.), *Functions of Language in the Classroom.* Teachers College Press, New York, 1972.

Hymes, D. Competence and performance in linguistic theory. In: R. Huxley and E. Ingram (eds.), *Language Acquisition: Models and Methods.* Academic Press, New York, 1971.

Idol, L., Paolucci-Whitcomb, P., and Nevin, A. *Collaborative Consultation.* Aspen Publishers, Inc., Rockville, MD, 1986.

Inhelder, B., and Piaget, J. *The Growth of Logical Thinking From Childhood to Adolescence-an Essay on the Construction of Formal Operational Structures.* Basic Books, New York, 1958.

Ivey, A. *Microcounseling: Innovation in Interviewing Techniques.* Charles C. Thomas, Springfield, IL, 1971.

Jackson, S. The growth of logical thinking in normal and subnormal children. *Br. J. Educ. Psychol.* 35:255-258, 1965.

Jastak, J., and Jastak, S. *The Wide Range Achievement Test: Manual of Instructions.* Jastak Assoc., Wilmington, DE, 1978.

Jencks, C., Smith, M., Acland, H., Bane, M., Cohen, D., Gintis, H., Heyns, B., and Michelson, S. *Inequality: A Reassessment of the Effect of Family and Schooling in America.* Basic Books, New York, 1972.

Jeweler, A. *Creative Strategy in Advertising.* Wadsworth Publishing Co., Belmont, CA, 1981.

Johnson, D. Using reading and writing to improve oral language skills. *Topics in Language Disorders* 5(3):55-69, 1985.

Johnson, D. *Language/learning disabilities in young adults.* Paper presented at the American Speech-Language-Hearing Association North Central Regional Conference, Milwaukee, WI, August 9-12, 1982.

Johnson, R. Creative thinking in the absence of language: Deaf versus hearing adolescents. *Child St. J.* 7(2):49-57, 1977.

Johnson, R., Greenspan, S., and Brown, G. *Children's ability to recognize and improve upon socially inept communications.* Paper presented at the Annual Convention of American Psychologists Association (88th), Montreal, September 1-5, 1980.

Johnson, W. *People in Quandries.* Harper and Row, New York, 1946.

Johnston, J. *Doing things with words.* Educational Teleconferencing Network, Madison, WI, Jan. 22, 29 and Feb. 5, 12, 1985.

Johnston, J. Discussion: Part 1: What is language intervention? The role of theory. In: J. Miller, D. Yoder, and R. Schiefelbusch (eds.), *Contemporary Issues in Language Intervention. ASHA Reports 12.* ASHA, Rockville, MD, 1983.

Johnston, J. Narratives: A new look at communication problems in older language-disordered children. *Lang. Speech & Hear. Serv. Sch.* 13(3):144-155, 1982.

Jones, P. Formal operational reasoning and the use of tentative statements. *Cog. Psychol.* 3:467-471, 1972.

Kagan, J., Rosman, B., Day, D., Albert, J., and Phillips, W. Information processing in the child: Significance of analytic and reflective attitudes. *Psychol. Monogr.* 78(1):1-37, 1964.

Kavanaugh, D. *Listen to Us!* Workman Publishing, New York, 1978.

Kearns, K. Flexibility of single-subject experimental designs. Part II: Design, selection and arrangement of experimental phases. *J. Speech & Hear. Dis.* 51(3),204-214, 1986.

Kett, J. *Rites of Passage: Adolescence in America, 1790 to the Present.* Basic Books, New York, 1977.

Killarney, G., and Lass, N. A survey of rural public awareness of speech-language pathology and audiology. *ASHA.* 23(6):415-419, 1981.

Killian, C. Cognitive development of college freshmen. *J. Res. in Sci. Teach.* 16:347-350, 1979.

King, R., Jones, C., and Lasky, E. In retrospect: A fifteen-year follow-up report of speech-language disordered children. *Lang. Speech & Hear. Serv. Sch.* 13:24-32, 1982.

Kirp, D. Student classification, public policy, and the courts: The rights of children. *Harvard Educ. R.* 44(1):7-52, 1974.

Kishta, M. Proportional and combinatorial reasoning in two cultures. *J. Res. Sci. Teach.* 16:439-443, 1979.

Klausmeier, H., and Allen, D. *Cognitive Development of Children and Youth.* Academic Press, New York, 1978.

Klausmeier, H., Jetter, J., and Nelson, N. *Tutoring Can Be Fun.* Wisconsin Research and Development Center for Cognitive Learning, Madison, WI, 1972.

Knapp, M. *Nonverbal Communication in Human Interaction.* Holt, Rinehart and Winston, New York, 1978.

Knight-Arest, I. Communicative effectiveness of learning disabled and normally achieving 10- to 13-year-old boys. *LD Quarterly* 7:237-245, 1984.

Knowles, M. *The Adult Learner: A Neglected Species.* Gulf Publishing, Houston, TX, 1973.

Kohlberg, L. The cognitive-developmental approach to moral education. *Phi Del. Kap.* 56(10):670-677, 1975.

Konopka, G. Requirements for healthy development of adolescent youth. *Adoles.* 8(3):291-316, 1973.

Konopka, G. Adolescence in the 1970's. *Child Wel.* 50(10):553-559, 1971.

Kosel, M., and Fish, M. *The Factory [Computer program].* Sunburst Communications Inc., Pleasantville, NY, 1984.

Koskinen, P., and Wilson, R. *Developing a Successful Tutoring Program.* Teachers College Press, Columbia University, New York, 1982a.

Koskinen, P., and Wilson, R. *Tutoring: A Guide to Success.* Teachers College Press, Columbia University, New York, 1982b.

Koskinen, P., and Wilson, R. *A Guide for Student Tutors.* Teachers College Press, Columbia University, New York, 1982c.

Kramer, P., Koff, E., and Luria, Z. The development of an exceptional language structure in older children and young adults. *Child Develop.* 43:121-130, 1972.

Kretschmer, E. *Korperbau und Character.* Springer-Verlag, Berlin, 1951.

Kroh, O. *Entwicklungspsychologic des Grundschulkindes.* Herman Beyer, Langensalza, 1944.

Labinowicz, E. *The Piaget Primer.* Addison-Wesley Publishing, Menlo Park, CA, 1980.

Labov, W. *The Study of Non-standard English.* Clearinghouse for Linguistics, Center for Applied Linguistics, New York, 1969.

Lakin, K., Hill, B., Hauber, F., and Bruininks, R. A response to the GAO report, "Disparities still exist in who gets special education". *Except. Child.* 50(1):30-36, 1983.

Lambert, R., Novak, J., and Dougherty, B. *Staying In...A Dropout Prevention Handbook K-12.* Wisconsin Vocational Studies Center, Madison, WI, 1981.

Larson, M., and Dittman, F. *Compensatory Education and Early Adolescence: Reviewing our National Strategy.* Stanford Research, Menlo Park, CA, 1975.

Larson, V. Lord, and McKinley, N. *Conversational development of adolescents with language disorders in two experimental conditions.* In preparation.

Larson, V. Lord, and McKinley, N. *Innovative service delivery models for adolescents with language disorders.* Paper presented at the American Speech-Language-Hearing Association Convention, Washington, DC, Nov. 22-25, 1985a.

Larson, V. Lord, and McKinley, N. General intervention principles with language impaired adolescents. *Topics in Language Disorders* 5(3):70-77, 1985b.

Larson, V. Lord, and Steiner, S. Language intervention using microcomputers. *Topics in Language Disorders* 6(1):41-55, 1985.

Lassman, F., Fisch, R., Vetter, D., and LaBenz, E. *Early Correlates of Speech, Language, and Hearing: The Collaborative Perinatal Project of the National Institute of Neurological and Communicative Disorders and Stroke.* PSG Publishing, Littleton, MA, 1980.

Lawson, A., and Wollman, W. Encouraging the transition from concrete to formal cognitive functioning—an experiment. *J. Res. Sci. Teach.* 13:413-430, 1976.

Leadbeater, B., and Dionne, J. The adolescent's use of formal operational thinking in solving problems related to identify resolution. *Adoles.* 16(61):111-121, 1981.

Lee, A., and Shapero-Fine, J. When a language problem is primary: Secondary school strategies. In G. Wallach and K. Butler (eds.), *Language Learning Disabilities in School-Age Children.* Williams and Wilkins, Baltimore, MD, 1984.

Lee, L. *Developmental Sentence Analysis.* Northwestern University Press, Evanston, IL, 1974.

Leiter, R. *Leiter International Performance Scale.* Stoetting, Chicago, IL, 1979.

Levin, J. What have we learned about maximizing what children learn? In: J. Levin and V. Allen (eds.), *Cognitive Learning in Children: Theories and Strategies.* Academic Press, New York, 1976.

Levine, M., and Sutton-Smith, B. Effects of age, sex, and task on visual behavior during dyadic interaction. *Develop. Psychol.* 9:400-405, 1973.

Lewin, K. Field theory and experiment in social psychology concepts and methods. *Am. J. Soc.* 44:868-897, 1939.

Lindquist, E., and Hieronymus, A. *Iowa Test of Basic Skills.* Houghton Mifflin, Boston, MA, 1971.

Lipscomb, D. The increase in prevalence of high frequency hearing impairment among college students. *Audiol.* 11:231-237, 1972.

Lipsitz, J. *Growing up Forgotten: A Review of Research and Programs Concerning Early Adolescence.* Transaction, New Brunswick, NJ, 1980.

Lipsitz, J. Adolescent development: Myths and realities. *Child. Today* 8(5):2-7, 1979.

Lissner, R. *Appleworks [Computer program].* Apple Computer, Cupertino, CA, 1985.

Loban, W. *Language Development: Kindergarten Through Grade Twelve.* National Council of Teachers of English, Urbana, IL, 1976.

Lochhead, J., and Clement, J. (eds.). *Cognitive Process Instruction: Research on Teaching Thinking Skills.* Franklin Institute Press, Philadelphia, PA, 1979.

Lund, N., and Duchan, J. *Assessing Children's Language in Naturalistic Contexts.* Prentice-Hall, Englewood Cliffs, NJ, 1983.

Luper, H., and Mulder, R. *Stuttering: Therapy for Children.* Prentice-Hall, Englewood Cliffs, NJ, 1964.

McCarthy, D. *The Language Development of the Preschool Child. (Institute of Child Welfare Monograph Series No. 4).* Univ. of Minnesota Press, Minneapolis, MN, 1930.

McFarlane, S., Fujiki, M., and Brinton, B. *Coping with Communication Handicaps: Resources for the Practicing Clinician.* Little Brown/College-Hill Press, San Diego, CA, 1984.

McGinnis, J. Prevention. *ASHA.* 26(8):22-24. 1984.

McKinley, N., and Larson, V. Lord. Neglected language disordered adolescent: A delivery model. *Lang. Speech & Hear. Serv. Sch.* 16(1):2-15, 1985.

McKinley, N., and Larson, V. Lord. *Adolescents' Communication: Development and Disorders—Update Pages.* Thinking Publications, Eau Claire, WI, 1984.

McKinley, N., and Larson, V. Lord. *Adolescents' conversations with a friend and an unfamiliar adult.* Paper presented at the American Speech-Language-Hearing Association Convention, Cincinnati, OH, Nov. 18-22, 1983.

McKinley, N., and Schwartz, L. *Referential Communication: Barrier Activities for Speakers and Listeners (Parts One and Two).* Thinking Publications, Eau Claire, WI, 1985.

McLean, J., and Snyder-McLean, L. *A Transactional Approach to Early Language Training.* Charles E. Merrill, Columbus, OH, 1978.

McReynolds, L., and Kearns, K. *Single-subject Experimental Designs in Communicative Disorders.* University Park Press, Baltimore, MD, 1983.

McReynolds, L., and Thompson, C. Flexibility of single-subject experimental designs. Part 1: Review of the basics of single-subject designs. *J. Speech & Hear. Dis.* 51(3):194-203, 1986.

Madden, R., Gardner, E., Rudman, H., Karlsen, B., and Merwin, J. *Stanford Achievement Tests.* Harcourt, Brace, Jovanovich, New York, 1973.

Mandler, J., and Johnson, N. Remembrance of things parsed: Story structure and recall. *Cog. Psychol.* 9:111-151, 1977.

Marge, M., The prevention of communication disorders. *ASHA.* 26(8):29-33, 1984.

Markgraf, B. An observational study determining the amount of time that students in the 10th and 12th grades are expected to listen in the classroom. In: S. Duker (ed.), *Listening Readings.* Scarecrow Press, New York, 1966.

Martorano, S. A developmental analysis of performance on Piaget's formal operations tasks. *Develop. Psychol.* 13(6):666-672, 1977.

Mathews, M., Whang, P., and Fawcett, S. Behavioral assessment of occupational skills of learning disabled adolescents. *J. Learn. Dis.* 15(1):38-41, 1982.

Maxwell, W. (ed.). *Thinking: The Expanding Frontier.* Franklin Institute Press, Philadelphia, PA, 1983.

Mead, M. *Coming of Age in Samoa.* New American Library, New York, 1950.

Mehrabian, A. Communication without words. *Psychol. Today* 2:51-52, 1968.

Mendelberg, H. Split and continuity in language use of Mexican-American adolescents of migrant origin. *Adoles.* 19(73):171-182, 1984.

Menyuk, P. The language-impaired child: Linguistic or cognitive impairment? *Ann. NY Acad. Sci.* 263:5-69, 1975.

Mercer, J. Psychological assessment and the rights of children. In: N. Hobbs (ed.), *Issues in Classification of Children, pp. 130-159, Vol. 1.* Jossey-Bass, San Francisco, CA, 1975.

Micropro International Corp. *Mailmerge [Computer program].* Micropro International Corp., San Rafael, CA, 1983.

Miller, J. *Assessing Language Production in Children: Experimental Procedures.* University Park Press, Baltimore, MD, 1981.

Miller, J., and Chapman, R. *Systematic Analysis of Language Transcripts (SALT) [Computer program].* Language Analyses Laboratory, Waisman Center on Mental Retardation and Human Development, University of Wisconsin-Madison, Madison, WI, 1983.

Miller, N., and Dollard, J. *Social Learning and Imitation.* Yale University Press, New Haven, CT, 1941.

Mind Puzzles [Computer program]. Minnesota Educational Computer Consortium, St. Paul, MN, 1983.

Mitchell, J. *Adolescent Psychology.* Holt, Rinehart and Winston of Canada Limited, Toronto, 1979.

Modgil, S., and Modgil, C. *Piagetian Research. Vol. 3: The Growth of Logic—Concrete and Formal Operations.* Humanities Press, Atlantic Highlands, NJ, 1976.

Moncur, J., and Brackett, I. *Modifying Vocal Behavior.* Harper and Row, New York, 1974.

Mordecai, D., Palin, M., and Palmer, C. *Lingquest 1: Computer Assisted Language Sample Analysis [Computer program].* Charles E. Merrill, Columbus, OH, 1985.

Morgan, D., and Guilford, A. *Adolescent Language Screening Test.* Modern Educational Corp., Tulsa, OK, 1984.

Morris, M., Leuenberger, J., and Aksamit, D. *Language learning disabled students in the college setting.* Paper presented at the American Speech-Language-Hearing Association Convention, Washington, DC, Nov. 22-25, 1985.

Morris, N., and Hawkins, G. *The Honest Politician's Guide to Crime Control.* University of Chicago Press, Chicago, IL, 1970.

Mowrer, D. *Methods of Modifying Speech Behaviors.* Charles E. Merrill, Columbus, OH, 1982.

Muma, J. *Language Handbook: Concepts, Assessment, Intervention.* Prentice-Hall, Englewood Cliffs, NJ, 1978.

Muuss, R. *Theories of Adolescence.* Random House, New York, 1975.

Myklebust, H. *The Psychology of Deafness.* Grune and Stratton, New York, 1960.

Myrick, R., and Erney, T. *Youth Helping Youth: A Handbook for Training Peer Facilitators.* Educational Media Corp., Minneapolis, MN, 1979.

Naisbitt, J. *Megatrends: Ten New Directions Transforming Our Lives.* Warner Books, New York, 1984.

National Commission on Excellence in Education. An open letter to the American people. A nation at risk: The imperative for educational reform. *Education Week.* April 27, 1983, pp. 12-16.

National Commission on Youth. *The Transition of Youth to Adulthood: A Bridge Too Long.* Westview Press, Boulder, CO, 1980.

National Youth Workers Conference, Washington, DC, July 5-8, 1982.

Neimark, E. Intellectual development in the exceptional adolescent as viewed within a Piagetian framework. *Except. Educ. Quarterly* 1(2):47-56, 1980.

Neimark, E. Current status of formal operations research. *Hum. Dev.* 22:60-67, 1979.

Nelson, M., Denny, E., and Brown, J. *The Nelson-Denny Reading Test: Vocabulary-Comprehension-Rate.* Houghton Mifflin, Boston, MA, 1960.

Nelson, N. Beyond information processing: The language of teachers and textbooks. In: G. Wallach and K. Butler (eds.), *Language Learning Disabilities in School-Age Children.* Williams and Wilkins, Baltimore, MD, 1984.

Nelson, N. *Dialect differences in language samples gathered from Black preschoolers: Interviewer effects and measurement procedures.* Paper presented at the American Speech and Hearing Association Convention, Houston, TX, Nov. 20-23, 1976.

Neville, M. Listening is an art: Practice it. *Elem. E.* 36:226-233, 1959.

Nichols, R., and Lewis, T. *Listening and Speaking: A Guide to Effective Oral Communication.* Wm. C. Brown, Dubuque, IA, 1954.

Nichols, R., and Stevens, L. Listening to people. *Harvard Bus. Rev.* 35(5):85-92, 1957.

Nisbet, J., Zanella, K., and Miller, J. An analysis of conversations among handicapped students and a non-handicapped peer. *Excep. Child.* 51(2):156-162, 1984.

Noel, M. Referential communication abilities of learning disabled children. *Learning Disab. Quarterly* 3:70-75, 1980.

Norman, J., and Harris, M. *The Private Life of the American Teenager.* Rawson, Wade Publishers, New York, 1981.

O'Connor, L., and Eldredge, P. *Communication Disorders in Adolescence: Program Planning, Diagnostics, and Practical Remediation Techniques.* Charles C. Thomas, Springfield, IL, 1981.

Offer, D., Ostrov, E., and Howard, K. The mental health professional's concept of the normal adolescent. *AMA Archives of General Psychiatry* 38(2):149-153, 1981a.

Offer, D., Ostrov, E., and Howard, K. *The Adolescent: A Psychological Self-Portrait.* Basic Books, New York, 1981b.

Offer, D., Ostrov, E., and Howard, K. *The Offer Self-Image Questionnaire for Adolescents: A Manual.* Michael Reese Hospital, Chicago, IL, 1977.

Oklahoma Project. *Exceptions: A Handbook for Teachers of Mainstream Students.* Project Mainstream in Cooperation with the Oklahoma Child Service Demonstration Center and Developer/Demonstrator Project, Cushing, OK, 1982.

Olver, R., and Hornsby, J. On equivalence. In: J. Bruner, R. Olver, and P. Greenfield (eds.), *Studies in Cognitive Growth.* John Wiley and Sons, New York, 1966.

Overton, W., and Meehan, A. Individual differences in formal operational thought: Sex role and learned helplessness. *Child Dev.* 53:1536-1543, 1982.

Page, J., and Stewart, S. Story grammar skills in school-age children. *Topics in Language Disorders* 5(2):16-30, 1985.

Papalia, D., and Olds, S. *A Child's World—Infancy Through Adolescence.* McGraw-Hill, New York, 1975.

Parrill-Burnstein, M. *Problem Solving and Learning Disabilities: An Information Processing Approach.* Grune and Stratton, New York, 1981.

Pearlstein, E., Russell, L., and Fink, R. *Speech/language pathology and audiology: The public's view.* Paper presented at the American Speech and Hearing Association Convention, Chicago, IL, Nov. 2-5, 1977.

Peck, M. Youth suicide. *Death Education* 6:29-47, 1982.

Peel, E. *The Nature of Adolescent Judgment.* Wiley-Interscience, New York, 1971.

Perls, F., Hefferline, R., and Goodman, P. *Gestalt Therapy.* Dell, New York, 1965.

Phelps-Terasaki, D., Phelps-Gunn, T., and Stetson, E. *Remediation and Instruction in Language.* Aspen Systems, Rockville, MD, 1983.

Piaget, J. Piaget's theory. In: P. Mussen (ed.), *Carmichael's Manual of Child Psychology, Volume 1.* John Wiley and Sons, New York, 1970.

Piaget, J. *The Language and Thought of the Child* (Reprint of 1926 edition). Routledge and Kegan Paul, London, 1959.

Piaget, J., and Inhelder, B. *The Psychology of the Child.* Basic Books, New York, 1969.

Prather, E. Developmental language disorders. In: A. Holland (ed.), *Language Disorders in Children.* Little Brown/College-Hill Press, San Diego, CA, 1984.

Prather, E., Beecher, S., Stafford, M., and Wallace, E. *Screening Test of Adolescent Language.* Univ. of Washington Press, Seattle, WA, 1980.

Project STILE. Draft copy. Lawrence High School, Lawrence, KS, 1979.

Prutting, C., and Kirchner, D. Applied pragmatics. In: T. Gallagher and C. Prutting (eds.), *Pragmatic Assessment and Intervention Issues in Language.* College-Hill Press, San Diego, CA, 1983.

Quigley, S., Steinkamp, M., Power, D., and Jones, B. *Test of Syntactic Abilities.* Dormac, Beaverton, OR, 1978.

Rank, O. *Will Therapy and Truth and Reality.* Knopf, New York, 1945.

Rankin, R. *The measurement of the ability to understand spoken language.* Unpublished doctoral dissertation, Univ. of Michigan, Ann Arbor, MI, 1926.

Raschke, D., and Dedrick, C. An experience in frustration: Simulations approximating learning difficulties. *Teach. Excep. Child.* 18(4):266-271, 1986.

Reed, N. *An analysis of comprehension levels of an ask/tell syntactic structure in a group of adolescents, aged ten to eighteen years.* Unpublished master's thesis, University of Cincinnati, Cincinnati, OH, 1977.

Rees, N. The speech pathologist and the reading process. *ASHA.* 16:255-258, 1974.

Rees, N., and Wollner, S. *A taxonomy of pragmatic abilities.* Educational Teleconferencing Network, Madison, WI, Feb. 1982.

Remplein, H. *Die Seelische Enturcklung in der Kindheit und Reifezeit.* Ernst Reinhard, Munchen, 1956.

Rhys, W. Geography and the adolescent. In: A. Floyd (ed.), *Cognitive Development in the School Years.* John Wiley and Sons, New York, 1979.

Rice, M. Contemporary accounts of the cognition/language relationship: Implications for speech-language clinicians. *J. Speech & Hear. Dis.* 48(4):347-359, 1983.

Riedlinger-Ryan, K., and Shewan, C. Comparison of auditory language comprehension skills in learning-disabled and academically achieving adolescents. *Lang. Speech & Hear. Serv. Sch.* 15(2):127-136, 1984.

Ripich, D., and Griffith, P. *Story structure, cohesion, and propositions in learning disabled children.* Paper presented at the American Speech-Language-Hearing Association Convention, Washington, DC, Nov. 22-25, 1985.

Ritter, E. Social perspective taking ability, cognitive complexity and listener adapted communication in early and late adolescence. *Commun. Monog.* 46:40-51, 1979.

Rivers, L., Henderson, D., Jones, R., Ladner, J., and Williams, R. Mosaic of labels for Black children. In: N. Hobbs (ed.), *Issues in the Classification of Children, Vol. 2.* Jossey-Bass, San Francisco, CA, 1975.

Robin, A., Kent, R., O'Leary, K., Foster, S., and Prinz, R. An approach to teaching parents and adolescents problem-solving communication skills: A preliminary report. *Behav. Ther.* 8:639-643, 1977.

Robinson, E. The child's understanding of inadequate messages and communication failure: A problem of ignorance or egocentrism? In: W. Dickson (ed.), *Children's Oral Communication Skills,* Academic Press, New York, 1981.

Roeber, E. *Development and Validation of Objective Referenced Test Instrument for Critical Listening: Grades, 4, 7 and 10.* Michigan Dept. of Education Technical Report, Lansing, MI, 1980.

Roesser, R. Industrial hearing conservation programs in high schools (Protect the ear before the 12th year). *Ear Hear.* 1:119-120, 1980.

Rogers, C. *On Becoming a Person: A Therapist's View of Psychotherapy.* Houghton Mifflin, Boston, MA, 1961.

Rosenbaum, J. *Making Inequality: The Hidden Curriculum of High School Tracking.* John Wiley and Sons, New York, 1976.

Rosenthal, D. Language skills and formal operations. *Merrill-Palmer Q.* 25(2):133-143, 1979.

Roth, F., and Spekman, N. Narrative disclosure: Spontaneously generated stories of learning-disabled and normally achieving students. *J. Speech & Hear. Dis.* 51(1):8-23, 1986.

Rowher, W. Prime time for education: Early childhood or adolescence? *Harvard Educ. R.* 41:316-341, 1971.

Rumelhart, D. Notes on a schema for stories. In: D. Bobrow and A. Collins (eds.), *Representation and Understanding: Studies in Cognitive Science.* Academic Press, New York, 1975.

Rutherford, R. Talk about pop. In: S. Rogers (ed.), *They Don't Speak our Language: Essays on the Language World of Children and Adolescents.* Edward Arnold, London, 1976.

Rutherford, R., Freeth, M., and Mercer, E. *Topics of Conversation in 15-Year-Old Children.* York, England, 1969.

Sanders, L. The comprehension of certain syntactic structures by adults. *J. Speech & Hear. Dis.* 14:739-745, 1971.

Schindler-Rainman, E. The poor and the PTA. *PTA Mag.* 61(8):4-5, 1967.

Schlesinger, I. The role of cognitive development and linguistic input in language acquisition. *J. Child Lang.* 4:153-169, 1977.

Schmitt, P. *Deaf children's comprehension and production of sentence transformations and verb tenses.* Unpublished doctoral dissertation, Univ. of Illinois, Chicago, IL, 1968.

Schumaker, J., Sheldon-Wildgen, J., and Sherman, J. *An Observational Study of the Academic and Social Behavior of Learning Disabled Adolescents in the Regular Classroom. (Research Report 22).* University of Kansas Institute for Research in Learning Disabilities, Lawrence, KS, 1980.

Schwartz, A. Microcomputer-assisted assessment of linguistic and phonological processes. *Topics in Language Disorders* 6(1):26-40, 1985.

Schwartz, L., and McKinley, N. *Daily Communication: Strategies for the Language Disordered Adolescent.* Thinking Publications, Eau Claire, WI, 1984.

Searle, J. What is a speech act? In: M. Black (ed.), *Philosophy in America.* Allen and Union, Cornell University Press, New York, 1965.

Semel, E., and Wiig, E. *Clinical Evaluation of Language Functions.* Charles E. Merrill, Columbus, OH, 1980.

Sequential Tests of Educational Progress (STEP). Series 11. Educational Testing Service, Trenton, NJ, 1958.

Shantz, C. The role of role-taking in children's referential communication. In: W. Dickson (ed.), *Children's Oral Communication Skills.* Academic Press, New York, 1981.

Sheehy, G. *Pathfinders: Overcoming the Crises of Adult Life and Finding Your Own Path to Well-being.* Bantam Books, New York, 1981.

Sheldon, A. On strategies for processing relative clauses: A comparison of children and adults. *J. Psycholin. Res.* 6:305-318, 1977.

Siegal, M. Kohlberg versus Piaget: To what extent has one theory eclipsed the other? *Merrill-Palmer Q.* 26(4):285-297, 1980.

Silliman, E. Interactional competencies in the instructional context: The role of teaching discourse in learning. In: G. Wallach and K. Butler (eds.), *Language Learning Disabilities in School-Age Children.* Williams and Wilkins, Baltimore, MD, 1984.

Simon, C. Functional-pragmatic evaluation of communication skills in school-aged children. *Lang. Speech & Hearing Serv. Sch.* 15(2):83-97, 1984.

Simon, C. *After is verbing: Then what?* Paper presented at the American Speech-Language-Hearing Association Convention, Los Angeles, CA, Nov. 20-23, 1981.

Simon, C. *Communicative Competence: A Functional-Pragmatic Language Program.* Communication Skill Builders, Tucson, AZ, 1980.

Simon, C. *Communicative Competence: A Functional-Pragmatic Approach to Language Therapy.* Communication Skill Builders, Tucson, AZ, 1979.

Simpson, R. *Conferencing Parents of Exceptional Children.* Aspen Publishers, Inc., Rockville, MD, 1982.

Sizer, T. High school reform: A need for engineering. *Phi Del. Kap.* 64(10):679-683, 1983.

Slavin, R. Learning together. *Am. Educ.* 10(2):6-13, 1986.

Slosson, R. *Slosson Intelligence Test.* Slosson Educational Pub., East Aurora, NY, 1963.

Spache, G. *Diagnostic Reading Scales.* California Test Bureau, Los Angeles, CA, 1963.

Speech Communication Association of America. *SCA Guidelines for Minimal Competencies in Speaking and Listening for High School Graduates.* Speech Commun. Assoc., Annandale, VA, 1979.

Spekman, N. A study of the dyadic verbal communication abilities of learning disabled and normally achieving 4th and 5th grade boys. *Learning Disab. Quarterly* 4:139-151, 1981.

Spranger, E. *Psychologie des Jugendalters. 24th Ed.* Quelle and Meyer, Heidelberg, 1955.

Springboard Software, Inc., *The Newsroom [Computer program].* Springboard Software, Inc., Minneapolis, MN, 1984.

Stein, N., and Glenn, C. An analysis of story comprehension in elementary school children. In: R. Freedle (ed.), *New Directions in Discourse Processing, Vol. 2.* Ablex, Norwood, NJ, 1979.

Strauss, S. *U-Shaped Behavioral Growth.* Academic Press, New York, 1982.

Strominger, A., and Bashir, A. *A nine-year follow-up of language-delayed children.* Paper presented at the American Speech and Hearing Association Convention, Chicago, IL, Nov. 2-5, 1977.

Sue, D. *Counseling the Culturally Different: Theory and Practice.* John Wiley and Sons, New York, 1981.

Tanner, J. Sequence and tempo in the somatic changes in puberty. In: M. Grumbach, G. Grave, and F. Mayer (eds.), *Control of the Onset of Puberty.* John Wiley and Sons, New York, 1974.

Task Force on Secondary Programs for the Speech-Language Impaired. *Project Adolang: Identification of Adolescent Language Problems and Implications for Education.* Bureau of Education for Exceptional Students, Florida Dept. of Education, April 1983.

Taylor, J. Speech-language services for youthful and adult offenders. *Federal Probation* 44(6):37-41, 1980.

Taylor, J. *The communicative abilities of juvenile delinquents: A descriptive study.* Unpublished doctoral dissertation, Univ. of Missouri, Columbia, MO, 1969.

Taylor, O., and Peters, C. Sociolinguistics and communication disorders. In: N. Lass, L. McReynolds, J. Northern, and D. Yoder (eds.), *Speech, Language, and Hearing: Vol. II Pathologies of Speech and Language.* W. B. Saunders, Philadelphia, PA, 1982.

Terman, L., and Merrill, M. *Stanford-Binet Intelligence Scale.* Houghton Mifflin, Boston, MA, 1960.

Tharp, R. The triadic model of consultation. In: C. Parker (ed.), *Psychological Consultation in the Schools: Helping Teachers Meet Special Needs.* Council for Exceptional Children, Reston, VA, 1975.

Tharp, R., and Wetzel, R. *Behavioral Modification in the Natural Environment.* Academic Press, New York, 1969.

Thinking Publications. *Problem Solving Communication Poster.* Thinking Publications, Eau Claire, WI, 1983.

Thomas, E., and Walmsley, S. *Some evidence of continuing linguistic acquisition in learning disabled adolescents.* Paper presented at the International Federation of Learning Disabilities, 3rd International Scientific Conference, Montreal, Aug. 9-13, 1976.

Thompson, J. *Using Role Playing in the Classroom.* The Phi Delta Kappa Educational Foundation, Bloomington, IN, 1978.

Thorndyke, P. Cognitive structures in comprehension and memory of narrative discourse. *Cog. Psych.* 9:77-110, 1977.

Thorpe, L., Lefever, D., and Naslund, R. *SRA Achievement Series.* Science Research Associates, Chicago, IL, 1968.

Thorum, A. *Fullerton Language Test for Adolescents.* Consulting Psychologists Press, Palo Alto, CA, 1980.

Tibbits, D. *Language Disorders in Adolescents.* Cliff Notes, Lincoln, NE, 1982.

Tiegs, E., and Clark, W. *California Achievement Test.* CTB/McGraw-Hill, Monterey, CA, 1963.

Torrance, E. *The Torrance Tests of Creative Thinking: Norms-Technical Manual.* Personnel Press, Lexington, MA, 1974.

Turner, J., and Helms, D. *Life Span Development.* W. B. Saunders, Philadelphia, PA, 1979.

Tyack, D., and Gottsleben, R. *Language Sampling, Analysis and Training: A Handbook for Teachers and Clinicians.* Consulting Psychologists Press, Palo Alto, CA, 1974.

Valens, E. *The Other Side of the Mountain.* Warner Books, Inc., New York, 1975.

Vallett, R. *Vallett Inventory of Critical Thinking Abilities.* Academic Therapy Publications, Novata, CA, 1981.

Valletutti, P., and Bender, M. *Teaching Interpersonal and Community Living Skills: A Curriculum Model for Handicapped Adolescents and Adults.* University Park Press, Baltimore, MD, 1982.

Vander Zanden, J., and Pace, A. *Educational Psychology in Theory and Practice. 2nd Ed.* Random House, New York, 1984.

Van Hattum, R. Public information: More is not enough. *ASHA.* 25(2):47-49, 1983.

Van Riper, C. *Speech Correction: Principles and Methods. 2nd Ed.* Prentice-Hall, Englewood Cliffs, NJ, 1947.

Vaughn-Cooke, F. Improving language assessment in minority children. *ASHA.* 25(9):29-34, 1983.

Velluntino, F. Toward an understanding of dyslexia: Psychological factors in specific reading disability. In: A. Benton and D. Pearl (eds.), *Dyslexia: An Appraisal of Current Knowledge.* Oxford University Press, New York, 1978.

Vermont Dept. of Education. *Basic Competencies: Teacher's Guide for Basic Competencies in Reasoning.* State Dept. of Education, Montpelier, VT, 1979.

Vermont Dept. of Education. *Basic Competencies: A Manual of Information and Guidelines for Teachers and Administrators.* State Dept. of Education, Montpelier, VT, 1977.

Vetter, D. Kluppel. Evaluation of clinical intervention: Accountability. *Seminars in Speech and Language* 6(1):55-64, 1985.

Vogel, S. Syntactic abilities in normal and dyslexic children. *J. Learn. Dis.* 7:47-53, 1974.

Vygotsky, L. *Thought and Language.* MIT Press, Cambridge, MA, 1962.

Waker, D. Sex differences in mental abilities, hemispheric lateralization, and rate of physical growth at adolescence. *Develop. Psychol.* 13:29-38, 1977.

Wasserman, R. Identifying the counseling needs of the siblings of mentally retarded children. *Pers. Guid. J.* 61(10):622-627, 1983.

Watson, B. Test-retest stability of the Hiskey-Nebraska Test of Learning Aptitude on a sample of hearing-impaired children and adolescents. *J. Speech & Hear. Dis.* 48(2):145-149, 1983.

Weaver, H. *Human Listening: Processes and Behavior.* Bobbs-Merrill, Indianapolis, IN, 1972.

Weaver, P., and Dickinson, D. Scratching below the surface structure: Exploring the usefulness of story grammars. *Discourse Processes* 5:225-243, 1982.

Webster, E. *Counseling with Parents of Handicapped Children: Guidelines for Improving Communication.* Grune and Stratton, New York, 1977.

Webster, E. *Professional Approaches with Parents of Handicapped Children.* Charles C. Thomas, Springfield, IL, 1976.

Wechsler, D. *Wechsler Intelligence Scale for Children (Revised).* Psychological Corp., New York, 1974.

Wechsler, D. *Wechsler Adult Intelligence Scale.* Psychological Corp., New York, 1955.

Weiner, P. The value of follow-up studies. *Topics in Language Disorders* 5(3):78-92, 1985.

Weiner, P. A language-delayed child at adolescence. *J. Speech & Hear. Dis.* 39(2):202-212, 1974.

Weiss, R., Hansen, K., and Heubelein, T. *Pragmatic psycholinguistic therapy for language disorders in early childhood.* Short course presented at the American Speech-Language-Hearing Association Convention, Atlanta, GA, Nov. 16-19, 1979.

Wellborn, S. Special report: Troubled teenagers. *U.S. News World Rep.* 41(24):40-43, 1981.

Wentworth, E. *Listen to Your Heart: A Message to Parents of Handicapped Children.* Houghton Mifflin, Boston, MA, 1974.

Werner, E. *A study of communication time.* Unpublished master's thesis, University of Maryland, College Park, MD, 1975.

Westby, C. Learning to talk—talking to learn: Oral-literate language differences. In: C. Simon (ed.), *Communication Skills and Classroom Success: Therapy Methodologies for Language-Learning Disabled Students.* Little Brown/College-Hill Press, San Diego, CA, 1985.

Westby, C. Development of narrative language abilities. In: G. Wallach and K. Butler (eds.), *Language Learning Disabilities in School-Age Children.* Williams and Wilkins, Baltimore, MD, 1984.

Wiig, E. *Assessment and development of social communication skills in adolescents with language-learning disabilities.* Educational Teleconferencing Network. Madison, WI, Oct. 25 and Nov. 1, 7, 14, 1983.

Wiig, E. *Identifying language disorders in adolescents.* Oral presentation at Gunderson Clinic, LaCrosse, WI, May 1982a.

Wiig, E. *Let's Talk: Developing Prosocial Communication Skills.* Charles E. Merrill, Columbus, OH, 1982b.

Wiig, E., and Becker-Caplan, L. Linguistic retrieval strategies and word-finding difficulties among children with language disabilities. *Topics in Language Disorders* 4(3):1-18, 1984.

Wiig, E., and Harris, S. Perception and interpretation of nonverbally expressed emotions by adolescents with learning disabilities. *Percept. & Motor Skills* 38:239-245, 1974.

Wiig, E., Kutner, S., Florence, D., Sherman, B., and Semel, E. Perception and interpretation of explicit negations by learning-disabled children and adolescents. *Percept. & Motor Skills* 44(3):1251-1257, 1977.

Wiig, E., and Semel, E. *Language Assessment and Intervention for the Learning Disabled.* Charles E. Merrill, Columbus, OH, 1980.

Wiig, E., and Semel, E. *Language Disabilities in Children and Adolescents.* Charles E. Merrill, Columbus, OH, 1976.

Wiig, E., and Semel, E. Productive language abilities in learning disabled adolescents. *J. of Learn. Dis.* 8(9):45-53, 1975.

Wiig, E., and Semel, E. Logicogrammatical sentence comprehension by adolescents with learning disabilities. *Percept. & Motor Skills* 38:1331-1334, 1974.

Wiig, E., and Semel, E. Comprehension of linguistic concepts requiring logical operations. *J. Speech & Hear. Res.* 16:627-636, 1973.

Wilkinson, A., Stratta, L., and Dudley, P. *Schools Council Oracy Project Listening Comprehension Tests.* MacMillan Education Ltd., London, 1974.

Wilson, D. *Voice Problems in Children. 2nd Ed.* Williams and Wilkins, Baltimore, MD, 1979.

Wolff, F., Marsnik, N., Tacey, W., and Nichols, R. *Perceptive Listening.* Holt, Rinehart and Winston, Chicago, IL, 1983.

Wolvin, A., and Coakley, C. *Listening.* W. C. Brown, Dubuque, IA, 1982.

Woodford, C. Notes on audiology in the public schools. *Hear. Aid J.* 33(7):5-9, 1980.

Woodford, C., and O'Farrell, M. High-frequency loss of hearing in secondary school students: An investigation of possible etiologic factors. *Lang. Speech & Hear. Serv. Sch.* 14:22-28, 1983.

Worden, P., Malmgren, I., and Gabourie, P. Memory for stories in learning disabled adults. *J. Learn. Dis.* 15(3):145-152, 1982.

Worden, P., and Nakamura, G. Story comprehension and recall in learning-disabled versus normal college students. *J. Ed. Psychol.* 74(5):633-641, 1982.

Ysseldyke, J. Current practices in making psychoeducational decisions about learning disabled students. *J. Learn. Dis.* 16(4):226-232, 1983.

Yuker, H., Block, J., and Younng, J. *The Measurement of Attitudes toward Disabled Persons. (Rehabilitation Series 3).* INA Mend Institute, Albertson, NY, 1970.

Zeller, W. *Konstitution und Entwicklung.* Psychologische Rundschau, Gottingen, 1952.

Zemlin, W. *Speech and Hearing Science, Anatomy and Physiology.* Prentice-Hall, Englewood Cliffs, NJ, 1968.

Zinsser, W. *On Writing Well: An Informal Guide to Writing Non-fiction.* Harper and Row, New York, 1985.

AUTHOR INDEX

SUBJECT INDEX